KT-441-655

Developmental Coordination Disorder and Its Consequences

EDITED BY JOHN CAIRNEY

STAFF LIBRARY
SINGLETON HOSPITAL
TEL: 01792 205666 EXT: 35281

UNIVERSITY OF TORONTO PRESS
Toronto Buffalo London

© University of Toronto Press 2015
Toronto Buffalo London
www.utppublishing.com

ISBN 978-1-4426-4939-2 (cloth)
ISBN 978-1-4426-2674-4 (paper)

Library and Archives Canada Cataloguing in Publication

Developmental coordination disorder and its consequences / edited
by John Cairney.

Includes bibliographical references and index.
ISBN 978-1-4426-4939-2 (bound).   ISBN 978-1-4426-2674-4 (pbk.)

1. Apraxia.   I. Cairney, John, 1968–, author, editor

RJ496.A63D49 2015   618.92′8552   C2014-908043-3

University of Toronto Press acknowledges the financial assistance to
its publishing program of the Canada Council for the Arts and the Ontario
Arts Council, an agency of the Government of Ontario.

     Canada Council   Conseil des Arts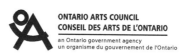
                  for the Arts   du Canada

University of Toronto Press acknowledges the financial support of the
Government of Canada through the Canada Book Fund for its publishing
activities.

This book is dedicated to Monique, Logan, and Morgan.
Time spent writing and editing this work meant time spent away
from them. Yet, they never complained, frequently and supportively
inquired as to my progress, and celebrated its completion with much
verve. I love each of you more than words can convey.

I would also like to dedicate this book to John "Alex" Cairney.
The subject matter of this book has allowed us to share a journey
together – mine of scientific exploration, his of self-discovery.
I am extremely proud of the young man you have become.

Contents

DEVELOPMENTAL COORDINATION DISORDER AND ITS CONSEQUENCES

SECTION ONE

Introduction

1 Developmental Coordination Disorder and Its Consequences: An Introduction to the Problem

JOHN CAIRNEY

This book is about children who are clumsy or physically awkward. Specifically, it is about the experiences that arise as a consequence of motor clumsiness. While the word "clumsy" has many negative (and potentially stigmatizing) connotations, it is a strikingly descriptive label, as are the words "physically awkward." In contemporary medical terminology, we refer to children who are clumsy or physically awkward with no apparent medical cause as having developmental coordination disorder, or DCD (American Psychiatric Association, 2000). Although DCD has become the dominant label, it is by no means the only one. Clumsy child syndrome (Gubbay, 1975), developmental dyspraxia (Dewey, 1995; Missiuna & Polatajko, 1995), perceptuo-motor dysfunction (Laszlo, Bairstow, & Bartrip, 1988), specific developmental disorder of motor function (World Health Organization, 1992), playground disability (Hay & Missiuna, 1998), minimal brain dysfunction (Clements, 1966), and *deficits in attention, motor control, and perception* (DAMP; Gillberg, 2003) are other names for the disorder. All of these labels refer to children who present with significant problems of motor function, problems that cause significant impairment and profoundly affect the quality of life of affected children and their families.

DCD, in contrast to some of these other labels, is relatively new, having first appeared in 1987 in the American Psychiatric Association's diagnostic manual (*Diagnostic and Statistical Manual of Mental Disorders, Third Edition*; APA, 1987). A group of experts who gathered in London, Ontario, Canada, in 1994, reached a consensus that DCD should be the preferred diagnostic label for children whose clumsiness has no known medical cause, and whose everyday social and academic functioning is significantly impaired (Polatajko, Fox, & Missiuna, 1995). Why the term first appeared in a diagnostic manual of psychiatric disorders remains unknown, but its inclusion in the official diagnostic manual of a powerful and influential medical organization gave it legitimacy as a diagnostic entity.

When we commenced work on this book, APA diagnostic criteria for DCD (hereafter DSM-IV criteria for DCD; see Table 1.1) required motor functioning well below that expected for the child's age. Problems in motor functioning also had to result in limitations to activities of daily living, and/or negatively affect school performance. So, for example, the child could experience problems with everyday activities like tying shoelaces or buttoning shirts, and also had to struggle with motor tasks related to schoolwork (e.g., printing, participating in physical education). At a functional level, the motor coordination problems had to negatively affect the child's life in order for the diagnosis to be given. If a child met diagnostic criteria for a neurological condition that affects movement, such as cerebral palsy, muscular dystrophy, or Prader-Willi syndrome, or if a child met the diagnostic criteria for pervasive developmental disorder, then the diagnosis of DCD was not advised. Finally, if mental retardation was present, then motor ability had to be assessed in relation to the child's intellectual age.[1]

While the DSM-IV criteria served a very important role in the London consensus statement, and in shaping research and clinical work in the field since that time, diagnostic criteria continue to be refined based on accumulated knowledge. From 2004 to 2005, Dr. David Sugden convened a series of seminars, known collectively as the Leeds Consensus working group, and produced a document that critically examined aspects of the DSM criteria based on the accumulated clinical and research knowledge in the span of time since the London meeting (Sugden, Chambers, & Utley, 2006). Many of the challenges of

---

1 Although in general the DSM criteria have become the standard for defining the disorder, consensus in the field of DCD research differs slightly with regard to this last point. According to the Leeds Consensus (Sugden, Chambers, & Utley, 2006) and the recently published European Academy of Childhood Disability Guidelines, a diagnosis would not normally be given in cases where the child's measured or assumed IQ is below 70 (Blank, Smits-Engelsman, Polatajko, & Wilson, 2012; Sugden et al., 2006). However, both the Leeds statement and the European guidelines do allow for a diagnosis of DCD in instances where a child's motor difficulties are in excess of those expected, given the child's IQ.

Table 1.1. DSM-IV and DSM-V Criteria for DCD

DSM-IV	DSM-V
Criterion A: Performance in daily activities that require motor coordination is substantially below that expected given the person's chronological age and measured intelligence. This may be manifested by marked delays in achieving motor milestones (e.g., walking, crawling, sitting), dropping things, "clumsiness," poor performance in sports, or poor handwriting.	Revised Criterion A: The acquisition and execution of coordinated motor skills is substantially below that expected given the individual's chronological age and opportunity for skill learning and use. Difficulties are manifested as clumsiness (e.g., dropping or bumping into objects) as well as slowness and inaccuracy of performance of motor skills (e.g., catching an object, using scissors or cutlery, handwriting, riding a bike, or participating in sports).
Criterion B: The disturbance in Criterion A significantly interferes with academic achievement or activities of daily living.	Revised Criterion B: The motor skills deficit in Criterion A significantly and persistently interferes with activities of daily living appropriate to chronological age (e.g., self-care and self-maintenance) and impacts academic/school productivity, prevocational and vocational activities, leisure, and play.
Criterion C: The disturbance is not due to a general medical condition (e.g., cerebral palsy, hemiplegia, or muscular dystrophy) and does not meet criteria for a Pervasive Developmental Disorder.	Revised Criterion C: Onset of symptoms is in the early developmental period.
Criterion D: If Mental Retardation is present, the motor difficulties are in excess of those usually associated with it.	Revised Criterion D: The motor skills deficits are not better explained by intellectual disability (intellectual developmental disorder) or visual impairment and are not attributable to a neurological condition affecting movement (e.g., cerebral palsy, muscular dystrophy, degenerative disorder).

operationalizing DSM-IV criteria for diagnosis are described in Sugden's document (see Chapter 7 for further discussion). More recently, the European Academy of Childhood Disability, under the direction of Dr. Rainer Blank, produced a set of clinical guidelines for the diagnoses, treatment, and management of DCD (Blank, Smits-Engelsman, Polatajko, & Wilson, 2012). Using systematic and meta-analytic methods, the guidelines are the first of their kind anywhere in the world. Finally, nearing the time of completion of this book, the DSM-V had only just been published. Not only is DCD included once again in this diagnostic manual but also some notable changes have been proposed. For example, children with pervasive developmental disorder will no longer be automatically excluded from receiving a diagnosis of DCD (see Chapter 7 for further discussion of DSM-V). Table 1.1 includes criteria from both DSM-IV and DSM-V for comparison.

For readers unfamiliar with DCD, however, these criteria – whether DSM or recent clinical guidelines – fall far short of describing children with this condition. To appreciate the nature of the disorder, descriptions that move beyond diagnostic criteria are required.

Describing Children with DCD

It is common in collected works such as this one to begin with a description of what DCD is like (e.g., Geuze, 2007; Sugden & Chambers, 2005). In fact, descriptions of the clumsy child have been in the published literature for some time (e.g., Orton, 1925; Walton, Ellis, & Court, 1962). These accounts are useful, for they help to paint a much more vivid picture of the affected child than is possible using clinical or technical terminology. At the same time, they reflect current understandings, and sometimes misunderstandings, about the condition. Rather than produce a new narrative account, I will review ones that already exist, showing how they are similar and how they differ.

One of the earliest modern descriptions, and one of the most colourful, appeared in the *British Medical Journal* in December 1962:

(The) so-called clumsy child, the child who is awkward in his movements, poor at games, hopeless in dancing and gymnastics, a bad writer, and defective in concentration. He is inattentive, cannot sit still, leaves his shoelaces untied, does buttons wrongly, bumps into furniture, breaks glassware, slips off his chair, kicks his legs against the desk, and perhaps reads badly. Some, she says, tend to make large sweeping movements when writing, to write with the whole body, with the tongue protruding and travelling from one side of the mouth to the other. Some are worse when they are anxious and being watched. Reprimands merely make the child worse and lead to a variety of behaviour problems – truancy, insecurity, aggressiveness, bullying, encopresis, enuresis, and day-dreaming. He cannot help it. (p. 1665)

The description is based largely on the work of Annell (1949), who considered the problem to be one of delay and felt that recovery was usually "spontaneous." As Gubbay (1975) noted, Annell and the authors of the editorial considered the problem of clumsiness to be quite common in children. They also went on to cite what appear to be other subtypes of clumsiness – however, types not entirely due to maturational delay. The main purpose of the editorial was to raise awareness of the problems clumsy children face, that is, to argue that the difficulties are real, significant, and deserving of medical intervention. Indeed, the authors expressed concern at the "sobering thought" that the child could be held responsible for behaviours resulting from poor coordination, not bad behaviour. Among the things the child could be held responsible for, such as neglect of homework, are several conditions the child could not possibly control but instead falls victim to, including "inherited personality," "errors in management" related to parenting, and "original sin."

One cannot help but notice that embedded within the description are externalizing behavioural problems (e.g., acting out), along with core symptoms of attention deficit hyperactivity disorder (ADHD; e.g., cannot sit still, slips off his or her chair). As ADHD was not recognized as such at the time this article was written, this is not surprising. The connection with ADHD symptoms is also reflected in many more recent descriptions of DCD. Indeed, many consider DCD and ADHD to be part of the same syndrome (Kaplan, Dewey, Crawford, & Wilson, 2001; Kaplan, Wilson, Dewey, & Crawford, 1998). Consider the following passage:

> Sara is a nine-year-old girl, attending primary school. Her father characterizes her motor skills as inaccurate, clumsy and somewhat poorly coordinated. When asked for more detail he mentions difficulties with buttoning and tying shoelaces, and putting in her earrings. She has irregular handwriting and no specific problems with physical education or games at school. Her school progress is average ... She is slightly hyperactive and distractible. (Geuze, 2007, p. 9)

The author went on to provide a score on the Movement ABC test (Henderson, Sugden, & Barnett, 2007), one of the most common assessment tools used to identify motor coordination problems in children (Blank et al., 2012). Not surprisingly, Sara scored in the clinically significant range, showing specific problems with manual dexterity and balance. It is unclear from the description whether the hyperactivity, described as slight, and the distractibility were the result of coordination problems or suggestive of another disorder.

Other recent descriptions, especially those written by practitioners sensitive to the differences between DCD and conditions like ADHD, make reference to the core symptoms of DCD and their impact on functioning, without reference to inattention or externalizing behaviours at all:

> Kyle is a six year old boy ... He has trouble doing up the button on his jeans, he can't hit a baseball, his teacher can't read his printing, and he can't tie his shoes ... Kyle's parents sense that there is something wrong with their son ... Morning routines and mealtimes are always stressful as Kyle seems to have trouble doing simple things like spreading jam or doing up his pants on his own. Kyle's teacher in Grade One is frustrated with him. Kyle seems to bright enough and can tell very interesting and complex stories, but he really seems to struggle whenever he has to do anything ... She tells him to focus and to try harder but it doesn't seem to make any difference. (Pollock, 2001, p. xiii)

Kyle's history also reveals that his pediatrician is not worried, having told Kyle's parents that the boy will eventually grow out of his motor coordination difficulties. Kyle's parents, however, are not convinced of this. As noted above, there is no mention of disruptive behaviour or hyperactivity. Instead the focus is on functional motor impairment and its consequences for everyday functioning. The theme of misattribution of the problem, from something present in the child and beyond his control to something behavioural and therefore remediable through focused attention and effort, is captured in the admonishments of the frustrated teacher.

These descriptions, of course, share some common themes. One is that motor coordination problems are the root cause of many negative secondary behaviours (e.g., disruptive behaviour in the classroom); however, these behaviours are not always viewed as being caused by dysfunction in motor control. When we consider the consequences or secondary problems associated with DCD, we must ask ourselves, if the cause of these problems is indeed related to poor motor coordination, will interventions that target other things (e.g., behaviour) be effective? Another common theme is that others in the child's life, be they parents, teachers, or physicians, do not seem to understand the problem and consider it to be transitory and self-correcting. This view has also been documented in the literature. Missiuna, Moll, Law, King, and King (2006) referred to the process of moving from awareness of the condition to receiving help in terms of "mysteries and mazes." For many children, and their families, frustration is the rule, not the exception, when dealing with the education and health care sectors.

Finally, the motor problems that children with DCD experience are highly variable. Many of the children described experience problems with fine motor control. This makes activities that involve manipulation with fingers and hands (e.g., printing, drawing, dressing oneself, using knives and forks when eating) extremely difficult. Fine motor problems are often not identified until the child attends school and begins to learn to print. It has been estimated that in primary school, 60 to 80 per cent of the time in the classroom is spent in activities that involve fine motor manipulation (e.g., printing, drawing, using scissors). However, children with DCD often have more pervasive motor problems, including problems with both fine and gross motor ability. In the examples above, problems negotiating movement around objects (e.g., bumping into furniture), participating in sport (e.g., hitting a baseball), and balancing (e.g., slipping off a chair) were also identified in these descriptions.

While these descriptions are not exhaustive of all the problems and experiences of children with DCD, they do provide a qualitative understanding of the main features of the disorder and the core issues (e.g., comorbidity with other disorders like ADHD) addressed throughout this book. Along with the diagnostic criteria, they help to capture what it is like to have DCD.

Understanding DCD as a Neurodevelopmental Disorder

In the research and clinical literature in this area, DCD is often described as a neurodevelopmental disorder (Henderson & Henderson, 2003). This implies that the observable functional problems characteristic of DCD are caused by dysfunction or pathology at a neurological level. It is important to note, however, that while neurological dysfunction is most likely a cause of poor motor coordination in children with DCD, researchers' understanding of motor coordination is rooted in theories that also consider other factors that influence human movement.

To many movement scientists, movement involves not only the brain and the muscles but also the environment. They use the term *dynamic systems theory* (e.g., Keogh & Sugden, 1985; Thelen & Smith, 1994; Wade, Johnson, & Mally, 2005) to describe an approach to understanding how people move that takes into account the complex interactions among factors intrinsic to the individual (e.g., nervous system, muscles), the task itself, and the environment. Dynamic systems researchers reject a top-down model where motor control is preprogrammed (Sugden, 2007). In a classic experiment, Thelen and her colleagues (Thelen, 1986) put 7-month-old infants onto a moving treadmill, supported high enough so their feet could just touch the moving belt. Even though these infants had not yet learned to walk (and were months away from being able to), once their feet touched the moving belt, their legs began to move in synchrony as if walking (i.e., alternating steps). By eliciting the "walking reflex" (something that disappears by 5 months of age) in these infants, the results of the experiment called into question maturational explanations of reflex inhibition and motor development. Of course, this result does not deny the existence or minimize the importance of innate neurological structures in the brain that coordinate action. Rather, it demonstrates that movement is a product of innate (neurological), biological, and environmental factors (stimuli).

The role that the environment plays in influencing movement is of critical importance to the child with DCD, both in relation to diagnosis (identification) and intervention. First, problems of coordination become evident only when environmental demands are not met. We do not know that a child cannot, for instance, learn to tie her shoelaces until the task is required. With regard to intervention, when motor coordination cannot be corrected, the environment can be modified to accommodate the child (see Chapter 7). We cannot separate the child from the environment, or the task, when we are dealing with problems with motor coordination.

The term *developmental*, the other part of the neurodevelopmental label, underscores the fact that the systems that govern or control movement in childhood are constantly changing. Consider the incredibly complex movement abilities that children acquire from birth to the age of 2 or 3. A newborn baby has extremely limited control over movement, being unable to lift her own head or manipulate objects with her fingers. But by about one year of age, most children can walk, hold objects in their hands, manipulate small toys, and carry out many other actions. Move forward to age 7, and most children can dress themselves (albeit not always in a manner acceptable to adults), have mastered eating with forks and spoons, and are beginning to play complex games with rules (again, fluid ones that may change often) that require the ability to coordinate movement in dynamic ("open") environments.

As the complexity of movement demands increases, coordination difficulties become evident. Consider the kicking of a ball during a soccer game.[2] The child has to be able not only to kick but also to judge distances and apply the right amount of force to make sure the ball moves to teammates or past the goalie to the back of the net – all in a matter of seconds, and often when the ball and the other players are moving. The act involves complex interactions among perception, proprioception (knowing where your body is in space), and muscle movement, getting the muscles to do what is required. Any readers who have seen 5-year-old children play soccer will know the intended act (e.g., scoring a goal) and the actual act do not always go together. But consider what the same game looks like when played by 10-year-old children, or by children who are 14 years of age. The level of coordination required becomes more and more complex. At some point, the child with DCD falls noticeably behind (Wall, 2004).

What is not captured thus far in this discussion is that while we can describe developmental changes in motor ability in terms of age, in fact, age is a relatively crude marker for developmental change. Every developmental variable of interest is imperfectly correlated with age. Height offers an example commensurate with common experience: The shortest child in a group of children at age 10 may not be the shortest at age 20. Each child follows a distinct trajectory, with growth spurts and plateaus, until the final height is reached. This is an important complication in questions of developmental disorder; it can be difficult to be sure, at least in mild cases, whether a delay is pathological or simply a temporary plateau.

Though a continuous process, development is often measured in terms of discrete milestones. In infancy and early childhood, for example, we note reaching, grasping, sitting up, standing, and walking as particularly important developmental markers. Failure to reach a milestone by a certain age raises concerns about possible delay. However, as with height, when individuals achieve these milestones varies considerably. For example, onset of walking typically occurs between 9 and 18 months (Largo et al., 1985) – a wide range that does not allow

---

2 The game to which I refer is, of course, football, for those readers who live in the United Kingdom, Europe, and indeed, the rest of the world.

us to identify cases of delay with much confidence. Other domains of motor development are equally variable. It is widely believed in the field that accurate assessment of motor coordination, using the tests currently available, is not feasible before the age of 3 (Henderson et al., 2007); older age cut-offs (e.g., 5 years of age) have also been proposed (Geuze, 2007).

Given the imperfect correlation between age and maturation, using age as a proxy for maturation will continue to pose significant problems for assessing motor development. Ideally, assessments of motor coordination should be repeated over time before diagnosing DCD; this will allow the clinician (or researcher) to take into account variability in rates of change within and between children.

To summarize, DCD is often described as a developmental disorder because children with the disorder cannot perform complex movements at the same level as their typically developing peers and may never catch up. The diagnosis is inherently comparative, and is based on an individual's failing to achieve age-appropriate norms in motor ability, notwithstanding the aforementioned limitations.

Having described what DCD is, I turn the attention to several important questions: (1) how common is DCD?; (2) what are the underlying physical causes of the disorder?; (3) is DCD a single disorder, or part of a syndrome that involves many different problems?; (4) which children are at risk for DCD?; and (5) is DCD a disorder of childhood or will the child eventually grow out of it? Addressing these points will set the stage for the more in-depth treatment of consequences and other issues that comprise the body of this book. I will conclude by briefly outlining each of the chapters.

How Common Is DCD?

It has been suggested that between 5 and 6 per cent of children between the ages of 4 and 11 have DCD (APA, 2000; Gibbs, Appleton, & Appleton, 2007; Maeland, 1992). However, the research on which this estimate is based varies tremendously in terms of sampling and case identification. Perhaps the biggest limitation is that not all studies use the same criteria for diagnosing the disorder. Indeed, while there is widespread endorsement in the field of DSM criteria, very few studies attempt to assess them fully. One exception is a recent prevalence study by Lingam, Hunt, Golding, Jongmans, and Emond (2009). Based on DSM-IV criteria, they estimated that 4.9 per cent of children show significant motor coordination problems, and 1.7 per cent have both motor delays and significant functional impairment. What makes this study so compelling, in addition to the large, population-based sample of children used to estimate prevalence, is the fact that full diagnostic criteria were applied. At the same time, as this was the first study to use contemporary criteria for operationalizing each component of the DSM criteria (Sugden et al., 2006), the researchers needed to make decisions about how best to measure each component, including the decision to use specific cut-offs (e.g., 10th percentile on the Activities of Daily Living [ADL] measure). These decisions do not and should not escape scrutiny (see Cairney, 2010). Among other concerns, their prevalence estimate was contingent on the cut point used to define problems with ADL. Adjustment of this threshold will of course increase or decrease prevalence depending on the level set. Because there is no currently agreed-upon criteria for determining such a threshold, their definition of caseness is left open to debate. Nevertheless, Lingam and colleagues have set a standard for epidemiological rigour for the estimation of prevalence that will have important implications for future studies in this area.

What Causes DCD?

Our understanding of the etiology of DCD is unfortunately rather limited. It is believed that the disorder has its origins very early in life, possibly in utero or soon after birth, as the fetal or infant brain is developing (Flouris, Faught, Hay, & Cairney, 2005; Gubbay, 1975). Exact causes are unclear and may vary from case to case. One possibility is that DCD results from a developmental insult during brain development, when the neural pathways responsible for governing motor control and coordination, and possibly other areas also involved in movement (e.g., sensory pathways), are being formed. This view is consistent with the high levels of comorbidity with ADHD and with the fact that the condition appears to be more or less localizable in the brain. Preterm birth has also been identified as a risk factor for DCD (Holsti, Grunau, & Whitfield, 2002). A genetic basis has also been posited, however, and has found some support (Gaines et al., 2008). In the end, DCD is probably one of several disorders that can be characterized as a deficit in brain functioning that can arise from various potential causes. This rather vague explanation is probably the best that can be provided at present.

Areas of the Brain Associated with DCD

Although many deficits in motor ability in children with DCD have been identified already in the literature (see Wilson & Butson, 2007), Geuze (2005) provides a useful typology of the problems that children with the disorder experience: (1) *poor postural control* or problems with both static and dynamic balance; (2) *poor sensorimotor coordination*, which, broadly, covers motor planning, timing, anticipating, and using feedback to respond to changes in the environment; and finally, (3) *problems with motor learning*, which involves learning novel skills, adapting to changes, and automatization (which allows one to focus on a task while other movements necessary for coordinated action occur with little or no conscious attention). In addition to displaying these characteristics, children with DCD have also been shown to be much slower than typically developing children when processing visuospatial information (Wilson & McKenzie, 1998). While there is obvious overlap among these categories, broadly, they capture the kinds of problems children with DCD experience.

Using this typology, Zwicker, Missiuna, and Boyd (2009) provide an excellent review of possible regions of the brain that affect each grouping of motor problems. For example, given the importance of the cerebellum to motor coordination and postural control, this area of the brain has been widely thought to play a role in the pathology of DCD (Cantin, Polatajko, Thach, & Jaglal, 2007; Visser, 2007). The cerebellum plays an important role, for example, in automatization processes (Kandel, Schwartz, & Jessell, 2000). Indeed, Visser (2007) has argued that the automatization deficit hypothesis, which comes from the literature on dyslexia (Fawcett & Nicolson, 1992), may be a useful model for understanding motor deficits in children with DCD. To get a better understanding of what is meant by automatization deficit, consider an example involving the execution of two tasks simultaneously. In brief, once a task (e.g., balancing on a beam) becomes automated, maintaining it requires little conscious or effortful attention. So, if a second, different task (e.g., counting backwards) is introduced and interferes with the first task (i.e., the child loses his or her balance), then the child is having difficulty with automatization. Obviously, the ability to automatize is a vital function for everyday life where we are often required to perform multiple tasks at the same time. Visser speculates that because children with DCD often present with comorbidities, including learning disabilities, problems with automatization resulting from cerebellar dysfunction are most likely part of the neuropathology of DCD.

Problems with visuospatial reasoning (Wilson & McKenzie, 1998), and deficits in motor planning that involve internal representational modelling (motor imagery), suggest the parietal lobe may also be part of the neuropathology of DCD. Wilson and his colleagues have shown across a series of studies that children are not only slower in the execution of motor tasks but are also slower in imagining execution of a motor task (e.g., Wilson, Maruff, Ives, & Currie, 2001; Wilson, Thomas, & Maruff, 2002). Complex visual cue recognition, for example, recognizing emotional cues from facial expressions, has also been shown to be poorer in children with DCD (Cummins, Piek, & Dyck, 2005). This kind of processing too has been linked to the parietal lobe.

Evaluating the evidence, Zwicker et al. (2009) concluded that given known patterns of comorbidity associated with DCD (e.g., ADHD, speech-language problems), and the kinds of problems commonly identified in children with DCD (postural control, timing, deficits in coordination of action), the evidence is strongest for cerebellar dysfunction. This finding certainly agrees with that of Visser (2007), who used a similar argument in support of the automatization deficit hypothesis as a means of understanding comorbidity patterns in children with DCD. However, given the complex and heterogeneous array of sensory processing and motor problems of children with DCD, likely more than one region of the brain is affected (Zwicker, Missiuna, & Boyd, 2009).

Most of the evidence implicating specific brain regions is indirect. The advent of technology such as functional magnetic resonance imaging (fMRI) allows researchers to pinpoint specific regions of the brain during functional tasks (e.g., manual rotation tasks), as well as imaged ones (e.g., mentally rotating an object in space), and thereby provide direct evidence of brain activation. While there is much work yet to be done, some evidence has started to find its way into the literature. Zwicker, Missiuna, Harris, and Boyd (2010b), for example, found that children with DCD had increased brain activity in the frontal, parietal, and temporal regions of the brain during a fine motor, trail-trace task, while typically developing children showed the greatest activation in the precuneus region. Using the same technique, but this time focusing on motor skill acquisition, the researchers found that children with DCD demonstrated underactivation in the cerebellar-parietal and cerebellar-prefrontal networks, as well as in the regions of the brain associated with visuospatial processing, when compared to typically developing children (Zwicker et al., 2010a). Functionally, children with DCD showed poorer accuracy overall in the tracing task overtime than did children without the condition.

Both of these studies suggest significant neurobiological differences between children with and without DCD. Children with DCD activate different regions of the brain and require much greater cognitive effort when completing the same task as typically developing children. Children with DCD also show little improvement following practice and rely on more areas of the brain to achieve cognitive control of movement. The latter findings, in particular, suggest that children with DCD have problems updating internal models of motor control. These data support the long-held view that children with DCD really do differ from typically developing children in terms of both functional motor performance and motor learning. These studies also support the hypothesis that cerebellar and parietal lobe dysfunction are likely part of the neuropathology of DCD. As noted earlier, however, DCD is a heterogeneous disorder, so it is unlikely that these two regions of the brain are the only areas that are affected.

One Disorder or Many?

In the preceding section, the issue of comorbidity in DCD was raised in relation to the role that the cerebellum may play in the pathology of the disorder. One of the most common co-occurring disorders is attention deficit hyperactivity disorder (ADHD) or attention deficit disorder (ADD). Studies have shown that half or more of children with ADHD/ADD also meet diagnostic criteria for DCD (Dewey, Kaplan, Crawford, & Wilson, 2002; Gillberg, 1995; Kadesjö & Gillberg, 1999). Reading disability (RD) and specific language impairment (SLI) are also common among children with DCD (Hill, 2001; Martini, Heath, & Missiuna, 1999; Miyahara, 1994).

There is an emergent literature on co-occurring mood and anxiety disorders in children with DCD (Cairney, Veldhuizen, & Szatmari, 2010). However, unlike ADHD, RD, and SLI, the co-occurrence of internalizing problems is often presented in the literature as an outcome or consequence of having DCD, rather than disorders that have a common underlying pathology. As an entire chapter of this volume is devoted to the mental health consequences of DCD (see Chapter 4), here I simply note that emotional problems are another kind of comorbidity commonly found in children with the disorder. In a similar vein, there is also increasing interest in overlap/co-occurrence of DCD with autism spectrum disorders (ASD; Reiersen, Constantino, & Todd, 2008). As with all the disorders identified above, it is unclear if ASD and DCD are distinct disorders, overlapping, or are causally related to the other. Given this uncertainty, the DSM-V has proposed allowing a joint diagnosis of ASD and DCD for the same child if, for example, the level of social impairment in a child with DCD is consistent with a diagnosis of ASD.

The high rate of concurrent problems observed in children with motor coordination problems raises at least the possibility that conditions such as DCD, RD, ADHD, SLI, and emotional-behavioural problems may not be separate disorders, but manifestations of a single, pervasive disorder. This is not a new idea. In the 1960s, the term *minimal brain dysfunction* (MBD) was used to describe cases of atypical development across multiple domains (Clements, 1966). As the label suggests, the underlying neuropathology was thought to be some kind of diffuse, rather than localized, abnormality. Gillberg and his colleagues (Gillberg Carlström, Rasmussen, & Waldenström, 1983; Gillberg & Rasmussen, 1982) replaced MBD with a more precise, clinical label, *deficits in attention, motor control, and perception* (DAMP). Kaplan, Wilson, Dewey, and Crawford (1998), meanwhile, have suggested *atypical brain development* (ABD).

In proposing these broader labels, researchers have sought to reconceptualize existing disorders as domains within a more general syndrome. This approach, however, remains controversial. There are many "pure" cases of DCD – for example, 45% of Kaplan et al.'s (1998) sample – and risk factors for conditions like DCD and ADHD appear to be different (Pearsall-Jones et al., 2008; Pearsall-Jones, Piek, Rigoli, Martin, & Levy, 2009). These results suggest that it may be more prudent at this time to retain the existing, separate diagnostic entities (Cairney et al., 2010). The high levels of comorbidity cannot be ignored, however, and stronger evidence on common etiologies, treatments, or patterns of deficits may yet tip the balance in the other direction.

Who Is at Risk of Developing DCD?

Much like our understanding of the neuropathology of DCD, our understanding of what places children at risk for DCD is limited. Unlike many other disorders of childhood, DCD appears *not* to be linked to socioeconomic status or ethnicity (Blank et al., 2012). DCD has been observed in many different cultures, suggesting that if culture plays a role, it will likely be in its response to the condition (how the condition is defined, how it is treated), not in its etiology.

While socioeconomic status and ethnicity do not appear to be risk factors for DCD, gender may be. However, its association with the disorder is complex. DCD has been described as a boys' disorder, with ratios of 2 or more to 1 in favour of males (Gibbs et al., 2007; Lingam, Hunt, Golding, Jongmans, & Edmodo, 2009; Maeland, 1992). This preponderance of boys seems, however, to be linked to sampling methods. In samples drawn from clinics, boys tend to outnumber girls significantly, while in general population samples the male–female ratio is closer to 1:1 (Cairney, Hay, Faught, Mandigo, & Flouris, 2005; Foulder-Hughes & Cooke, 2003; Skinner & Piek, 2001; but see Lingam et al., 2009). This difference implies that a referral bias may be responsible for greater numbers of boys seen in clinical settings. Some evidence suggests that motor coordination problems are regarded as less problematic in girls (Gillberg, 2003; Taylor, 1990). High levels of comorbidity with ADHD may also be responsible, however, as this disorder is more commonly identified in males (e.g., Rhee, Waldman, Hay, & Levy, 2001), and entering care for ADHD may lead to subsequent identification of DCD. The possibility of under-identification of girls with DCD should be a concern for researchers and practitioners and is an area of research that requires much more attention.

The only other clinical risk factors associated with DCD are perinatal: extremely low birth weight (Holsti et al., 2002); preterm birth (Foulder-Hughes & Cooke, 2003); mild damage to the developing brain, especially in preterm infants (Jongmans, Henderson, de Vries, & Dubowitz, 1993); and complications during birth, particularly those involving neonatal hypoxia (Pearsall-Jones, Piek, & Levy, 2010b). More severe oxygen profusion problems, including hypoxia and placental difficulties, are also associated with cerebral palsy (CP; e.g., Thorngren-Jerneck, & Herbst, 2006), and it has been suggested that DCD may, in fact, be a mild form of CP (Pearsall-Jones, Piek, & Levy, 2010b).

Evidence on genetic factors is mixed, with some indications that DCD is less strongly influenced by genetics than is ADHD (Pearsall-Jones et al., 2008; Pearsall-Jones et al., 2009). Conversely, case histories have shown that DCD can occur in siblings and parents in the same family (Gaines et al., 2008), suggesting at some level a role for genetic heritability. Our current understanding of the genetics of DCD is limited; yet, the phenotype of DCD is likely the result of both genetic and environmental factors.

Do Children Grow Out of DCD?

DCD is sometimes described in terms of "delay," which implies that children with DCD may eventually catch up to typically developing children. Developmental disparity is also true of other conditions, however, and this view is often optimistic.

The literature on DCD broadly supports the view that DCD persists into adolescence, and perhaps adulthood, but not in all cases. Evidence comes largely from two longitudinal studies. Cantell, Smyth, and Ahonen (1994, 2003) followed a cohort of children ($n = 81$) with delayed motor development from age 5. At age 11, 65% of the children continued to show motor coordination problems. By age 17, this proportion dropped to 46%. Geuze and Borger (1993) also found that about 50% of cases of children with motor problems identified at 7 to 12 years of age continued to exhibit problems 5 years later (ages 12 to 17). Such studies must contend, however, with issues of case ascertainment; even studies that perform assessments very close together in time (e.g., to assess the test–retest reliability of an instrument) find less-than-perfect agreement, and any bias on levels of persistence will be downward, being affected by false positives at baseline and false negatives at follow-up.

Qualitative data, meanwhile, suggest that adults who had DCD when they were children continued to have problems with motor coordination in adulthood (Fitzpatrick & Watkinson, 2003). Moreover, most of these reflected on the negative experiences they had as children, suggesting that the impact of DCD extends well beyond childhood.

As with other areas we have reviewed, there is more need for research on the natural history of DCD. The aforementioned studies use small, nonrepresentative samples, so our picture of the long-term stability of the disorder is very limited. Available evidence does suggest that for many children, particularly those with quite severe levels of motor impairment (Knuckey & Gubbay, 1983), DCD is not a transient problem that resolves on its own.

What Makes This Book Unique? A Focus on Consequences

There have been other collected works on DCD (e.g., Cermak & Larkin, 2002; Geuze, 2007; Sugden & Chambers, 2005), and there will be some overlap in content between this work and the others. It is difficult, for example, to produce a volume on DCD and not describe the disorder, characterize its main features, discuss possible etiology, and the like, as

I have done in this opening chapter. Research articles that have stood the test of time are cited throughout this book. However, this book differs from other works in two important ways. First, the work was conceived and written several years after the last edited collection was published (Geuze, 2007), and it will therefore include relevant studies that have appeared in the interim. In this chapter alone I have cited a number of important articles published since 2007. In a rapidly changing field such as DCD research, it is perhaps past time for a new collection.

Of much greater importance, however, is that this book has a more specific focus than previous collected works. This book is about consequences. It is not clumsiness per se but its consequences that draw attention to the disorder and fuel concerns among parents, teachers, clinicians, and researchers. The issue of successful execution of motor skills could be understood solely in terms of aesthetics; some children perform complex motor tasks with more accuracy, speed, and grace than do others. For those who do not, however, surely the problem is not medical? If physical awkwardness leads to ridicule from peers, results in less engagement in motor-based activities, and leads thereby to obesity, or if clumsiness itself prevents a child from performing simple everyday tasks necessary for normal social interaction and functioning, then the problem is more than a matter of aesthetics. We care about DCD because we are concerned about the negative effects it has on children. Clinicians, researchers, and those who have DCD or who have a loved one with DCD need no convincing that the disorder has negative consequences for the child. The same is not necessarily true of the broader medical and health sciences research communities. As many have noted, DCD is a hidden disorder, not often recognized, and poorly understood by teachers, health care professionals, and parents (Missiuna et al., 2006). It is critically important that we raise awareness of the problems associated with DCD. Books such as this can serve an important role in this regard.

In addition, this book goes beyond consequences, providing the reader with current information and recommendations related to screening and identification of children with DCD, methodological issues relevant to research on the consequences of DCD, and outlining a comprehensive range of treatment options for children with DCD. The evidence base for DCD is growing every day, informing clinical practice and advancing our understanding of the causes and consequences of this disorder. The information here is relevant to all students of the discipline, be they established researchers or those new to the field, clinicians with years of experience or those who are just embarking on their careers. A book that fails to consider measurement and research challenges, or the implications that our understanding of secondary consequences has for intervention, is simply incomplete.

The Organization of This Book

The remaining chapters in this book are divided into three sections. The first section includes four chapters that cut to the heart of the matter: the secondary consequences associated with DCD. Chapter 2, by Batya Engel-Yeger, broadly explores the impact of DCD across a number of different domains. Here readers see the pervasive impact of the disorder, not only on physical activity but also on school-based tasks and recreational pursuits. Chapter 3, my contribution to this section, narrows the focus, concentrating specifically on participation in physical play and its consequences for fitness and physical health. In Chapter 4, Jan Piek and Daniela Rigoli review what is known about the psychosocial and mental health consequences related to DCD. Chapter 5, by Peter Wilson, concludes the first section and focuses on neurocognitive deficits. Here the focus is at a neurological level, so readers can begin to understand the brain processes that underlie the condition.

The second section consists of two chapters focused on issues related to identification and methodology. Having established the pervasive, secondary consequences associated with DCD, it is important to consider what must be done. Chapter 6 is Marina Shoemaker and Brenda Wilson's review on screening for DCD. As noted earlier, DCD continues to be a hidden problem, and the challenges of identifying children with the disorder are formidable. The authors of this chapter review what is known about screening for DCD, especially in community- or population-based settings. Chapter 7, by Scott Veldhuizen and John Cairney, focuses on research methods. Based on what we have learned from the preceding chapters, what we know and what is not known, the authors consider a key question: What kinds of research methods are required to better understand secondary consequences? The authors also address methodological issues, particularly ways to identify children with DCD.

The third and final section of the book contains two chapters. Chapter 8 addresses the problem of intervention, or what clinicians might do to address the secondary consequences that arise from DCD. Cheryl Missiuna, Helene Polatajko, and Nancy Pollock discuss this problem, arguing for a population-based approach that addresses the problems of long waiting lists and a scarcity of clinical providers. Finally, the last chapter, Chapter 9, offers reflections on the future of work in this area based on what has been presented in this collection.

Together, the chapters in this collection review what we currently know about the possible short- and long-term, direct and indirect, consequences of DCD, provide directions for further work, discuss the challenges facing researchers, and suggest interventions to address these problems early, before they take hold and negatively affect the child's quality of life.

REFERENCES

American Psychiatric Association. (1987). *Diagnostic and statistical manual of mental disorders* (3rd ed.). Arlington, VA: American Psychiatric Publishing.

American Psychiatric Association. (2000). *Diagnostic and statistical manual of mental disorders* (4th ed., text rev.). Washington, DC: Author

Annell, A.L. (1949, Oct). School problems in children of average or superior intelligence: A preliminary report. *Journal of Mental Science, 95*(401), 901–909. Medline:15396383

Blank, R., Smits-Engelsman, B., Polatajko, H., Wilson, P., & European Academyof Childhood Disability. (2012, Jan). European Academy of Childhood Disability (EACD): Recommendations on the definition, diagnosis and intervention of developmental coordination disorder (long version). *Developmental Medicine and Child Neurology, 54*(1), 54–93. http://dx.doi.org/10.1111/j.1469-8749.2011.04171.x Medline:22171930

British Medical Journal. (1962). Clumsy children. *British Medical Journal*, 1665–1666.

Cairney, J. (2010). Diagnostic criteria and case ascertainment of DCD in epidemiological studies: Does DSM help? [E-letter]. *Pediatrics* (6 January 2010), http://pediatrics.aappublications.org/content/123/4/e693/reply#pediatrics_el_49177

Cairney, J., Hay, J.A., Faught, B.E., Mandigo, J., & Flouris, A. (2005). Developmental coordination disorder, self-efficacy toward physical activity and participation in free play and organized activities: Does gender matter? *Adapted Physical Activity Quarterly; APAQ, 22*(1), 67–82.

Cairney, J., Veldhuizen, S., & Szatmari, P. (2010, Jul). Motor coordination and emotional-behavioral problems in children. *Current Opinion in Psychiatry, 23*(4), 324–329. http://dx.doi.org/10.1097/YCO.0b013e32833aa0aa Medline:20520549

Cantell, M., Smyth, M.M., & Ahonen, T.P. (1994). Clumsiness in adolescence: Educational, motor and social outcomes of motor delay detected at 5 years. *Adapted Physical Activity Quarterly; APAQ, 11,* 115–129.

Cantell, M.H., Smyth, M.M., & Ahonen, T.P. (2003, Nov). Two distinct pathways for developmental coordination disorder: Persistence and resolution. *Human Movement Science, 22*(4-5), 413–431. http://dx.doi.org/10.1016/j.humov.2003.09.002 Medline:14624826

Cantin, N., Polatajko, H.J., Thach, W.T., & Jaglal, S. (2007, Jun). Developmental coordination disorder: Exploration of a cerebellar hypothesis. *Human Movement Science, 26*(3), 491–509. http://dx.doi.org/10.1016/j.humov.2007.03.004 Medline:17509709

Cermak, S.A., & Larkin, D. (2002). *Developmental coordination disorder.* Albany, NY: Delmar Thompson Learning.

Clements, S.D. (1966, Mar). The child with minimal brain dysfunction: A multidisciplinary catalyst. *Lancet, 86*(3), 121–123. Medline:5904645

Cummins, A., Piek, J.P., & Dyck, M.J. (2005, Jul). Motor coordination, empathy, and social behaviour in school-aged children. *Developmental Medicine and Child Neurology, 47*(7), 437–442. http://dx.doi.org/10.1017/S001216220500085X Medline:15991862

Dewey, D. (1995, Dec). What is developmental dyspraxia? *Brain and Cognition, 29*(3), 254–274. http://dx.doi.org/10.1006/brcg.1995.1281 Medline:8838385

Dewey, D., Kaplan, B.J., Crawford, S.G., & Wilson, B.N. (2002, Dec). Developmental coordination disorder: Associated problems in attention, learning, and psychosocial adjustment. *Human Movement Science, 21*(5-6), 905–918. http://dx.doi.org/10.1016/S0167-9457(02)00163-X Medline:12620725

Fawcett, A.J., & Nicolson, R.I. (1992, Oct). Automatisation deficits in balance for dyslexic children. *Perceptual and Motor Skills, 75*(2), 507–529. http://dx.doi.org/10.2466/pms.1992.75.2.507 Medline:1408614

Fitzpatrick, D., & Watkinson, E.J. (2003). The lived experience of physical awkwardness: Adults; retrospective views. *Adapted Physical Activity Quarterly; APAQ, 20,* 279–297.

Flouris, A.D., Faught, B.E., Hay, J., & Cairney, J. (2005, Jul). Exploring the origins of developmental disorders. *Developmental Medicine and Child Neurology, 47*(7), 436. http://dx.doi.org/10.1017/S0012162205000848 Medline:15991861

Foulder-Hughes, L.A., & Cooke, R.W. (2003). Developmental co-ordination disorder in preterm children born <32 weeks gestational age. *Dyspraxia Foundation Professional Journal, 2*, 3–13.

Gaines, R., Collins, D., Boycott, K., Missiuna, C., Delaat, D., & Soucie, H. (2008, Nov). Clinical expression of developmental coordination disorder in a large Canadian family. *Paediatrics & Child Health (Oxford), 13*(9), 763–768. Medline:19436536

Geuze, R.H. (2005). Postural control in children with developmental coordination disorder. *Neural Plasticity, 12*(2-3), 183–196, discussion 263–272. http://dx.doi.org/10.1155/NP.2005.183 Medline:16097486

Geuze, R.H. (Ed.). (2007). *Developmental coordination disorder: A review of current approaches*. Marseille, France: Solal.

Geuze, R.H., & Borger, H. (1993). Children who are clumsy, five years later. *Adapted Physical Activity Quarterly; APAQ, 10*, 10–21.

Gibbs, J., Appleton, J., & Appleton, R. (2007, Jun). Dyspraxia or developmental coordination disorder? Unravelling the enigma. *Archives of Disease in Childhood, 92*(6), 534–539. http://dx.doi.org/10.1136/adc.2005.088054 Medline:17515623

Gillberg, C. (1995). Deficits in attention, motor control and perception, and other syndromes attributed to minimal brain dysfunction. In C. Gillberg (Ed.), *Clinical child neuropsychiatry* (pp. 138–172). New York, NY: Cambridge University Press. http://dx.doi.org/10.1017/CBO9780511570094.009

Gillberg, C. (2003, Oct). Deficits in attention, motor control, and perception: A brief review. *Archives of Disease in Childhood, 88*(10), 904–910. http://dx.doi.org/10.1136/adc.88.10.904 Medline:14500312

Gillberg, C., Carlström, G., Rasmussen, P., & Waldenström, E. (1983, Jan). Perceptual, motor and attentional deficits in seven-year-old children: Neurological screening aspects. *Acta Paediatrica Scandinavica, 72*(1), 119–124. http://dx.doi.org/10.1111/j.1651-2227.1983.tb09675.x Medline:6858674

Gillberg, C., & Rasmussen, P. (1982, Jan). Perceptual, motor and attentional deficits in six-year-old children: Screening procedure in pre-school. *Acta Paediatrica Scandinavica, 71*(1), 121–129. http://dx.doi.org/10.1111/j.1651-2227.1982.tb09382.x Medline:7136607

Gillberg, C., Rasmussen, P., Carlström, G., Svenson, B., Waldenström, E. (1982, Apr). Perceptual, motor and attentional deficits in six-year-old children. Epidemiological aspects. *Journal of Child Psychology and Psychiatry, 23*(2) 131–144. http://dx.doi.org/ 10.1111/j.1469-7610.1982.tb00058.x

Gubbay, S.S. (1975). *The clumsy child: A study in developmental apraxia and agnosic ataxia*. London, England: W.B. Saunders.

Hay, J., & Missiuna, C. (1998). Motor proficiency in children reporting low levels of participation in physical activity. *Canadian Journal of Occupational Therapy, 65*(2), 64–71. http://dx.doi.org/10.1177/000841749806500203

Henderson, S.E., & Henderson, L. (2003). Toward an understanding of Developmental Mental Coordination Disorder: terminological and diagnostic issues. *Neural Plasticity, 10* (1–2), 1–13.

Henderson, S.E., Sugden, D.A., & Barnett, A. (2007). *Movement Assessment Battery for Children* (2nd ed.). London, England: Pearson.

Hill, E.L. (2001, Apr–Jun). Non-specific nature of specific language impairment: A review of the literature with regard to concomitant motor impairments. *International Journal of Language & Communication Disorders, 36*(2), 149–171. http://dx.doi.org/10.1080/13682820010019874 Medline:11344592

Holsti, L., Grunau, R.V.E., & Whitfield, M.F. (2002, Feb). Developmental coordination disorder in extremely low birth weight children at nine years. *Journal of Developmental and Behavioral Pediatrics, 23*(1), 9–15. http://dx.doi.org/10.1097/00004703-200202000-00002 Medline:11889346

Jongmans, M., Henderson, S., de Vries, L., & Dubowitz, L. (1993, Jul). Duration of periventricular densities in preterm infants and neurological outcome at 6 years of age [Special issue]. *Archives of Disease in Childhood, 69*(1), 9–13. http://dx.doi.org/10.1136/adc.69.1_Spec_No. 9 Medline:8346967

Kadesjö, B., & Gillberg, C. (1999, Jul). Developmental coordination disorder in Swedish 7-year-old children. *Journal of the American Academy of Child and Adolescent Psychiatry, 38*(7), 820–828. http://dx.doi.org/10.1097/00004583-199907000-00011 Medline:10405499

Kandel, E.R., Schwartz, J.H., & Jessell, T.M. (2000). *Principles of neural science.* New York, NY: McGraw-Hill Professional Publishing.

Kaplan, B.J., Dewey, D.M., Crawford, S.G., & Wilson, B.N. (2001, Nov–Dec). The term comorbidity is of questionable value in reference to developmental disorders: Data and theory. *Journal of Learning Disabilities, 34*(6), 555–565. http://dx.doi.org/10.1177/002221940103400608 Medline:15503570

Kaplan, B.J., Wilson, B.N., Dewey, D., & Crawford, S.G. (1998). DCD may not be a discrete disorder. *Human Movement Science, 17*(4-5), 471–490. http://dx.doi.org/10.1016/S0167-9457(98)00010-4

Keogh, J.F., & Sugden, D.A. (1985). *Movement skill development.* New York, NY: Macmillan.

Knuckey, N.W., & Gubbay, S.S. (1983, Mar). Clumsy children: A prognostic study. *Australian Paediatric Journal, 19*(1), 9–13. Medline:6191748

Largo, R.H., Molinari, L., Weber, M., Comenale Pinto, L., & Duc, G. (1985, Apr). Early development of locomotion: Significance of prematurity, cerebral palsy and sex. *Developmental Medicine and Child Neurology, 27*(2), 183–191. http://dx.doi.org/10.1111/j.1469-8749.1985.tb03768.x Medline:3996775

Laszlo, J., Bairstow, P., & Bartrip, J. (1988). A new approach to treatment of perceptuo-motor dysfunction: Previously called "clumsiness." *Support for Learning, 3*(1), 35–40. http://dx.doi.org/10.1111/j.1467-9604.1988.tb00068.x

Lingam, R., Hunt, L., Golding, J., Jongmans, M., & Emond, A. (2009, Apr). Prevalence of developmental coordination disorder using the DSM-IV at 7 years of age: A UK population-based study. *Pediatrics, 123*(4), e693–e700. http://dx.doi.org/10.1542/peds.2008-1770 Medline:19336359

Maeland, A.F. (1992). Identification of children with motor coordination problems. *Adapted Physical Activity Quarterly; APAQ, 9*, 330–342.

Martini, R., Heath, N., & Missiuna, C. (1999). A North American analysis of the relationship between learning disabilities and developmental coordination disorder. *International Journal of Learning Disabilities, 14*, 46–58.

Missiuna, C., & Polatajko, H. (1995, Jul-Aug). Developmental dyspraxia by any other name: Are they all just clumsy children? *American Journal of Occupational Therapy., 49*(7), 619–627. http://dx.doi.org/10.5014/ajot.49.7.619 Medline:7573332

Missiuna, C., Moll, S., Law, M., King, S., & King, G. (2006, Feb). Mysteries and mazes: Parents' experiences of children with developmental coordination disorder. *Canadian Journal of Occupational Therapy, 73*(1), 7–17. Medline:16570837

Miyahara, M. (1994). Subtypes of students with learning disabilities based on gross motor functions. *Adapted Physical Activity Quarterly; APAQ, 11*, 368–382.

Orton, S.T. (1925). "Word-blindness" in school children. *Archives of Neurology and Psychiatry, 14*(5), 581–615. http://dx.doi.org/10.1001/archneurpsyc.1925.02200170002001

Pearsall-Jones, J.G., Piek, J.P., & Levy, F. (2010a, Apr). Etiological pathways for developmental coordination disorder and attention-deficit/hyperactivity disorder: Shared or discrete? *Expert Review of Neurotherapeutics, 10*(4), 491–494. http://dx.doi.org/10.1586/ern.10.20 Medline:20367201

Pearsall-Jones, J.G., Piek, J.P., & Levy, F. (2010b, Oct). Developmental coordination disorder and cerebral palsy: Categories or a continuum? *Human Movement Science, 29*(5), 787–798. http://dx.doi.org/10.1016/j.humov.2010.04.006 Medline:20594606

Pearsall-Jones, J.G., Piek, J.P., Martin, N.C., Rigoli, D., Levy, F., & Hay, D.A. (2008). A monozygotic twin design to investigate etiological factors for DCD and ADHD. *Journal of Pediatric Neurology, 6*(3), 209–219.

Pearsall-Jones, J.G., Piek, J.P., Rigoli, D., Martin, N.C., & Levy, F. (2009, Aug). An investigation into etiological pathways of DCD and ADHD using a monozygotic twin design. *Twin Research and Human Genetics, 12*(4), 381–391. http://dx.doi.org/10.1375/twin.12.4.381 Medline:19653839

Polatajko, H., Fox, M., & Missiuna, C. (1995). An international consensus on children with developmental coordination disorder. *Canadian Journal of Occupational Therapy, 62*, 3–6.

Pollock, N. (2001). Preface. In C.A. Missiuna (Ed.), *Children with developmental coordination disorder: Strategies for success* (p. xiii). Binghamton, NY: Haworth Press.

Reiersen, A.M., Constantino, J.N., & Todd, R.D. (2008, Jun). Co-occurrence of motor problems and autistic symptoms in attention-deficit/hyperactivity disorder. *Journal of the American Academy of Child and Adolescent Psychiatry,* 47(6), 662–672. http://dx.doi.org/10.1097/CHI.0b013e31816bff88 Medline:18434922

Rhee, S.H., Waldman, I.D., Hay, D.A., & Levy, F. (2001). Aetiology of the sex difference in the prevalence of DSM-III-R ADHD: A comparison of two models. In F. Levy & D.A. Hay (Eds.), *Attention, genes and ADHD* (pp. 139–156). Hove, England: Brunner-Routledge.

Skinner, R.A., & Piek, J.P. (2001, Mar). Psychosocial implications of poor motor coordination in children and adolescents. *Human Movement Science,* 20(1-2), 73–94. http://dx.doi.org/10.1016/S0167-9457(01)00029-X Medline:11471399

Sugden, D.A. (2007). Dynamic management of developmental coordination disorder. In R.H. Geuze (Ed.), *Developmental coordination disorder: A review of current approaches* (pp. 183–209). Marseille, France: Solal.

Sugden, D.A., & Chambers, M. (Eds.). (2005). *Children with developmental coordination disorder.* London, England: Whurr Publishers.

Sugden, D.A., Chambers, M., & Utley, A. (2006). Leeds Consensus Statement. Available online at http://dcd.canchild.ca/en/dcdresources/consensusstatements.asp (downloaded 14 May 2011).

Taylor, M.J. (1990). Marker variables for early identification of physically awkward children. In G. Doll-Tepper, C. Dahms, B. Doll, & H. von Selzam (Eds.), *Adapted physical activity* (pp. 379–386). Berlin, Germany: Springer-Verlag. http://dx.doi.org/10.1007/978-3-642-74873-8_57

Thelen, E. (1986, Dec). Treadmill-elicited stepping in seven-month-old infants. *Child Development,* 57(6), 1498–1506. http://dx.doi.org/10.2307/1130427 Medline:3802974

Thelen, E., & Smith, L.B. (1994). *A dynamic systems approach to the development of cognition and action.* Cambridge, MA: Massachusetts Institute of Technology Press.

Thorngren-Jerneck, K., & Herbst, A. (2006, Dec). Perinatal factors associated with cerebral palsy in children born in Sweden. *Obstetrics and Gynecology,* 108(6), 1499–1505. http://dx.doi.org/10.1097/01.AOG.0000247174.27979.6b Medline:17138786

Visser, J. (2007). Substypes and co-morbidities. In R.H. Geuze (Ed.), *Developmental coordination disorder: A review of current approaches* (pp. 83–110). Marseille, France: Solal.

30   John Cairney

Wade, M.G., Johnson, D., & Mally, K. (2005). A dynamical systems perspective of developmental coordination disorder. In D.A. Sugden & M. Chambers (Eds.), *Children with developmental coordination disorder* (pp. 72–92). London, England: Whurr Publishers.

Wall, A.E. (2004). The developmental skill-learning gap hypothesis: Implications for children with movement difficulties. *Adapted Physical Activity Quarterly; APAQ, 21*(3), 197–218.

Walton, J.N., Ellis, E., & Court, S.D.M. (1962, Sep). Clumsy children: Developmental apraxia and agnosia. *Brain, 85*(3), 603–612. http://dx.doi.org/10.1093/brain/85.3.603 Medline:13998739

Wilson, P., & Butson, M. (2007). Deficits underlying DCD. In R.H. Geuze (Ed.), *Developmental coordination disorder: A review of current approaches* (pp. 111–138). Marseille, France: Solal.

Wilson, P.H., Maruff, P., Ives, S., & Currie, J. (2001, Mar). Abnormalities of motor and praxis imagery in children with DCD. *Human Movement Science, 20*(1-2), 135–159. http://dx.doi.org/10.1016/S0167-9457(01)00032-X Medline:11471394

Wilson, P.H., & McKenzie, B.E. (1998, Sep). Information processing deficits associated with developmental coordination disorder: A meta-analysis of research findings. *Journal of Child Psychology and Psychiatry, and Allied Disciplines, 39*(6), 829–840. http://dx.doi.org/10.1017/S0021963098002765 Medline:9758192

Wilson, P.H., Thomas, P.R., & Maruff, P. (2002, Jul). Motor imagery training ameliorates motor clumsiness in children. *Journal of Child Neurology, 17*(7), 491–498. http://dx.doi.org/10.1177/088307380201700704 Medline:12269727

World Health Organization. (1992). *The ICD-10 classification of mental and behavioural disorders: Clinical Descriptions and diagnostic guidelines.* Geneva, Switzerland: Author.

Zwicker, J.G., Missiuna, C., & Boyd, L.A. (2009, Oct). Neural correlates of developmental coordination disorder: A review of hypotheses. *Journal of Child Neurology, 24*(10), 1273–1281. http://dx.doi.org/10.1177/0883073809333537 Medline:19687388

Zwicker, J.G., Missiuna, C., Harris, S.R., & Boyd, L.A. (2010a, Apr). Brain activation associated with motor skill practice in children with developmental coordination disorder: An fMRI study. *International Journal of Developmental Neuroscience, 29*(2), 145–152. http://dx.doi.org/10.1016/j.ijdevneu.2010.12.002 Medline:21145385

Zwicker, J.G., Missiuna, C., Harris, S.R., & Boyd, L.A. (2010b, Sep). Brain activation of children with developmental coordination disorder is different than peers. *Pediatrics, 126*(3), e678–e686. http://dx.doi.org/10.1542/peds.2010-0059 Medline:20713484

SECTION TWO

Personal, Social, Physical, and Mental Health Consequences

2 Developmental Coordination Disorder and Participation

BATYA ENGEL-YEGER

"It's difficult for me to button my shirt and to tie my shoes." "I don't know how to use the fork and the knife." "I stay in class after all other children because I don't succeed copying the assignments the teacher wrote on the board." "Sports activities like running and jumping are difficult for me. I can hardly breathe when performing them." "Some kids ask me: Why are you so slow when you get out of the car?" "Kids laugh at me in sports class; they do not want me to play football with them." "If I play, I prefer to be the goalie." "Actually, I prefer playing soccer on the Sony Play Station."

These are only a few examples of the experiences of a boy I know with developmental coordination disorder (DCD). His experiences not only reflect the motor difficulties that disrupt daily living activities but also show how DCD may affect social interactions, academic life, and family relationships. The comments capture the emotional distress that children with DCD often experience, distress that may affect their self-esteem and general well-being. These experiences also exemplify the challenges of managing DCD difficulties, evident in the boy's choice of activities and how he prefers to participate.

Taking into account that DCD is not an inconsequential condition, but one that can have immediate and long-term psychological and physical morbidity (Poulsen, Ziviani, & Cuskelly, 2008), researchers need to use a broad perspective to understand the motor difficulties associated with DCD and the consequences they have on children who live with the condition. We might ask: How does DCD affect participation at school or in leisure time? What are the consequences of DCD on social relationships with friends and family members? Does DCD influence relationships with significant others (e.g., teachers)? What are the impacts of DCD on self-concept, such as self- confidence and self-efficacy? How does the child deal with these difficulties and their emotional outcomes? How do these difficulties affect development, health status, and well-being? Such questions focus attention on social and personal consequences associated with DCD and the broad impact this condition has on children's quality of life. They also direct us to consider the important roles that both the child and others (e.g., family, teachers, clinicians) may play in managing the DCD.

In this chapter I will discuss DCD within just such a broad perspective, focusing on the physical, social, academic, and emotional difficulties and their relationships to activity performance and participation. I will review existing theoretical models and existing studies. I will also consider the practical implications associated with the consequences of DCD to participation.

What Does Participation Mean, and Why Is It Important for the Child's Function and Development?

According to the World Health Organization (WHO), participation refers to the nature and extent of a person's involvement in life situations, including personal maintenance, mobility, information exchange, social relationships, home life, education, work and employment, economic life, and community, social, and civic life (WHO, 2001).

In 2001 the WHO introduced a classification system for understanding health and disability, the International Classification of Functioning, Disability and Health (hereafter the IFC model). This model refers to *body function and structure* (impairment), *activity* (activity limitations), and *participation* (participation restrictions) and highlights that the level of body function or structure influences a person's ability to perform activities and to participate in everyday life. Functional outcomes are conceptualized as the result of interactions among these components (see Figure 2.1). Health is achieved, supported, and maintained when individuals are able to engage in occupations and in activities that allow desired or needed participation in home, school, workplace, and community settings (AOTA, 2002, p. 611). Thus, participation is essential for psychological and emotional well-being, as well as for skill development, and contributes to one's life satisfaction and overall sense of competence.

The increasing emphasis on participation by international organizations such as the WHO, and by national governments and health and social welfare systems, makes it all the more important that we understand participation, what it means, what facilitates it, and how

Figure 2.1. The conceptual framework adopted by the ICF. From the International Classification of Functioning, Disability and Health (WHO, 2001, p. 18). Copyright 2001 by the World Health Organization.

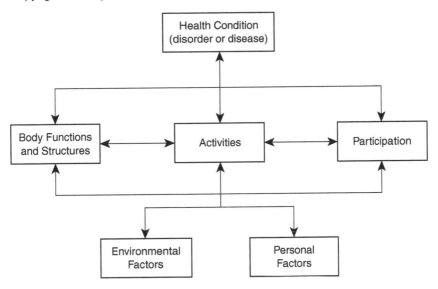

best to measure it (Law, 2002). In the sections that follow I will outline how the major domains identified in the model affect a child's participation.

What Affects Participation?

Environmental and personal factors may affect individual choices (Law, 2002; Law & Dunn, 1994). Therefore, when evaluating what affects participation, it is necessary to consider person–environment fit.

Environmental factors include elements of the physical and social environments. Physical elements include the natural environment (e.g., light, temperature) and geographical structures (e.g., physical accessibility of buildings). Social environmental elements include social/cultural attitudes, legal and social structures, attitudes of community members, and familial factors such as income, availability of opportunities, values, role models, psychosocial support, children's care and training, family preferences (Law, 2002; Law et al., 2004; Osterweil & Nagano, 1991), supportive modelling, familial routines, cultural background, and attitudes regarding children (e.g., behaviours and skills to be encouraged and developed; Katz, Kizony, & Parush, 2002; Rosenblum, Katz, Hahn-Markowitz, Mazor-Karsenty, & Parush, 2000).

Personal factors are individual-level elements that include body functions and abilities (motor, sensory, mental, etc.), as well as other health conditions, gender, age, social background, education, overall behaviour pattern, character style, and coping styles (Law et al., 2006; Sherwood, Story, Neumark-Sztainer, Adkins, & Davis, 2003; WHO, 2001).

The Various Dimensions of Participation

In order to have a thorough understanding of the child's participation profile, it is important to consider various dimensions of participation: (1) types of activities (diversity), (2) intensity of participation, (3) individuals with whom the child participates, (4) places the child participates, (5) child's enjoyment level when participating in the activity, and (6) child's preferred activities (Larson & Verma, 1999; Law, 2002). When assessing participation or, in the context of research, measuring it, researchers need to consider all these dimensions. By using this model, researchers will better understand what shapes participation, and what they learn will help them plan interventions to enhance participation or to design effective policies and programs at a broader, systems level (Law et al., 2003).

According to the literature, several activity types have been identified: recreational activities, active play or physical activities, social activities, skill-based activities, and self-improvement and educational activities (King et al., 2004). These activities can be further categorized under two broad domains: formal activities, which are structured, have rules and organization, involve leaders, and often require preplanning (e.g., music or art lessons, organized sports, youth groups); and informal activities, such as reading, talking on the phone, or doing a puzzle, which are typically more spontaneous, occur with less planning, and have only a few rules (King, Law, King, Rosenbaum, Kertoy, & Young, 2003).

Participation of Children with DCD

For children, participating in everyday activities is vital. There is widespread recognition that being involved in an activity has a positive influence on the development of skills and competencies, building social relationships, and establishing long-term mental and physical health (Caldwell, 1990; Forsyth & Jarvis 2002; Larson & Verma, 1999; Lyons, 1993; Simeonsson, Carlson, Huntington, McMillen, & Brent, 2001). Thus, the participation of children with DCD is a topic of increasing interest in research and practice.

Defined as a condition where motor ability is below that expected for age and cognitive ability, DCD is not attributable to any diagnosed sensory or neurological problems (see Chapter 1 for the complete diagnostic criteria). To fit the DCD rubric, the motor coordination difficulties must significantly interfere with academic achievement or participation in everyday activities (American Psychiatric Association, 2000).

It is well established that movement allows children to meet basic needs, to communicate, to learn, and to participate effectively in activities of daily living (Summers, Larkin, & Dewey, 2008) and, thus, is essential for healthy physical and mental development (Poulsen et al., 2008). Children with DCD manifest deficits in almost every motor domain. They are slower than their typically developing peers (Schoemaker et al., 2001); they are likely to experience difficulty with flexibility and adaptability (Wilson, Ruddock, Smits-Engelsman, Polatajko, & Blank, 2013), which are required for activities related to gross motor movements such as running, jumping, throwing, and catching, as well as fine motor movements such as writing or managing buttons and zippers (Polatajko, 1999). They are known to struggle in sports requiring complex spatial and temporal coordination of action (e.g., baseball, football, hockey; Sekaran, Reid, Chin, Ndiaye, & Licari, 2012).

It is also well established that meaningful participation in an activity depends on perceptions of choice or control, a sense of challenge, enjoyment, and perceived self-efficacy (Allison, 1996; Simeonsson et al., 2001). Children with DCD struggle to learn new motor skills, and this often leads to a pattern of avoidance that results in fewer practice opportunities (Engel-Yeger, Hanna Kasis, & Rosenblum, 2012). These experiences may limit a child's participation in school activities and age-appropriate activities of daily living (Mandich, Polatajko, & Rodger, 2003; Missiuna, Moll, King, King, & Law, 2007; Rodger et al., 2003; Rosenblum, 2006; Smyth & Anderson, 2000). Parents of children with DCD emphasized that "achieving competency in the everyday activities of childhood is a rite of passage for children, and failure in these seemingly unimportant activities can be devastating" (Mandich et al., 2003, p. 588). Low involvement in activities and restricted participation of children with DCD may also be affected by comorbid conditions associated with DCD, such as nonverbal learning disabilities, speech and articulation difficulties, and attention deficit disorder (Hill, 2001; Polatajko, 1999).

Through the application of the ICF model to children with DCD, it is reasonable to assume that limitations in activity performance and participation would affect the children's physical and mental health, as well as their overall sense of well-being (Mandich et al., 2003). Yet, researchers and clinicians lack information about the physical and mental health outcomes associated with the restricted participation of children with DCD, and also about the interrelationships between these aspects and the children's well-being. The existing literature mostly discusses the effects of participation (or lack of participation) in physical and sports activities and social activities (e.g., Cairney, 2008; Sylvestre, Nadeau, Charron, Larose, & Lepage, 2013). Information about other participation dimensions and other activity types is less common.

Participation in Physical Activities

Children with DCD participate less in physical activities when compared to their typically developing peers. Because of their motor difficulties, they may withdraw from performing physical activities, avoid environments where physical activity is promoted, such as the school playground (Faught, Hay, Cairney, & Flouris, 2005), and spend less time accomplishing physical tasks. In the sections that follow I will provide a brief overview of some of the major issues associated with this aspect of participation (a comprehensive review of the association between DCD, inactivity, and health-related outcomes is covered in Chapter 3).

Children with DCD who try to participate in physical activities often make unsuccessful attempts to engage in sports, particularly in team sports such as soccer, baseball, and hockey (Poulsen, Ziviani, Cuskelly, & Smith, 2007b). In the last decade or so, studies have highlighted that low participation in physical activity in children with DCD may lead to a host of negative secondary impairments. Reduced strength and endurance, for example, may lead to increased body fat and reduced cardiorespiratory fitness in the child with DCD (Raynor, 2001; Hay, Cairney, Faught, & Flouris, 2003; Cairney, Hay, Faught, Flouris, & Klentrou, 2007). The lower cardiorespiratory fitness of children with DCD may persist over time and thus lower their physical health status (Cairney, Hay, Veldhuizen, & Faught, 2010; Watkinson et al., 2001).

Numerous studies have referred to the participation patterns of boys with DCD and to the effects of restricted physical activity on their participation in other domains (e.g. Missiuna et al., 2007; Watkinson et al., 2001). This may be because boys with DCD have disproportionately higher referral rates for intervention than do girls with the disorder (Poulsen et al., 2008). Moreover, previous studies on typically developing children, as well as on children with disabilities, have emphasized that gender is a major predictor of participation in physical activities, including sporting and other gregarious activities (Engel-Yeger, 2009). Boys have been reported to be more physically active than girls (Dessing et al., 2013; Nettlefold et al., 2011). Boys are often more involved in active, forceful play (Fabes, Martin, & Hanish, 2003a; Fabes et al., 2003b) and usually play in groups that produce more conflicts and competition. Girls, conversely, spend less time in competitive games (Blatchford, 1998) and prefer jumping rope, singing, and playing clapping games. The differences between genders in physical activities were also reported in different age groups: Offord (2001) found that typically developing girls ages 6 to 11 years participated less in organized sports and physical activity than did boys. Posner and Vandell (1999) found that among typically developing children 8 to 10 years of age, girls were more likely to engage in academic activities and socializing, whereas boys were more likely to play coached sports. In a study conducted by Higgins, Gaul, Gibbons, and Van Gyn (2003), using data from the 1996–1997 Canadian National Population Health Survey of youth 12 to 24 years old, the authors found that girls were significantly less physically active than boys. More recently, results from the Canadian Health Measures Survey (2007 to 2009), which used accelerometers to measure physical activity, showed that boys were much more likely than girls to attain the recommended 60 minutes of moderate-to-vigorous physical activity per day, for at least 6 days per week (Colley, Garriguet, Janssen, Craig, Clarke, & Tremblay, 2011).

Cairney and his colleagues (2005) reported that boys with DCD have significantly lower participation in recreational physical activity than do typically developing boys. The higher involvement of typically developing boys in physical activities suggests that restrictions in physical participation among boys with DCD may impair their self-confidence, interpersonal relationships (Missiuna et al., 2007; Watkinson et al., 2001), and social participation. Yet, it is important to emphasize that although most of these studies referred to boys, the possible restricted participation in physical activities of girls with DCD, and its impacts on their social experiences, should not be ignored.

Participation in Social Activities

Social participation includes children's interactions with important others such as parents, teachers, peers, classmates, and siblings and other family members within the accessible contexts of school, home, and community (Simeonsson et al., 2001). Coster (1998) emphasized that the social context is crucial for growth enhancement. As mentioned above, most of the existing research on social participation of children with DCD focuses on boys. Previous studies reported that boys with DCD have significantly lower participation in social and physical activities than do boys without DCD (Poulsen, Ziviani, & Cuskelly, 2007a). Low participation means that boys with DCD miss out on opportunities for enjoyable social and physical experiences. By limiting their participation, however, these children may also be avoiding negative experiences such as teasing and offending. Parents of children with DCD perceive social participation difficulties to be of greater concern than any other area of functioning for their child (Cohn, 2001). Parents of children with DCD indicate that their children are often isolated, introverted, and socially immature (Gibson, 1996; Stephenson & Chesson, 2008).

Social Participation in the Context of School

School provides children not only with academic training but also with opportunities to develop and practice the skills necessary to support a healthy, engaged lifestyle (Booth & Samdal, 1997), with social benefits resulting from social interaction with classmates and teachers. Smyth and Anderson (2000) examined participation in physical play as well as in social play in the school playground among 6–10-year-old children with DCD. These authors found that children with DCD spent more time alone as onlookers and were excluded from particular types of play, especially those involving motor skill. These authors noted that boys with DCD tended to play formal games in large groups less often than boys without DCD, while girls with DCD played informal games in large groups less often than typically developing girls. Other studies also highlighted how children with DCD avoided participating in playground activities and had fewer positive social interactions with classmates than did typically developing children (Smyth & Anderson, 2000). Children with DCD also demonstrate educational underachievement, poor concentration, and disorganization as compared to typically developing children (Cantell, Smyth, & Ahonen, 2003;

Wocadlo & Rieger, 2008). Teachers indicate that a relatively high proportion of children with DCD exhibit behavioural problems (Losse et al., 1991; Wang, Tseng, Wilson, & Hu, 2009). Such difficulties, in turn, may exacerbate withdrawal from social situations. As a result, children with DCD often report low levels of social acceptance (Hillier, McIntyre, & Plummer, 2010).

Social Participation at Home

The difficulties that children with DCD experience may have a major effect on family life and result in limiting family social activities (Chia, 1997; Novak, Lingam, Coad, & Emond, 2012). In many cases, routine activities as well as occasional activities have to be adjusted to accommodate the special needs of children with DCD (Chesson, Mckay, & Stephenson, 1990). Children and adolescents with DCD do not participate in household work such as cooking, cleaning, and washing dishes as much as their parents expect or would like (Cogle & Tasker, 1982). The children's motor difficulties may affect their performance quality and lower their motivation to participate in such household tasks (May-Benson, Ingolia, & Koomar, 2002). This means that other family members will likely complete a larger share of household work (Chen & Cohn, 2003). Siblings of children with DCD may feel frustrated, neglected, or resentful that they receive less attention than their sibling with DCD (Chesson et al., 1990; Gibson, 1996). These feelings may contribute to increased conflict at home.

Social Participation in the Community

The primary and secondary difficulties of DCD, including the poor self-perception that children and adolescents with DCD often experience, may explain why individuals with DCD are less involved in community activities than their peers. Community-based activities often involve both formal and informal leisure activities (King et al., 2003). Leisure activities pursued outside of school involve over half of a child's waking hours and provide opportunities for psychological need fulfilment (Poulsen et al., 2008). Meeting leisure needs for enjoyment, creativity, and relationships contributes to overall leisure satisfaction. Leisure satisfaction itself is positively associated with global life satisfaction (Ellis & Witt, 1994).

Only a few studies have examined community-based leisure activities among children with DCD. Longitudinal research has shown that children as well as adolescents with DCD participate less in leisure or out-of-school activities than do typically developing peers (Jarus, Lourie-Gelberg, Engel-Yeger, & Bart, 2011; Poulsen, Ziviani, & Cuskelly, 2006; Poulsen et al., 2007b). These studies highlighted that low participation may contribute to low global life satisfaction (Poulsen et al., 2006) and to the loneliness of children with DCD (Poulsen et al., 2007b). For example, Berguno, Leroux, McAinsh, and Shaikh (2004) reported that boys who reluctantly participate in or eventually withdraw from popular and socially sanctioned activities are more likely to be lonely and may experience negative reactions from adults and peers, such as irritation, a lack of empathy, bullying, and victimization. In addition to the loneliness and social dissatisfaction that boys with DCD may experience, they also show lower global life satisfaction in comparison to boys without DCD (Poulsen et al., 2008).

As the previous sections show, although much of the literature on participation of children with DCD focuses on physical and social activities, there is a need to move beyond these activities to further examine participation of children with DCD across various dimensions of participation in the specific contexts where they are performed – at home, in school, and within the community. Moreover, additional research is needed regarding the interrelationships between participation and other psychosocial aspects of children with DCD.

Psychosocial Aspects of DCD and Their Relation to Participation

The complex, multidimensional nature of DCD makes it necessary to consider not only the disorder's primary movement difficulties but also its consequences. Special attention should be given to the negative emotional and behavioural consequences of DCD (Cantell & Kooistra, 2002) and their relation to the child's daily performance, social life, and participation in various environments. This is most important because these negative outcomes are known to have long-term effects on performance and participation across the lifespan (Lingam, Novak, Emond, & Coad, 2014; Kirby, Williams, Thomas, & Hill, 2013). Because most studies refer to the participation of children with DCD in social and physical/sports activities (e.g., Cairney, 2008), most explanations for the psychosocial aspects related to DCD are based on physical-social associations. On the other hand, Mandich, Polatajko, and Rodger (2003) reported that once children with DCD were able to participate in activities with their peers, it changed their lives. The children gained confidence as they mastered their goals; as a result, they were willing to try new activities because they believed they could master them now.

Children with DCD are particularly at risk of negative internal and external appraisals of their ability (Poulsen et al., 2008), including negative self-perceptions, especially perceived competency and self-esteem, when compared to typically developing children (Faught, 2005; Faught, Hay, Flouris, Cairney, & Hawes, 2002; Hay et al., 2003). Vicious cycles may exist between the motor difficulties children with DCD experience and the children's self-perception and self-worth. Studies show that children with DCD, even as young as five years old, frequently report that they do not feel competent in performing daily activities (Dunford, Missiuna, Street, & Sibert, 2005). Specifically, they perceive themselves as less competent than their coordinated peers in the domains of athletic competence, scholastic competence, physical appearance, and social acceptance (Engel-Yeger & Hanna Kasis, 2010; Piek, Dworcan, Barrett, & Coleman, 2000; Skinner & Piek, 2001). This low self-perception or self-worth can greatly influence their motivation to practice motor skills (Skinner & Piek, 2001) and may contribute to a reduction in or withdrawal from leisure activities (Causgrove Dunn & Watkinson, 2002; Smyth & Anderson, 2000). Mandich et al. (2003) highlighted that performance competency plays an important role among individuals with DCD in their being accepted by peers and being able "to be part of the group." On the other hand, loneliness and social dissatisfaction in childhood, which may be accompanied by boredom and aimlessness, contribute to feelings of depression and anxiety, limited participation, and possibly even suicide (Pratt & Hill, 2011; Skinner & Piek, 2001).

Recent studies of children with DCD have shown that their restricted patterns of participation may also be related to their low *perceived freedom in leisure* (PFL; Poulsen et al., 2007a), a cognitive motivational construct where perceptions of leisure competence and control over leisure experiences, satisfaction of leisure needs and depth of involvement, influence leisure behaviour and global life satisfaction (Ellis & Witt, 1994). This term has received growing attention in recent studies because PFL has a positive influence on the relationships between motor ability, participation, and global life satisfaction (Poulsen et al., 2007a). In this context PFL was studied mainly in regard to sports-related activities. According to Poulsen et al. (2008), there is a need to identify PFL when planning treatment interventions and preventive programs aimed at increasing life satisfaction and reducing loneliness for boys with DCD.

However, it is also essential to explore the relationship between PFL and participation in other activities to establish whether specific types of activities or contexts related to participation are related to positive PFL. This information will further assist clinicians in designing intervention programs that target the child's strengths and elevate the child's sense of self-competency.

In order to achieve a more complete understanding of participation of children with DCD, researchers must consider children's ability to evaluate their own capacity to perform a task competently, often referred to as self-efficacy (Harter, 1986). Self-efficacy has been shown to influence choice of activities, persistence, and skill acquisition (Bandura, 1997). Children with low self-efficacy may avoid certain tasks, whereas children who see themselves as efficacious participate more frequently and are more likely to persist when tasks become difficult (Schunk, 1991). Engel-Yeger and Hanna Kasis (2010) examined the relationship between the self-efficacy of children with DCD and their preference to participate in activities during their free time outside school hours. This study relied on self-reports from the child, following the principles of client-centred practice (Law, 1998; Missiuna, 1998), which argues that participation in any occupation is best understood from the perspective of the person who engages in it (Primeau & Ferguson, 1999). It is interesting that the negative impacts of DCD on participation are often determined using parent reports (Summers et al., 2008). In this study, the child's report was obtained by using the Perceived Efficacy and Goal Setting System (PEGS; Missiuna, Pollock, & Law, 2004) and the Preference for Activities of Children (PAC), which is a part of the Children's Assessment of Participation and Enjoyment (CAPE; King et al., 2004). The CAPE measures participation in daily activities performed outside mandated school hours, whereas the PAC measures preference to participate in activities regardless of actual participation in a given activity (King et al., 2004). This study had three major findings: (1) Children with DCD exhibited lower self-efficacy than their typically developing peers did, not only in physical activities but also in activities requiring self-care, relating to school or productivity, and involving leisure time. Moreover, the lower their motor performance, the lower their self-efficacy was in regard to these activities. (2) Children with DCD expressed lower preference, as compared to their typically developing peers, to participate not only in physical and social activities but also in other types such as recreational activities, skill-based activities, and self-improvement activities. (3) Significant relationships were found between the child's self-efficacy and the child's preferred activities. For example, children with higher self-efficacy in leisure occupations showed a higher preference to engage in active physical activities, self-improvement activities, and formal activities. Children with higher self-efficacy in self-care activities demonstrated a higher preference for self-improvement and informal activities. Children with higher self-efficacy in school or productivity activities showed a higher preference to participate in self-improvement activities.

These results show that children with DCD may experience positive self-efficacy when performing activities that do not necessarily involve intensive motor abilities. For example, when participating in self-improvement activities, such as writing letters, reading, and shopping, the children felt safer than in other activities because they did not necessarily need to expose their motor abilities to peers. As Cairney (2008) noted, children with DCD learn to conceal their problems by avoiding activities that expose their coordination difficulties. Informal activities (e.g., doing puzzles or crafts, drawing, colouring, playing computer or video games, gardening, fishing) are less constricted and organized by rules, and may also be performed alone. Another important result of this study to consider in research and intervention is that children with DCD are aware of their difficulties and how they affect their participation, and are able to report them.

Persistence of Limited Participation of Children with DCD

Cantell and Kooistra (2002) emphasized that because of the complex, multidimensional nature of the disorder, there is a need to explore "how the experiential impact of DCD changes from childhood to adolescence" (p. 38). Although there is evidence that a subgroup of children with DCD may catch up to their peers during adolescence (Cantell et al., 2003), many children with DCD do not outgrow their difficulties. The psychosocial difficulties and low participation, for example, in social and physical leisure activities, may persist well into adolescence and adulthood (Cantell et al., 2003; Hill & Brown, 2013; Rasmussen & Gillberg 2000).

Physical and social environments also change as individuals age, and these changes can influence how individuals with DCD manage their difficulties. In the school environment, for example, children with DCD often struggle with handwriting or the demands of physical education class. As the children grow older, these activities may be less of an issue. Specifically, by high school age, students may need to type assignments rather than write by hand, and for many students physical education becomes optional. At the same time, during adolescence new tasks, such as driving or meeting the motor demands of a new job, may replace earlier challenges (Missiuna, Moll, King, Stewart, & Macdonald, 2008).

One of the main persistent problems for individuals with DCD is social participation. Social acceptance and support from peers continue to be important for physical and emotional well-being, especially during adolescence. Studies report that similar to young children, adolescents with DCD have emotional difficulties associated with their poor movement ability, difficulties reflected in lower self-perceptions of physical appearance, athletic competence, and global self-worth (Piek, Baynam, & Barrett, 2006). Adolescents with DCD also generally have lower ratings of their social competence and self-worth when compared to their classmates (Lingam et al., 2014; Skinner & Piek, 2001).

Reflecting on their lives, adults self-described as "being physically awkward" focused on the adverse experiences and social dissatisfaction associated with all physical activities (Fitzpatrick & Watkinson, 2003). Examples of these issues are found in another study, which examined the life experiences of young adults with coordination difficulties (Missiuna et al., 2008). Using in-depth interviews in which participants were asked to retrospectively recall their experiences during adolescence, the researchers found several key themes: managing coordination differences through avoidance, withdrawal, and adaptation; seeking compatible activities; using humour; and persevering. Here is one example: "If you have the coordination difficulty ... you're not in the 'in crowd.' You're marginalized, so you're already kind of made to feel socially uncomfortable because you're not in the cool group. Especially for guys with sports and things like that" (p. 161). In this study, some participants described family members' specific expectations that were difficult to meet (such as getting involved in extracurricular activities) and noted their parents' overall disappointment or frustration when they did not live up to the expectations. Participants also described strategies they used to deal with their difficulties and reduce barriers that limited their participation. The most frequent strategy participants reported was to avoid or withdraw from activities demanding physical coordination. Some individuals tried to find activities they were good at, those that matched their abilities to the demands of the task, such as music, drama, and art, or to jobs that were not physically demanding.

Another strategy was to use humour to deflect attention from their poor motor abilities. They explained that rather than being upset or frustrated, they were able to minimize the importance of their coordination difficulties by learning to laugh at themselves or make a joke about it. They also identified taking on alternative roles as an effective strategy. These alternative roles enabled them to participate even in a sports activity, where, for example, an individual might take on the role of scorekeeper. Others engaged in additional practice in order to improve their skill.

The central message of the study by Missiuna et al. (2008) is that the young adults with DCD may continue to experience the negative consequences of their poor motor skills. Yet, growing older, together with changes in environmental demands, may enable adolescents and adults with DCD to perceive a greater ability to influence and create more positive situations for themselves and to feel more in control of their education, lifestyle, and work choices. This research in particular contains important information for intervention and highlights that to facilitate participation in motivating activities, therapists should help adolescents with DCD to recognize and optimize their strengths.

Implications for Intervention for Children with DCD

While previous interventions for children with DCD focused primarily on physical activities related to remediating gross and fine motor deficits (Mandich, Polatajko, Macnab, & Miller, 2001), the literature review above suggests the need for a new orientation to DCD in clinical settings or in research, one that needs to be based on a comprehensive understanding of the disorder's pervasive impact (see Chapter 7 for one example of such an approach). This review also emphasizes the need to apply the ICF model (WHO, 2001) in the evaluation and intervention process for children and adolescents with DCD. Thus, therapists should move beyond impairment-based approaches to more ecological or environmental interventions (Stewart, Stavness, King, Antle, & Law, 2006). They should consider an individual's performance in all levels of the ICF model with participation in life situations (in home, community, and school) as an ultimate goal of intervention (Polatajko, Mandich, Miller, & Macnab, 2001; Watter et al., 2008).

Clinicians and scholars should pay particular attention to the reciprocal causal pathways between DCD and participation: Difficulties related to DCD may limit participation, and limited participation may reduce involvement in activities, thus affecting the development of skills as well as physical and emotional well-being. The harmful consequences of DCD may worsen and have a greater impact on participation over time.

Therapists should also be aware that DCD is not limited to the childhood years, but that negative consequences may persist into adulthood and possibly worsen with age. Thus, a child with DCD should be evaluated as early as possible, and ongoing attention to the pathways connecting motor ability, activity, and participation, which illuminate the child–activity–environment fit (Mandich et al., 2003; Missiuna, 2001; Missiuna et al., 2001), should be reevaluated over time.

Evaluation and intervention should start from understanding the child's concerns, problems, and risks: (1) How do the child's performance skills (i.e., motor skills such as postures, mobility, coordination, strength) relate to the child's performance in various areas of relevant occupations (i.e., daily activities, school, leisure activities, social settings)? (2) What occupations and activities enhance the child and what inhibits him or her? (3) What are the child's own priorities and targeted outcomes? (4) What are the child's weaknesses and strengths? Is he or she aware of them? (5) How do they affect the child's engagement in occupations and support the child's participation?

When measuring participation in children with DCD, researchers need to provide data not only about the children's choice of occupations and areas of interest but also about their patterns of participation in various dimensions, including how intensely they participate, where and with whom they participate, and how well they enjoy the activity (Law, 2002).

It is also important for clinicians to examine the relationship between the child's actual participation and the child's preferred activities. This information may assist clinicians in building intervention programs according to the child's interest. Focusing treatment on the activities the children have identified as goals may provide the children with a new sense of efficacy and help them achieve far more than simple acquisition of a skill (Mandich et al., 2003).

It is of most importance that the evaluation of and intervention for children with DCD be based on the client-centred approach (Law, 1998). Specifically, considering that adults and children do not always have the same priorities (McGavin, 1998; Pollock & Stewart, 1998; Taber, 2010), it is important to refer in the evaluation and intervention to the child's point of view. Children hold a view of themselves that is unique, valid, and stable over time (Sturgess, Rodger, & Ozanne, 2002). Participation in an occupation is best understood from the perspective of the child who engages in it (Engel-Yeger, Jarus, Anaby, & Law, 2009; Primeau & Ferguson, 1999). Self-report assessments give children a greater voice in their therapy and assist the clinician in the determination of personal treatment goals related to their specific needs and interests. As such, children with DCD can provide valuable input into the assessment and determination of their own goals (Dunford, 2011; Dunford et al., 2005; Sturgess et al., 2002). This process may enhance a child's involvement in therapy and lead to better therapy results. The CAPE and the PAC, which are self-report tools, may serve as suitable tools for measuring a child's actual participation and its relationship to the child's preferred activities (Jarus et al., 2011).

Yet, assessing participation patterns is not enough. According to the ICF model, clinicians need to consider personal and environmental factors that may support or interfere with meaningful activity engagement and gauge the extent to which contexts help or hinder children's development (Simeonsson et al., 2001) and participation. For example, clinicians should identify the personal, physical, and emotional characteristics of the child. That is, in addition to improving the motor coordination of children with DCD and encouraging them to participate in various environments, clinicians should also address the psychological impact of DCD on children and adolescents. For example, how motivated is the child to participate in the intervention process? What is his or her self-perception? Does the child hold negative perceptions of self-efficacy? Are negative self-evaluations associated with anxiety or other emotional difficulties? Clinicians should also ask themselves what knowledge should be imparted to the child's social network in order to enhance the youngster's social involvement.

Since participation may be facilitated or restricted by the nature and accessibility of the environment (Simeonsson et al., 2001), clinicians should consider the multifaceted environmental aspects that influence participation; they should notice not only the child's potentially problematic activities but also the features of the activities themselves that may support or prevent the child's participation. Therapists should look at accommodation, through creative adaptations of traditional roles, and find suitable tasks and settings that will foster the will to participate (Missiuna et al., 2008).

The intervention process should also evaluate the involvement of important others in the child's life. For example, in the family, parents are the most important decision makers in arranging the daily routines and family recreation. The values and attitudes of parents towards their children's coordination disorders may influence the children's social life (Cohn, 2001). Thus, information gathering as well as goal setting should involve family members. In school, teachers and peers should receive information about difficulties that children with DCD may experience as well as guidelines for assisting them in participating in class and playground activities with friends.

Polatajko, Mandich, Miller, and Macnab (2001) recommend applying the Cognitive Orientation to daily Occupational Performance (COOP) approach as well as providing social skill training for children with DCD in order to encourage their participation in social activities at school. Intervention with children with DCD should include leisure counseling to direct children to activities most likely to offer them a sense of competence (Engel-Yeger & Hanna Kasis, 2010). Moreover, in addition to considering environmental accommodations and educational processes as integral to the intervention goals for the child and significant others, therapists should verify that the modifications are related to the context in which the child participates – for example, personal context (age, gender, socioeconomic status); cultural background; relationship to the child's habits, routines, and roles; temporal context (stage of life, time of year); and social context.

Finally, throughout the intervention process, clinicians should explore a number of questions: Are the relevant outcomes of intervention achieved? Is the child satisfied? Does the child feel competent? How does the intervention affect quality of life?

In summary, because of the complexity of DCD, evaluation and intervention processes for children with DCD require a broad perspective, incorporating personal and environmental factors. The application of the ICF model is recommended. It is important to consider the interaction between the child's difficulties, activity performance, and participation. In making an evaluation and planning intervention, clinicians should take into account personal factors and other mediators, such as external environmental barriers, that may affect participation. Clinicians should also consider the interactions among the child's physical ability, life satisfaction, perceived quality of life, and leisure activity participation patterns (Poulsen et al., 2007a). Evaluation and intervention should be client centred and family centred. Family members, professionals in the education system, and individuals in the community should be given guidance about what to expect from the individual with DCD and what strategies to adopt (Missiuna et al., 2008).

Implications for Further Research on Children with DCD

Further research on DCD is needed to support existing intervention strategies and to develop new ones. Researchers from various disciplines (e.g., occupational therapists, psychologists, physicians, physiotherapists) should conduct studies on DCD based on the constructs included in the ICF model. These studies should further illuminate how personal factors, including physical and emotional difficulties of children with DCD, interact with activity performance and participation, and how context and environment may further affect these associations. Studies should also elucidate how the interaction between DCD, activity performance, and participation patterns affects children's self-efficacy, life satisfaction, quality of life, and well-being. To get an authentic point of view, researchers should use evaluations that are client centred and based on the subjects' self-reports. Another important aspect that should receive increased attention in research is the perspective of family members of children with DCD. Because DCD affects not only the child but also the child's family, researchers need to examine how parents and siblings perceive the child's difficulties, how these difficulties affect them, their social life, their performance in daily situations, and their relationships with the child. When trying to shape and enhance the child's participation, clinicians should gather data from teachers and other relevant individuals in the community who may assist in removing barriers and enhance the child's participation in community activities. It is important that these studies be based not only on quantitative data but also on qualitative data such as interviews and videos, because in comparison to other sources these may provide a deeper, more authentic perspective about the consequences of DCD.

Missiuna and her colleagues (2008) emphasized that it is critical to consider, simultaneously, the relationship between body functions (activity) and participation, the impact of contextual and environmental factors, and the need to implement a client- and family-centred approach: "I always felt like I was less than other people because I couldn't do stuff properly. I couldn't write properly and I couldn't play sports properly and I was always spilling things or breaking things. It just makes me feel so – like you're so different from other people, and nobody can ever really understand. It would make me feel like there was something wrong with me personally, when really I couldn't really help it" (p. 162).

By elucidating the individual's strengths, enhancing his or her self-confidence and feelings of belonging, clinicians will help the individual manage DCD difficulties and optimize participation, and thus elevate the individual's life satisfaction and well-being.

REFERENCES

Allison, K.R. (1996, Sep-Oct). Predictors of inactivity: An analysis of the Ontario Health Survey. *Canadian Journal of Public Health, 87*(5), 354–358. Medline:8972972

American Psychiatric Association. (2000). *Diagnostic and statistical manual of mental disorders* (4th ed., text rev.). Washington, DC: Author.

AOTA. (2002, Nov-Dec). Occupational therapy practice framework: Domain and process. *American Journal of Occupational Therapy., 56*(6), 609–639. http://dx.doi.org/10.5014/ajot.56.6.609 Medline:12458855

Bandura, A. (1997). *Self-efficacy: The exercise of control.* New York, NY: Freeman.

Berguno, G., Leroux, P., McAinsh, K., & Shaikh, S. (2004). Children's experience of loneliness at school and its relation to bullying and the quality of teacher interventions. *Qualitative Report, 9,* 483–499.

Blatchford, P. (1998). *Social life in school.* London, England: Falmer.

Booth, M.L., & Samdal, O. (1997). Health-promoting schools in Australia: Models and measurement [Special issue]. *Australian and New Zealand Journal of Public Health, 21*(4), 365–370. http://dx.doi.org/10.1111/j.1467-842X.1997. tb01716.x Medline:9308200

Cairney, J. (2008, Aug). What should we do to help children with DCD? *Developmental Medicine and Child Neurology, 50*(8), 566. http://dx.doi. org/10.1111/j.1469-8749.2008.03056.x Medline:18754891

Cairney, J., Hay, J.A., Faught, B.E., Flouris, A., & Klentrou, P. (2007, Feb). Developmental coordination disorder and cardiorespiratory fitness in children. *Pediatric Exercise Science, 19*(1), 20–28. Medline:17554154

Cairney, J., Hay, J., Veldhuizen, S., & Faught, B.E. (2010). Trajectories of cardiorespiratory fitness in children with and without developmental coordination disorder: A longitudinal analysis. *British Journal of Sports Medicine, 45*(15) 1196–1201. Medline:20542967

Caldwell, L.L. (1990). Leisure, health, and disability: A review and discussion. *Canadian Journal of Community Mental Health, 9,* 111–122.

Cantell, M., & Kooistra, L. (2002). Long-term outcomes of developmental coordination disorder. In S. Cermak & D. Larkin (Eds.), *Developmental coordination disorder* (pp. 23–38). Albany, NY: Delmar.

Cantell, M.H., Smyth, M.M., & Ahonen, T.P. (2003, Nov). Two distinct pathways for developmental coordination disorder: Persistence and resolution. *Human Movement Science, 22*(4-5), 413–431. http://dx.doi.org/10.1016/j.humov.2003.09.002 Medline:14624826

Chen, H.F., & Cohn, E.S. (2003). Social participation for children with developmental coordination disorder: Conceptual, evaluation and intervention considerations. *Physical & Occupational Therapy in Pediatrics, 23*(4), 61–78. Medline:14750309

Chesson, R., McKay, C., & Stephenson, E. (1990, Mar-Apr). Motor/learning difficulties and the family. *Child: Care, Health and Development, 16*(2), 123–138. http://dx.doi.org/10.1111/j.1365-2214.1990.tb00644.x Medline:2335016

Chia, S.H. (1997). The child, his family and dyspraxia. *Professional Care of Mother and Child, 7*(4), 105–107. Medline:9348971

Cogle, F.L., & Tasker, G.E. (1982). Children and housework. *Family Relations, 31*(3), 395–399. http://dx.doi.org/10.2307/584172

Cohn, E.S. (2001, May-Jun). Parent perspectives of occupational therapy using a sensory integration approach. *American Journal of Occupational Therapy., 55*(3), 285–294. http://dx.doi.org/10.5014/ajot.55.3.285 Medline:11723969

Coster, W. (1998, May). Occupation-centered assessment of children. *American Journal of Occupational Therapy, 52*(5), 337–344. http://dx.doi.org/10.5014/ajot.52.5.337 Medline:9588258

Colley, R.C., Garriguet, D., Janssen, I., Craig, C.L., Clarke, J., Tremblay, M.S. (2011). Physical activity of Canadian children and youth: Accelerometer results from the 2007 to 2009 Canadian Health Measures Survey. Health Reports, 22(1), 15–23. Medline:21510586

Dessing, D., Pierik, F.H., Sterkenburg, R.P., van Dommelen, P., Maas, J., & de Vries, S.I. (2013). Schoolyard physical activity of 6-11 year old children assessed by GPS and accelerometry. *The International Journal of Behavioral Nutrition and Physical Activity, 14*(10), 97. doi: 10.1186/1479-5868-10-97.

Dunford, C. (2011, Aug). Goal-orientated group intervention for children with developmental coordination disorder. *Physical & Occupational Therapy in Pediatrics, 31*(3), 288–300. http://dx.doi.org/10.3109/01942638.2011.565864 Medline:21488710

Dunford, C., Missiuna, C., Street, E., & Sibert, J. (2005). Children's perceptions of the impact of developmental coordination disorder on activities of daily living. *British Journal of Occupational Therapy, 68*(5), 207–214.

Dunn, J.C., & Watkinson, E.J. (2002). Considering motivation theory in the study of developmental coordination disorder. In S.A. Cermak & D. Larkin (Eds.), *Developmental coordination disorder* (pp. 185–199). Albany, NY: Delmar Thomson Learning.

Ellis, G.D., & Witt, P.A. (1994). Perceived freedom in leisure and satisfaction: Exploring the factor structure of the perceived freedom components of the leisure diagnostic battery. *Leisure Sciences, 16*(4), 259–270. http://dx.doi.org/10.1080/01490409409513236

Engel-Yeger, B. (2009, Jan-Feb). Sociodemographic effects on activities preference of typically developing Israeli children and youths. *American Journal of Occupational Therapy., 63*(1), 89–95. http://dx.doi.org/10.5014/ajot.63.1.89 Medline:19192731

Engel-Yeger, B., & Hanna Kasis, A. (2010, Sep). The relationship between developmental co-ordination disorders, child's perceived self-efficacy and preference to participate in daily activities. *Child: Care, Health and Development, 36*(5), 670–677. http://dx.doi.org/10.1111/j.1365-2214.2010.01073.x Medline:20412146

Engel-Yeger, B., Hanna Kasis, A., & Rosenblum, S. (2012, Jul-Aug). Can gymnastic teacher predict leisure activity preference among children with developmental coordination disorders (DCD)? *Research in Developmental Disabilities, 33*(4), 1006–1013. http://dx.doi.org/10.1016/j.ridd.2012.01.005 Medline:22502824

Engel-Yeger, B., Jarus, T., Anaby, D., & Law, M. (2009, Jan-Feb). Differences in patterns of participation between youths with cerebral palsy and typically developing peers. *American Journal of Occupational Therapy, 63*(1), 96–104. http://dx.doi.org/10.5014/ajot.63.1.96 Medline:19192732

Fabes, R.A., Martin, C.L., & Hanish, L.D. (2003a, May-Jun). Young children's play qualities in same-, other-, and mixed-sex peer groups. *Child Development, 74*(3), 921–932. http://dx.doi.org/10.1111/1467-8624.00576 Medline:12795398

Fabes, R.A., Martin, C.L., Hanish, L.D., Anders, M.C., & Madden-Derdich, D.A. (2003b, Sep). Early school competence: The roles of sex-segregated play and effortful control. *Developmental Psychology, 39*(5), 848–858. http://dx.doi.org/10.1037/0012-1649.39.5.848 Medline:12952398

Faught, B.E., Hay, J.A., Cairney, J., & Flouris, A. (2005, Nov). Increased risk for coronary vascular disease in children with developmental coordination disorder. *Journal of Adolescent Health, 37*(5), 376–380. http://dx.doi.org/10.1016/j.jadohealth.2004.09.021 Medline:16227122

Faught, B., Hay, J., Flouris, A., Cairney, J., & Hawes, R. (2002). Diagnosing developmental coordination disorder using the CSAPPA scale. *Canadian Journal of Applied Physiology, 27*, S17.

Fitzpatrick, D.A., & Watkinson, E.J. (2003). The lived experience of physical awkwardness: Adults' retrospective views. *Adapted Physical Activity Quarterly; APAQ, 20*, 279–297.

Forsyth, R., & Jarvis, S. (2002, Jul). Participation in childhood. *Child: Care, Health and Development, 28*(4), 277–279. http://dx.doi.org/10.1046/j.1365-2214.2002.00272.x Medline:12190818

Gibson, R.C. (1996). The effects of dyspraxia on family relationships. *British Journal of Therapy and Rehabilitation, 3*(2), 101–105. http://dx.doi.org/10.12968/bjtr.1996.3.2.14861

Harter, S. (1986). Processes underlying the construction, maintenance, and enhancement of the self-concept in children. In J. Suls & A.G. Greenwald (Eds.), *Psychology perspectives on the self* (pp. 136–182). Hillsdale, NJ: Erlbaum.

Hay, J.A., Cairney, J., Faught, B.E., & Flouris, A. (2003). The contribution of clumsiness to risk factors of coronary vascular disease in children. *Portuguese Journal of Sport Science, 3*(2), 127–129.

Higgins, J.W., Gaul, C., Gibbons, S., & Van Gyn, G. (2003, Jan-Feb). Factors influencing physical activity levels among Canadian youth. *Canadian Journal of Public Health, 94*(1), 45–51. Medline:12583679

Hill, E.L. (2001, Apr-Jun). Non-specific nature of specific language impairment: A review of the literature with regard to concomitant motor impairments. *International Journal of Language & Communication Disorders, 36*(2), 149–171. http://dx.doi.org/10.1080/13682820010019874 Medline:11344592

Hill, E.L., & Brown, D. (2013, Aug). Mood impairments in adults previously diagnosed with developmental coordination disorder. *Journal of Mental Health (Abingdon, England), 22*(4), 334–340. http://dx.doi.org/10.3109/09638237.2012.745187 Medline:23323694

Hillier, S., McIntyre, A., & Plummer, L. (2010, May). Aquatic physical therapy for children with developmental coordination disorder: A pilot randomized controlled trial. *Physical & Occupational Therapy in Pediatrics, 30*(2), 111–124. http://dx.doi.org/10.3109/01942630903543575 Medline:20367516

Jarus, T., Lourie-Gelberg, Y., Engel-Yeger, B., & Bart, O. (2011, Jul-Aug). Participation patterns of school-aged children with and without DCD. *Research in Developmental Disabilities, 32*(4), 1323–1331. http://dx.doi.org/10.1016/j.ridd.2011.01.033 Medline:21324639

Katz, N., Kizony, R., & Parush, S. (2002). Visuomotor organization and thinking operations performance of school-age Ethiopian, Bedouin, and mainstream Israeli children. *Occupational Therapy Journal of Research, 22*, 34–43.

King, G. Law, M., King, S., Hurley, P., Hanna, S., Kertoy, M., … Young, N. (2004). *Children's Assessment of Participation and Enjoyment (CAPE) and Preferences for Activities of Children (PAC)*. San Antonio, TX: Harcourt Assessment.

King, G., Law, M., King, S., Rosenbaum, P., Kertoy, M.K., & Young, N.L. (2003). A conceptual model of the factors affecting the recreation and leisure participation of children with disabilities. *Physical & Occupational Therapy in Pediatrics, 23*(1), 63–90. http://dx.doi.org/10.1080/J006v23n01_05 Medline:12703385

Kirby, A., Williams, N., Thomas, M., & Hill, E.L. (2013, Apr). Self-reported mood, general health, wellbeing and employment status in adults with suspected DCD. *Research in Developmental Disabilities, 34*(4), 1357–1364. http://dx.doi.org/10.1016/j.ridd.2013.01.003 Medline:23417140

Larson, R.W., & Verma, S. (1999, Nov). How children and adolescents spend time across the world: Work, play, and developmental opportunities. *Psychological Bulletin, 125*(6), 701–736. http://dx.doi.org/10.1037/0033-2909.125.6.701 Medline:10589300

Law, M.C. (1998). Client-centered occupational therapy. In M. Law (Ed.), *Client-centered occupational therapy* (pp. 1–18). Thorofare, NJ: Slack.

Law, M. (2002, Nov-Dec). Participation in the occupations of everyday life. *American Journal of Occupational Therapy, 56*(6), 640–649. http://dx.doi.org/10.5014/ajot.56.6.640 Medline:12458856

Law, M., & Dunn, W. (1994). Perspectives on understanding and changing the environments of children with disabilities. *Physical & Occupational Therapy in Pediatrics, 13*(3), 1–17. http://dx.doi.org/10.1080/J006v13n03_01

Law, M., Hanna, S., King, G., Hurley, P., King, S., Kertoy, M., & Rosenbaum, P. (2003, Sep). Factors affecting family-centred service delivery for children with disabilities. *Child: Care, Health and Development, 29*(5), 357–366. http://dx.doi.org/10.1046/j.1365-2214.2003.00351.x Medline:12904243

Law, M., Finkelman, S., Hurley, P., Rosenbaum, P., King, S., King, G., & Hanna, S. (2004). Participation of children with physical disabilities: Relationships with diagnosis, physical function, and demographic variables. *Scandinavian Journal of Occupational Therapy, 11*(4), 156–162. http://dx.doi.org/10.1080/11038120410020755

Law, M., King, G., King, S., Kertoy, M., Hurley, P., Rosenbaum, P., … Hanna, S. (2006, May). Patterns of participation in recreational and leisure activities among children with complex physical disabilities. *Developmental Medicine and Child Neurology, 48*(5), 337–342. http://dx.doi.org/10.1017/S0012162206000740 Medline:16608540

Lingam, R.P., Novak, C., Emond, A., & Coad, J.E. (2014, May). The importance of identity and empowerment to teenagers with developmental co-ordination disorder. *Child: Care, Health and Development, 40*(3), 309–318. Medline:23781846

Losse, A., Henderson, S.E., Elliman, D., Hall, D., Knight, E., & Jongmans, M. (1991, Jan). Clumsiness in children – Do they grow out of it? A 10-year follow-up study. *Developmental Medicine and Child Neurology, 33*(1), 55–68. http://dx.doi.org/10.1111/j.1469-8749.1991.tb14785.x Medline:1704864

Lyons, R.F. (1993). Meaningful activity and disability: Capitalizing upon the potential of outreach recreation networks in Canada. *Canadian Journal of Rehabilitation, 6,* 256–265.

Mandich, A.D., Polatajko, H.J., Macnab, J.J., & Miller, L.T. (2001). Treatment of children with developmental coordination disorder: What is the evidence? *Physical & Occupational Therapy in Pediatrics, 20*(2-3), 51–68. http://dx.doi.org/10.1080/J006v20n02_04 Medline:11345512

Mandich, A.D., Polatajko, H.J., & Rodger, S. (2003, Nov). Rites of passage: Understanding participation of children with developmental coordination disorder. *Human Movement Science, 22*(45), 583–595. http://dx.doi.org/10.1016/j.humov.2003.09.011 Medline:14624835

May-Benson, T., Ingolia, P., & Koomar, J. (2002). Daily living skills and developmental coordination disorder. In S.A. Cermak & D. Larkin (Eds.), *Developmental coordination disorder* (pp. 140–156). Albany, NY: Delmar Thomson Learning.

McGavin, C. (1998). Planning rehabilitation: A comparison of issues for parents and adolescents. *Physical & Occupational Therapy in Pediatrics, 18*(1), 69–82.

Missiuna, C. (1998). Development of "All About Me," a scale that measures children's perceived motor competence. *Occupational Therapy Journal of Research, 18*(2), 85–108.

Missiuna, C. (2001). Strategies for success: Working with children with developmental coordination disorder. *Physical & Occupational Therapy in Pediatrics, 20*(2–3), 1–4. Medline:11345505

Missiuna, C., Mandich, A.D., Polatajko, H.J., & Malloy-Miller, T. (2001). Cognitive Orientation to daily Occupational Performance (CO-OP): Part I, Theoretical foundations. *Physical & Occupational Therapy in Pediatrics, 20*(2-3), 69–81. http://dx.doi.org/10.1080/J006v20n02_05 Medline:11345513

Missiuna, C., Moll, S., King, S., King, G., & Law, M. (2007). A trajectory of troubles: Parents' impressions of the impact of developmental coordination disorder. *Physical & Occupational Therapy in Pediatrics, 27*(1), 81–101. Medline:17298942

Missiuna, C., Moll, S., King, G., Stewart, D., & Macdonald, K. (2008, Jun). Life experiences of young adults who have coordination difficulties. *Canadian Journal of Occupational Therapy, 75*(3), 157–166. http://dx.doi.org/10.1177/000841740807500307 Medline:18615927

Missiuna, C., Pollock, N., & Law, M. (2004). *Perceived Efficacy and Goal Setting System (PEGS).* San Antonio, TX: Psychological Corporation.

Nettlefold, L., McKay, H.A., Warburton, D.E., McGuire, K.A., Bredin, S.S., & Naylor, P.J. (2011). The challenge of low physical activity during the school day: At recess, lunch and in physical education. British Journal of Sports Medicine, 45(10), 813–819.

Novak, C., Lingam, R., Coad, J., & Emond, A. (2012, Nov). "Providing more scaffolding": Parenting a child with developmental co-ordination disorder, a hidden disability. Child: Care, Health and Development, 38(6), 829–835. http://dx.doi.org/10.1111/j.1365-2214.2011.01302.x Medline:21848938

Offord, D. (2001). Four hypotheses about the public policy significance of youth recreation: Lessons from a literature review and data analysis on "Learning through Recreation." Ottawa, ON: Canadian Policy Research Networks.

Osterweil, Z., & Nagano, K.N. (1991). Maternal view on autonomy: Japan and Israel Journal of Cross-Cultural Psychology, 22(3), 362–375. http://dx.doi.org/10.1177/0022022191223003

Piek, J.P., Baynam, G.B., & Barrett, N.C. (2006, Feb). The relationship between fine and gross motor ability, self-perceptions and self-worth in children and adolescents. Human Movement Science, 25(1), 65–75. http://dx.doi.org/10.1016/j.humov.2005.10.011 Medline:16442171

Piek, J.P., Dworcan, M., Barrett, N., & Coleman, R. (2000). Determinants of self-worth in children with and without developmental coordination disorder. International Journal of Disability Development and Education, 47(3), 259–272. http://dx.doi.org/10.1080/713671115

Polatajko, H. (1999). Developmental coordination disorder (DCD): Alias the clumsy child. In K., Whitmore, H. Hart, & G. Willems (Eds.), A neurodevelopmental approach to specific learning disorders. London, England: MacKeith Press.

Polatajko, H.J., Mandich, A.D., Miller, L.T., & Macnab, J.J. (2001). Cognitive Orientation to daily Occupational Performance (CO-OP): Part II, The evidence. Physical & Occupational Therapy in Pediatrics, 20(2-3), 83–106. http://dx.doi.org/10.1080/J006v20n02_06 Medline:11345514

Pollock, N., & Stewart, D. (1998). Occupational performance needs of school-aged children with physical disabilities in the community. Physical & Occupational Therapy in Pediatrics, 18(1), 55–68. http://dx.doi.org/10.1080/J006v18n01_04

Posner, J.K., & Vandell, D.L. (1999, May). After-school activities and the development of low-income urban children: A longitudinal study. Developmental Psychology, 35(3), 868–879. http://dx.doi.org/10.1037/0012-1649.35.3.868 Medline:10380876

Poulsen, A.A., Ziviani, J.M., & Cuskelly, M. (2006, Dec). General self-concept and life satisfaction for boys with differing levels of physical coordination: The role of goal orientations and leisure participation. Human Movement

Science, 25(6), 839–860. http://dx.doi.org/10.1016/j.humov.2006.05.003 Medline:16859792

Poulsen, A.A., Ziviani, J.M., & Cuskelly, M. (2007a, Jul). Perceived freedom in leisure and physical co-ordination ability: Impact on out-of-school activity participation and life satisfaction. *Child: Care, Health and Development*, 33(4), 432–440. http://dx.doi.org/10.1111/j.1365-2214.2007.00730.x Medline:17584399

Poulsen, A.A., Ziviani, J.M., & Cuskelly, M. (2008). Leisure time physical activity energy expenditure in boys with developmental coordination disorder: The role of peer relations self-concept perceptions. *OTJR: Occupation, Participation and Health*, 28(1), 30–39. http://dx.doi.org/10.3928/15394492-20080101-05

Poulsen, A.A., Ziviani, J.M., Cuskelly, M., & Smith, R. (2007b, Jul-Aug). Boys with developmental coordination disorder: Loneliness and team sports participation. *American Journal of Occupational Therapy.*, 61(4), 451–462. http://dx.doi.org/10.5014/ajot.61.4.451 Medline:17685178

Pratt, M.L., & Hill, E.L. (2011, Jul-Aug). Anxiety profiles in children with and without developmental coordination disorder. *Research in Developmental Disabilities*, 32(4), 1253–1259. http://dx.doi.org/10.1016/j.ridd.2011.02.006 Medline:21377831

Primeau, L.A., & Ferguson, J.M. (1999). Occupational frame of reference. In P. Kramer & J. Hinojosa (Eds.), *Frames of reference for pediatric occupational therapy* (pp. 469–516). Philadelphia, PA: Williams & Wilkins.

Rasmussen, P., & Gillberg, C. (2000, Nov). Natural outcome of ADHD with developmental coordination disorder at age 22 years: A controlled, longitudinal, community-based study. *Journal of the American Academy of Child and Adolescent Psychiatry*, 39(11), 1424–1431. http://dx.doi.org/10.1097/00004583-200011000-00017 Medline:11068898

Raynor, A.J. (2001, Oct). Strength, power, and coactivation in children with developmental coordination disorder. *Developmental Medicine and Child Neurology*, 43(10), 676–684. http://dx.doi.org/10.1017/S0012162201001220 Medline:11665824

Rodger, S., Ziviani, J., Watter, P., Ozanne, A., Woodyatt, G., & Springfield, E. (2003, Nov). Motor and functional skills of children with developmental coordination disorder: A pilot investigation of measurement issues. *Human Movement Science*, 22(4-5), 461–478. http://dx.doi.org/10.1016/j.humov.2003.09.004 Medline:14624828

Rosenblum, S. (2006, Nov). The development and standardization of the Children Activity Scales (ChAS-P/T) for the early identification of children with developmental coordination disorder. *Child: Care, Health and*

Development, 32(6), 619–632. http://dx.doi.org/10.1111/j.1365-2214. 2006.00687.x Medline:17018039

Rosenblum, S., Katz, N., Hahn-Markowitz, J., Mazor-Karsenty, T., & Parush, S. (2000, Apr). Environmental influences on perceptual and motor skills of children from immigrant Ethiopian families. *Perceptual and Motor Skills, 90*(2), 587–594. http://dx.doi.org/10.2466/pms.2000.90.2.587 Medline:10833758

Schoemaker, M.M., van der Wees, M., Flapper, B., Verheij-Jansen, N., Scholten-Jaegers, S., & Geuze, R.H. (2001, Mar). Perceptual skills of children with developmental coordination disorder. *Human Movement Science, 20*(1-2), 111–133. http://dx.doi.org/10.1016/S0167-9457(01)00031-8 Medline:11471393

Schunk, D.H. (1991). Self-efficacy and academic motivation. *Educational Psychologist, 26*(3-4), 207–231. http://dx.doi.org/10.1080/00461520.1991.9653133

Sekaran, S.N., Reid, S.L., Chin, A.W., Ndiaye, S., & Licari, M.K. (2012, May). Catch! Movement kinematics of two-handed catching in boys with developmental coordination disorder. *Gait & Posture, 36*(1), 27–32. http://dx.doi.org/10.1016/j.gaitpost.2011.12.010 Medline:22464636

Sherwood, N.E., Story, M., Neumark-Sztainer, D., Adkins, S., & Davis, M. (2003, Nov). Development and implementation of a visual card-sorting technique for assessing food and activity preferences and patterns in African American girls. *Journal of the American Dietetic Association, 103*(11), 1473–1479. http://dx.doi.org/10.1016/j.jada.2003.08.028 Medline:14576711

Simeonsson, R.J., Carlson, D., Huntington, G.S., McMillen, J.S., & Brent, J.L. (2001, Jan 20). Students with disabilities: A national survey of participation in school activities. *Disability and Rehabilitation, 23*(2), 49–63. http://dx.doi.org/10.1080/096382801750058134 Medline:11214716

Skinner, R.A., & Piek, J.P. (2001, Mar). Psychosocial implications of poor motor coordination in children and adolescents. *Human Movement Science, 20*(1-2), 73–94. http://dx.doi.org/10.1016/S0167-9457(01)00029-X Medline:11471399

Smyth, M.M., & Anderson, H.I. (2000). Coping with clumsiness in the school playground: Social and physical play in children with coordination impairments. *British Journal of Developmental Psychology, 18*(3), 389–413. http://dx.doi.org/10.1348/026151000165760

Stephenson, E.A., & Chesson, R.A. (2008, May). "Always the guiding hand": Parents' accounts of the long-term implications of developmental co-ordination disorder for their children and families. *Child: Care, Health and Development, 34*(3), 335–343. http://dx.doi.org/10.1111/j.1365-2214.2007.00805.x Medline:18410640

Stewart, D., Stavness, C., King, G., Antle, B., & Law, M. (2006). A critical appraisal of literature reviews about the transition to adulthood for youth with disabilities. *Physical & Occupational Therapy in Pediatrics, 26*(4), 5–24. http://dx.doi.org/10.1080/J006v26n04_02 Medline:17135067

Sturgess, J., Rodger, S., & Ozanne, A. (2002). A review of the use of assessment with young self-report children. *British Journal of Occupational Therapy, 65*(3), 108–116.

Summers, J., Larkin, D., & Dewey, D. (2008, Apr). Activities of daily living in children with developmental coordination disorder: Dressing, personal hygiene, and eating skills. *Human Movement Science, 27*(2), 215–229. http://dx.doi.org/10.1016/j.humov.2008.02.002 Medline:18348898

Sylvestre, A., Nadeau, L., Charron, L., Larose, N., & Lepage, C. (2013, Oct). Social participation by children with developmental coordination disorder compared to their peers. *Disability and Rehabilitation, 35*(21), 1814–1820. http://dx.doi.org/10.3109/09638288.2012.756943 Medline:23600713

Taber, S.M. (2010, Dec). The veridicality of children's reports of parenting: A review of factors contributing to parent–child discrepancies. *Clinical Psychology Review, 30*(8), 999–1010. http://dx.doi.org/10.1016/j.cpr.2010.06.014 Medline:20655135

Wang, T.N., Tseng, M.H., Wilson, B.N., & Hu, F.C. (2009, Oct). Functional performance of children with developmental coordination disorder at home and at school. *Developmental Medicine and Child Neurology, 51*(10), 817–825. http://dx.doi.org/10.1111/j.1469-8749.2009.03271.x Medline:19416344

Watkinson, E.J., Causgrove Dunn, J., Cavaliere, N., Calzonetti, K., Wilhelm, L., & Dwyer, S. (2001). Engagement in playground activities as a criterion for diagnosing developmental coordination disorder. *Adapted Physical Activity Quarterly; APAQ, 18*, 18–34.

Watter, P., Rodger, S., Marinac, J., Woodyatt, G., Ziviani, J., & Ozanne, A. (2008). Multidisciplinary assessment of children with developmental coordination disorder: Using the ICF framework to inform assessment. *Physical & Occupational Therapy in Pediatrics, 28*(4), 331–352. http://dx.doi.org/10.1080/01942630802307093 Medline:19042476

Wilson, P.H., Ruddock, S., Smits-Engelsman, B., Polatajko, H., & Blank, R. (2013, Mar). Understanding performance deficits in developmental coordination disorder: A meta-analysis of recent research. *Developmental Medicine and Child Neurology, 55*(3), 217–228. http://dx.doi.org/10.1111/j.1469-8749.2012.04436.x Medline:23106668

Wocadlo, C., & Rieger, I. (2008, Nov). Motor impairment and low achievement in very preterm children at eight years of age. *Early Human Development, 84*(11), 769–776. http://dx.doi.org/10.1016/j.earlhumdev.2008.06.001 Medline:18639396

World Health Organization. (2001). *The international classification of functioning, disability and health* [Introduction]. Retrieved 17 July 2007 from World Health Organization website: http://www.who.int/classifications/icf?myurl=introduction.html&mytitle=

3 Developmental Coordination Disorder, Physical Activity, and Physical Health: Results from the PHAST Project

JOHN CAIRNEY

In this chapter I begin with a familiar narrative in the literature on DCD in children: As a result of their motor coordination problems, children with DCD struggle with everyday tasks, including play.[1] Gross motor problems associated with balance, deficits in hand–eye coordination, and basic skills such as kicking and catching make both organized sports and free play extremely difficult. The result is that when they can, children with DCD avoid such activities. The resultant inactivity is thought to have both social and physical consequences. Children who do not play with other children miss important opportunities for socialization: Play is where children learn to problem solve, deal with conflict, and generally master the complex ebb and flow of social interaction. Children who cannot play successfully with others tend to play alone. The isolation that follows can in turn lead to psychological consequences such as depression.

The second consequence is related to physical health, especially obesity and cardiovascular health. When play is vigorous, involving large muscle groups, and when there is physical exertion (e.g., increased respiration, sweating), as is the case with activities such as running and jumping or in structured activities such as sports, then play can be classified as physical activity or even exercise. Physical activity is associated with numerous health benefits, chronic inactivity with numerous health problems. Among other things, it is an important determinant of obesity in all children (Janssen & LeBlanc, 2010). Given that the prevalence of pediatric

---

1 An earlier version of this chapter was presented as an invited presentation at the 9th International Developmental Coordination Disorder Scientific Conference in Lausanne, Switzerland, in June 2011.

obesity has risen dramatically in Western countries over the past few decades, obesity and associated metabolic concerns are of grave importance (Shields, 2006; Tremblay et al., 2010). What is perhaps most disturbing in relation to this is the increasing incidence of metabolic-related pathology in children: Conditions that were once mostly restricted to adulthood, including hypertension, hyperlipidemia (Dietz, 1998; Maggio et al., 2008; Sorof & Daniels, 2002), accelerated atherosclerosis (Berenson et al., 1998), insulin resistance (Chiarelli & Marcovecchio, 2008), Type 2 diabetes mellitus (Marcovecchio, Mohn, & Chiarelli, 2005), and metabolic syndrome (Andersen et al., 2008) are increasingly found in children. The inactivity associated with DCD has been linked to many of these problems, especially obesity. The difference between children with DCD and other children lies in what we believe to be the cause of inactivity. For typically developing children, inactivity has been linked to increasing dependence on "screen" activities (e.g., computer games, TV) as the main sources of recreation, as well as decreased active transport (e.g., walking to and from school), which is largely blamed on environments (and therefore lifestyles) that are structured around passive modes of transportation. Diet and stress also play a role, as does socioeconomic status of the family (Powell, Han, & Chaloupka, 2010). While these same conditions affect children with DCD, it is poor motor coordination, not motivation, lack of interest in physical activity, or passive transport that is suspected to be the root cause. If true, the intervention to address inactivity in this population could be quite different than would be the case for children without motor coordination difficulties. Whether the focus is on social or physical consequences – and, although the two are certainly interdependent, very little research has explored these linkages – the prognosis for children with DCD is not good.

That is the narrative, but we may ask, What is the validity of these claims? What evidence is there to support what seems to be widely held in the field? Addressing these questions is the purpose of this chapter. However, some caveats must first be acknowledged. First, this chapter is not a systematic review of the available evidence. Such reviews are already available (e.g., Hands & Larkin, 2002; Rivilis, Hay, Cairney, Klentrou, Liu, & Faught, 2011), so I will not repeat what these reviews already provide. Second, while the consequences of DCD surely affect participation in a broad range of domains, participation in active play, and the physical health consequences associated with physical inactivity, mostly cardiovascular related outcomes, will be the focus of discussion. Mental health consequences and participation in activities outside active play or physical activity are reviewed in detail elsewhere in this volume (see Chapters 2 and 4).

This chapter will review a body of research that comes from what is certainly the largest, and arguably most comprehensive, study of motor coordination, inactivity, and cardiovascular health conducted in this field to date, the Physical Health Activity Study Team, or PHAST. I had the privilege of being one of the principal investigators (along with Drs. John Hay and Brent Faught from Brock University) of that study from its inception in 2003. In reviewing key findings from this study, I will answer the question, What do we know about the relationship between inactivity and physical health in relation to DCD? In addition, I will also identify what we still do not know about these associations and what we need to do next to fill in the gaps in our knowledge. This chapter will also draw on research and contributions from studies other than PHAST where appropriate.

The Theoretical Context for Linking Motor Coordination to Physical Health through Inactivity

Before proceeding with a discussion of PHAST, let me set the theoretical context for this problem. Although it is not always so, scientific inquiry should begin with a set of theoretical propositions that are used for the generation of testable hypotheses. Kurt Lewin is often credited with the saying, "There is nothing quite as useful as a good theory." Theory itself is refined on the basis of the empirical testing of hypotheses, which in turn leads to new studies, and so on. So, we may ask, What theory exists to guide inquiry in this particular field of inquiry?

The Activity Deficit Hypothesis, the Skill Gap Hypothesis, and the Influence of Age (Development) on the Inactivity Gap between Children with DCD and Typically Developing Children

In the literature on inactivity or hypo-activity in children with DCD, Oded Bar-Or (1983) is usually credited with identifying the "activity deficit," which itself is a more general descriptive hypothesis regarding the impact of gross motor problems on physical activity in children. Quite simply, children with conditions that impair gross motor function are less physically active, when compared to typically developing children; they are inactive because of physical disabilities that affect fundamental movement. Bar-Or was a physician and a pediatric exercise physiologist who was concerned clinically with conditions that affected a child's ability to be physically active. He viewed physiological factors as core determinants of activity, among other factors (e.g., motivation). The activity deficit, then, is not specific to children with DCD but includes a wide range of conditions that are unified not by a common underlying pathology but, rather, by a common functional limitation – they all affect the child's ability to move (e.g., cerebral palsy, idiopathic juvenile arthritis).

Wall (2004) is also frequently cited in the DCD literature in relation to the activity deficit. He can be credited with furthering our understanding of the hypothesis by focusing specifically on motor skill, and by placing the activity deficit in an explicitly developmental context. Unlike Bar-Or, whose focus was on medical conditions that lead to physical disability, Wall was interested in children he viewed as having a motor learning problem (one of the ways in which DCD is sometimes conceptualized; see Chapter 8 of this volume). If untreated, a motor learning disability would retard or prevent the acquisition of fundamental skills necessary to be successful at physical activity. The result, like the activity deficit, is a gap in motor skill ability between those with and without motor learning disability. In terms of development, this gap would increase or widen as children grow. Among very young children, differences would be very slight, as most children early in their development struggle with gross motor tasks like catching or kicking a ball. However, in the absence of specific training or intervention, children with motor learning problems may never fully develop core skills such as catching and kicking. With age, the gap between their ability and that of their unaffected peers becomes increasingly noticeable. Most children develop motor skills not through specific training but through explorative play. The consequence for the child with a motor learning disability is that she falls further and further behind her peers as active play becomes more demanding and complex. The process repeats in a negative cycle or feedback loop: The child whose motor skill does not develop withdraws from activity; inactivity does not allow the child to develop motor skill, which in turn leads to further inactivity; and so on. Of course, the widening gap in motor skill would also produce a similar gap in activity participation. Lacking the fundamental skills to participate would, in turn, lead a child with motor coordination problems to increasing levels of inactivity over time.

While intuitive, studies that actually test these theories are scarce. Wall (2004) presented data that show differences in motor skill, assessed under different experimental conditions, between children with and without motor learning problems. There is evidence showing larger differences in skill among older, as compared to younger, children. Relying instead on field data where the focus is on participation in active play, Bouffard et al. (1996) and Cairney et al. (2006) also studied differences between children with high and low levels of motor competence. The former study used observational techniques in a specific context – recess during school hours – while the latter collected self-report data on participation from the children themselves. Both studies were cross-sectional. It is interesting that neither study was able to provide evidence that participation rates differ to a greater or lesser extent when the age of the child is taken into account. In other words, contrary to the activity deficit hypothesis, there is no age-related effect on differences in active play between children with and without motor coordination difficulties. As we will see below, longitudinal data from PHAST has been used to explore the divergence with age in activity deficit. To my knowledge, it is the first and only study to do so.

Inactivity and Health-Related Consequences

A concern of both the activity deficit and skill gap hypotheses is the impact of motor coordination on participation in active play or physical activity. Thus, while inactivity is commonly linked to outcomes such as obesity, poor physical fitness, and other cardiovascular risk factors, the association of motor coordination with these outcomes through inactivity is at best implied rather than specified in these theoretical perspectives. The following two theoretical models make explicit links between motor coordination or motor skill and outcomes such as obesity.

Hands and Larkin (2002) described a negative feedback loop to characterize the relationship between motor coordination, hypo-activity, and physical fitness. A version of the model is provided in Figure 3.1. Similar to Wall's (2004) conception of motor skill and activity in the skill gap hypothesis, Hands and Larkin emphasize the mutually reinforcing processes between these constructs. In their model, motor coordination leads to hypoactivity, which in turn leads to poor physical or health-related fitness (obesity is included in this construct, along with cardiorespiratory fitness and other components of fitness such as strength and flexibility). The double-headed arrows suggest that deterioration in one domain can be a cause of deterioration in another. Poor fitness itself can lead to both inactivity (e.g., children with muscles that are tight and inflexible will

Figure 3.1. Hands and Larkin's (2002) continuous negative feedback loop.

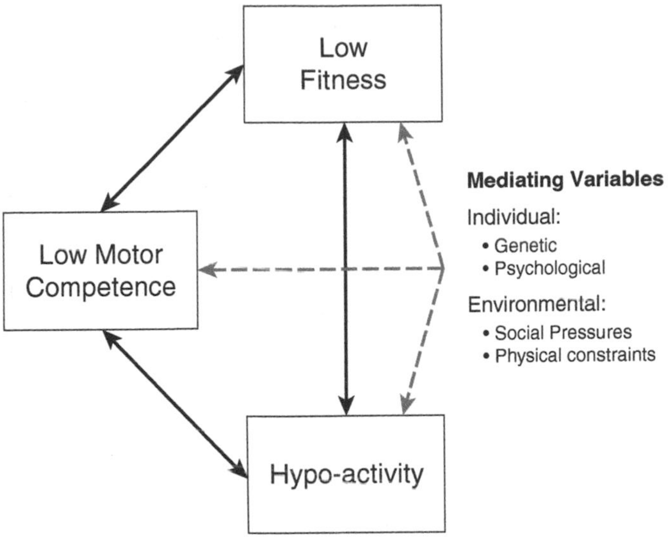

Note: Adapted from the original (Hands & Larkin, 2002).

find it difficult, even painful to be physically active) and poorer coordination (e.g., children with poor aerobic fitness will be unlikely to persist
at games involving physical exertion, which affects the ability to develop
key motor skills). And so the loop continues, resulting in continued
declines in motor coordination, fitness, and activity as the child grows.

In addition to the bidirectional associations between the core domains
identified in the model, Hands and Larkin (2002) also theorized about
the role individual and environmental factors play in the associations
between factors. For example, there are potentially important properties of the child (and the environment) that may influence the pathways
between low motor competence, physical inactivity, and physical fitness. Cardiorespiratory or aerobic fitness – the efficiency with which
oxygen can be delivered from the lungs to the mitochondria for the
production of energy to sustain activity over time – is genetically and
environmentally determined (Rowland, 1996). While low motor competence can negatively affect aerobic fitness, principally by decreasing
a child's participation in physical activity (and therefore, the opportunity to train at a level that confers aerobic benefit), this effect will

also be constrained by limits to fitness that are genetically determined. Environmental effects can also influence pathways in this model. Children with low motor competence who have supportive parents who value the importance of physical activity may act as a positive source of motivation that may help, at least in some cases, to compensate for poor motor coordination. A child with DCD who is encouraged and properly supported is more likely to engage and persist in activities that challenge his motoric abilities.

The particular strengths of this model lie in the explicit recognition of the bidirectional associations between motor competence, physical fitness, and inactivity over time. The implications of this for the interpretation of study results, particularly those based on cross-sectional data, are far from trivial. The model suggests that we need to be careful about the attribution of causality, as there is not a straightforward, linear cause-and-effect relationship between these constructs. At the same time, if these are truly mutually reinforcing effects, then perhaps the issue is not what comes first (precedence); rather, the challenge is to recognize the inherent interdependencies between these constructs as time unfolds. It does not matter which construct researchers target for intervention: Improvement in any domain should positively affect the others. Another strength of the model is that at both the individual level and the environmental level it incorporates potentially moderating influences that can alter the associations between physical inactivity, fitness, and motor competence. These are particularly helpful because a better understanding of these influences will provide useful information for the design of interventions at the individual and ecological levels.

There are ways, however, in which we can enhance the framework to aid us in inquiries about the impact of motor coordination on activity and fitness. For example, although there is a developmental perspective embedded in this model – captured by the conceptualization of the negative feedback loop – there is more room for theorizing about how the relationships between these constructs may change over time as the child develops. I have tried to capture this diagrammatically in Figure 3.2.

In this model, time is depicted on the x-axis and risk of poor cardiovascular health – for example, obesity, poor physical fitness, elevated blood cholesterol levels – is shown on the y-axis. The arrow that cuts across the top represents a developmental trajectory over time. The dots demarcate critical developmental periods, where the interconnections between fitness, activity, and motor competence interact to

Figure 3.2. Continuous negative feedback loop over time.

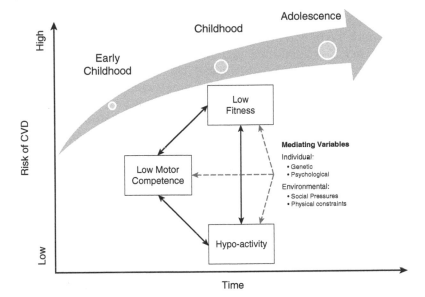

produce health risks. The widening of the arrow (and dots) over time is intended to represent the relative impact of the core process – the negative feedback loop including motor coordination, fitness, and hypoactivity – on the risk of poor cardiovascular health as a function of time. If left unchecked and unaltered, this process will increase risk over time. If we imagine assessment of these three constructs at any one point in time (imagine a line passing through the dot from the top of the figure through the x-axis), we would capture only the correlations among the three constructs. Depending on the age of the child, the relative risk of poor motor coordination, fitness, and/or hypoactivity will vary: Older children will be at greater risk than younger children if we assume that the longer the child is exposed to these effects, the more deleterious the effects on health will be. If left unaltered, the negative spiral between these constructs will significantly increase over time.

The final model I would like to briefly consider is from Stodden and his colleagues (2008). There is considerable overlap between this model, and the one by Hands and Larkin (2002). The core of the model, the link between motor competence, physical fitness, and physical activity, is essentially the same. Indeed, all the core constructs are comparable across models – the difference is in presentation, not substance. Unlike the Hands and Larkin model, which uses a broad category, health-related fitness, to include a number of different variables (e.g., fitness, body composition), Stodden and his colleagues specify a specific health-related outcome – obesity – that is both a cause and consequence of motor incompetence. Their model also specifies an ongoing role for perceived and actual motor competence in moderating the association between motor ability and risk of obesity. Even in the face of increased risk of obesity, positive perceptions of competence can serve as a protective factor that may ultimately reverse or prevent unhealthy weight gain.

Notwithstanding these minor deviations, Stodden and his colleagues (2008) make no direct reference to DCD, nor do they reference the Hands and Larkin (2002) model. This reflects, I think, a kind of disciplinary myopia that will ultimately hinder theoretical and empirical work in this field. Stodden and his colleagues are writing for physical activity researchers and physical educators, who view motor competence from the perspective of normative development of fundamental motor skills (mostly gross motor) and their importance to physical activity, and not as a result of pathology (neurodevelopmental disorders like DCD). While this is not unique to this area of research, it is nevertheless unfortunate, as this discipline-specific approach limits potentially meaningful exchanges between disciplines. It is clear that regardless of whether we view motor incompetence as arising from a disease process, or from the point of view of typical development, the processes that we hypothesize connect motor coordination problems to other behaviours and health-related outcomes are, for all intents and purposes, the same.

Having established a conceptual basis hypothesizing a relationship between motor coordination problems (whether it is described in terms of motor skills or motor competence), physical activity, physical fitness, and, in turn, health-related outcomes such as obesity, I now turn to a review of the empirical evidence to support these associations.

The Physical Health and Activity Study Team

As mentioned at the outset, this chapter is not a systematic review of the literature on DCD, physical activity, and health-related fitness. Instead, I focus principally on evidence generated from what is arguably the largest prospective study on this topic in existence today – the physical health and activity study team (PHAST). Although details of the study design (Cairney, Hay, Veldhuizen, Missiuna, & Faught, 2010a), and some of the challenges of doing large school-based studies of this kind have been published previously (Cairney, Hay, & Faught, 2009), it is important in this context to review the core features of the design again.

Why PHAST?

The purpose of PHAST was to better understand the secondary consequences related to physical activity and physical health arising from DCD. When we began to design and implement the study, the current state of understanding regarding the impact of DCD (and motor coordination more generally) on physical activity and health was limited in the following ways. First, although there were many studies, including some from our own investigative team, showing that children with DCD were less likely to be physically active (Bouffard et al., 1996; Cairney et al., 2005b; Cairney et al., 2005c; Castelli & Valley, 2007; Causgrove Dunn & Dunn, 2006; Christiansen, 2000; Fisher et al., 2005; Hay & Missiuna, 1998; Poulsen, Ziviani, & Cuskelly, 2006, 2007a, 2008; Poulsen, Ziviani, Cuskelly, & Smith, 2007b; Mandich, Polatajko, & Rodger, 2003; Schott, Alof, Hultsch, & Meermann, 2007; Ulrich, 1987; Visser, Geuze, & Kalverboer, 1998; Wrotniak, Epstein, Dorn, Jones, & Kondilis, 2006), more likely to be overweight or obese (Cairney et al., 2005a; Haga, 2008a, 2008b; Hands & Larkin, 2006; Tsiotra et al., 2006; Schott et al., 2007; Wrotniak et al., 2006), less likely to be physically fit (Castelli & Valley, 2007; Hands & Larkin, 2002, 2006), especially in relation to cardiorespiratory fitness (Cairney, Hay, Faught, Flouris, & Kentrou, 2007a; Castelli & Valley, 2007; Faught, Hay, Cairney, & Flouris, 2005; Kanioglou, 2006; Schott et al., 2007; Tsiotra et al., 2006), when compared to children who were typically developing (at least in regard to motor development), most of these studies used cross-sectional designs. While these studies are informative, they cannot address issues of causality or be used to better understand stability and change over time. Although PHAST is not the only study in existence today to explore the association between motor coordination problems, physical activity, and physical health longitudinally (e.g., Cantell, Smyth, & Ahonen, 1994; Hands, 2008; Visser, Geuze, & Kalverboer, 1998; Li, Wu, Cairney, & Hsieh, 2011), when we began, it was clear that the field was in need of prospective studies, a situation that largely remains to this day.

Second, many studies in the field were limited by small sample sizes. This not only made exploring differences between typically developing children and those with DCD challenging, it also made exploring within-group differences very difficult. Within-group differences can refer to the presentation of the disorder, heterogeneity in the kinds of motor coordination deficits children with DCD present with (Visser, 2007), and other characteristics of the child. Of the latter, one of the most important is gender or sex. Although DCD is commonly thought of as a "boys'" disorder, where boys may be two or more times as likely as girls to have the condition (Gibbs et al., 2007), there is compelling evidence to suggest that gender differences may actually be due to systematic differences in the way children are diagnosed (see Chapter 1 for a discussion). Studies where children are sampled from clinical settings show a two- or more fold difference in prevalence favouring boys, whereas community- or school-based samples, where children are screened or tested directly for DCD, typically report similar prevalences among boys and girls (Cairney et al., 2005b; Foulder-Hughes & Cooke, 2003; Skinner & Piek, 2001). The possibility that boys are detected more often than girls, but that girls are affected at about the same rate, has important implications for understanding the impact of the disorder on physical activity and on health-related fitness in this population. It is commonly observed in typically developing children that boys are much more physically active than girls, especially during adolescence (Kimm et al., 2005). Girls with DCD may find it easier socially to withdraw from activity and therefore may, in turn, be at even greater risk of poor health. Small samples of children with DCD – and indeed, samples drawn exclusively from clinical settings – will make examination of gender differences difficult. It is interesting that the question of whether heterogeneity of motor deficits or different clinical subtypes of DCD affect participation in physical activity differentially remains an understudied area that also, of course, requires relatively large numbers of children with the condition.

Third, existing research examining physical activity and physical fitness in children with DCD was largely limited to what researchers might call field-based assessments. So, in the case of cardiorespiratory fitness, for example, the 20-metre shuttle run test had been used to assess VO_2 in children with and without DCD (e.g., Cairney et al., 2007a; Kanioglou, 2006; Mata, Ruiz, & Hay, 2007; Schott et al., 2007; Tsiotra et al., 2006). Body mass index (BMI) had been used in many studies to estimate overweight and obesity (e.g., Cairney et al., 2005c; Hands, 2008; Schott et al., 2007; Tsiotra, Nevill, Lane, & Koutedakis, 2009). While these kinds of measures are quite often used in studies of weight and aerobic fitness in children, there is concern about the validity of these assessments, especially when used on children with DCD. Similarly, while activity deficits between children with and without DCD have been measured using observational methods (e.g., Bouffard et al., 1996) and self-report questionnaires (e.g., Cairney et al., 2005b; Mandich, Polatajko, & Rodger, 2003; Poulsen et al., 2006, 2007a; Poulsen et al., 2007b; Poulsen, Ziviani, & Cuskelly, 2008), other techniques, such as accelerometers, are much less common. There was ample need therefore to replicate the results of earlier work with more sensitive (and in some cases different) measures of physical activity, fitness, and body composition to ensure that what was observed before was not purely an artefact of measurement.

Finally, if there is compelling evidence confirming associations between DCD, inactivity, overweight or obesity, and physical fitness, and these health-related outcomes are themselves risk factors for cardiovascular disease, then it stands to reason that children with DCD may also be at greater risk for cardiovascular disease. Very little research had examined this relationship (Cantell, Crawford, & Tish Doyle-Baker, 2008), none of which was available when PHAST was designed and implemented.

PHAST: Design, Sample, and Measures

The PHAST project is, in fact, two studies: a prospective cohort study tracking a large sample of children, and a longitudinal case-control study involving a subsample of children from the larger cohort study who were asked to participate in a lab-based study. The target sample comprised all children enrolled in Grade 4 (ages 8 and 9) in the public school board of the Niagara Region, a large, geographically, socioeconomically, and ethnically diverse region of the province of Ontario. The public school board is the largest school board in the district, serving children in kindergarten through Grade 12. Grade 4 was selected as the baseline grade because we wanted to evaluate children's competence with regard to physical activity and their perceptions of their motor ability; children younger than 8 would not have been able to complete many of the self-reported measures included in our test battery.

After receiving approval from the school board, we next had to seek consent from individual school administrators for access to students. Details of this, and how consent was obtained from individual students (and their families), have been described in detail in previous publications (Cairney et al., 2010b; Cairney, Hay, & Faught, 2009). Out of a total of 92 schools in the region, we received approval to test in 75 (a school-level response of 81.5%). In these 75 schools, the total number of students enrolled in Grade 4 in 2004 was 2,378. Of these, we obtained parental consent for 2,297, or 95.4%, all of whom completed the first (baseline) assessment. In order to develop the systems required to assess more than 2,000 students located in 75 schools scattered throughout the region, we conducted a pilot data collection project in the fall (September to November) of 2004. The first baseline assessment occurred in the spring of 2005, near the end of the school year. Thereafter, testing occurred twice per year, once in the fall near the beginning of the academic year (September to October), and then again in the spring (May to June), towards the end of the same academic year. In total, from 2005 to 2007, there were five time points, following children from the end of their Grade 4 year through to the end of Grade 6. A list of the key measures relevant to this chapter is provided in Table 3.1. This period of the study I refer to as PHAST I.

While most of the core measures listed in Table 3.1 were administered at each time point, motor coordination testing followed a slightly different protocol, owing to both time and monetary constraints. Motor testing was conducted on each child only once during this phase of this study. All 75 schools were randomized into three blocks (25 schools in each block), and motor testing was conducted in each block separately over the first 2.5 years of the study. Trained research assistants, blind to the results of the other assessments, conducted testing in the schools using the short form of the *Bruininks-Oseretsky Test of Motor Proficiency*

Table 3.1. Core Measures Included in PHAST

Variables of Interest	Measures
Motor coordination	Bruininks-Oseretsky Test of Motor Proficiency, short form (Bruininks, 1978)
Body composition	Height and weight, obtained using a medical stadiometer; waist circumference
Cardiorespiratory fitness	20-m shuttle run test (Léger & Lambert, 1982)
Generalized self-efficacy towards physical activity	Children's Self-Appraisal of Adequacy in and Predilection for Physical Activity (CSAPPA; Hay, 1992)
Participation in active free play and organized sports or activities	Participation questionnaire (Hay, 1992)

(BOTMP-sf; Bruininks, 1978), one of the most commonly used tools to assess DCD in North America (Faught et al., 2005). As noted above, motor testing, when added to the other measures we were assessing, would have been too expensive and potentially too burdensome to our subjects. More important, we were using the BOTMP-sf to identify children with significant motor coordination problems (below the 6th percentile, based on population norms). In the absence of any direct intervention, there would be no reason to assume that a child's motor proficiency would change substantially over the course of the study. Indeed, we hypothesized, based on the literature, that motor coordination scores would remain relatively stable over time for most children. In the spring of 2007 we tested this assumption by retesting 340 children, all randomly selected from 5 schools from the first block of 25 that was tested in the spring of 2005. The correlation between scores was 0.70, suggesting that our assumption was generally correct.

Identification of Children with Motor Coordination Problems

In total, we identified 111 children in PHAST I who scored below the 6th percentile on the BOTMP-sf, 65 girls (58.6%) and 46 boys (41.4%). These children were classified as having possible DCD (pDCD), because we did not assess all of the diagnostic criteria for the disorder. However, we were concerned about who was being classified into this group, given that the motor test was based on a short-form measure administered in field conditions by trained research assistants, not clinicians. At the end of each motor testing block, 10 children – 8 who scored below the 6th percentile on the BOTMP-sf and 2 who scored above this cut-off – were randomly selected from the pool of subjects. An occupational therapist (OT), trained on the second edition of the Movement ABC (MABC-2; Henderson, Sugden, & Barnett, 2007), the most commonly used clinical tool used to assess motor coordination problems in children and adolescents, administered the test to each child individually; the OT also administered a test called the Kaufman Brief Intelligence Test (K-BIT; Kaufman & Kaufman, 2004) to assess intelligence. The OT was blind to the results of the first assessment. The inclusion of two children scoring above the 6th percentile was to prevent the OT from becoming test wise (i.e., only seeing children with significant motor problems). Overall, agreement between test scores was very good. Of the 24 children identified as pDCD in the field, 21 (87%) children scored below the 15th percentile of the M-ABC-2, a positive predictive value of 0.88 (95% CI = 0.69 to 0.96).

PHAST II: Design and Measures

In 2007, fully two and one-half years into the study, we secured additional funding from the same granting agency (the Canadian Institutes of Health Research) to continue to track the original cohort of children and to add another component or substudy to the existing design. Specifically, we initiated a nested, prospective case-control study, following a subset of children with possible DCD and a group of sex- and school-matched controls in order to further explore health-related fitness and cardiovascular health using a series of lab-based tests. We began by contacting all of the children who scored below the 10th percentile on the BOTMP-sf in PHAST I ($n = 67$), and inviting them to participate; 80 children who scored above the 10th percentile were also invited. All 147 were reassessed and classified as possible DCD or non-DCD based on the results of the protocol described in the next paragraph. A total of 63 children, 53 out of 67 children (79%) who scored below the 10th percentile on the BOTMP-sf and who provided consent to participate, and 10 children (12.5%) from the group who scored above the 10th percentile (also with consent), all met the criteria for possible DCD. These children were then school and age matched on all remaining children who did not meet criteria for DCD. All 126 children were assessed at baseline (spring of 2007) and again in the winter of 2008, and 2009 (3 times points in total). Sample attrition resulted in a loss of 41 children (32.5%) by the third year.

All children invited to the lab were reassessed by a trained occupational therapist, who was blind to the results of the field study (the BOTMP-sf), on the M-ABC-2, and the K-BIT. Children scoring below the 16th percentile on the M-ABC-2 and who had no existing medical condition that would exclude them from a diagnosis of DCD were classified as having DCD. Children scoring above this threshold were classified as typically developing controls. In addition, each child received a comprehensive body composition analysis, including height and weight measurements and waist circumference, but also body fat estimation using bioelectrical impedance, and total body volume estimation using whole body, air displacement plethysmography (Nuñez et al., 1999). Children underwent cardiorespiratory fitness testing using a programmable cycle ergometer. The protocol involved a continuous and incremental exercise protocol until the participant reached maximal volitional fatigue. Respiratory gases were collected and analysed using a metabolic cart (Model S-3A, AEI Technologies, Pittsburgh, Pennsylvania). Heart rate was monitored continuously throughout the test. Further details of the protocol have been described in a previous publication (Cairney et al., 2010a). Finally, children also underwent electrocardiography to estimate left ventricular mass and carotid artery thickness, as well as other functional component estimates of heart function (e.g., stroke volume, cardiac output). As part of this procedure, resting heart rate and blood pressure were also assessed, using standardized protocols for this population. Details of these specific procedures are also provided in previous publications (Chirico et al., 2011).

While children were completing the lab assessment, parents were asked to complete a series of surveys regarding their child's health status and use of medical services, as well as a family health history. They also completed a questionnaire (Conners, Sitarenios, Parker, & Epstein, 1998) to assess attentional difficulties and hyperactivity in their child. Between assessments, children also completed questionnaires regarding their beliefs, perceptions, and actual behaviours in relation to physical activity.

At the conclusion of the lab visit, the child was fitted with an accelerometer and both the parent and child were instructed on its use. As well, the parent was provided with an accelerometer logbook and instructed how to complete it. Finally, arrangements were made for a time when one of our trained research assistants would travel to the subject's home to collect the accelerometer and logbook. Within 8 to 10 days after the lab visit, a trained research assistant visited the home of the child early in the morning before breakfast. Each child had been instructed to fast for 8 to 10 hours prior to the visit. A pin-prick test for blood glucose and fats was conducted. Also, the parent and child were provided with Tanner staging images (Taylor et al., 2001), and the maturational stage of the child was determined. Finally, the accelerometer and logbook were collected and brought back to the lab for analysis.

In addition to the lab study, we continued to track the whole cohort of children in the field. Instead of two assessments per year, however, we tested children in the schools only once in the fall each year. All children who participated in the lab were also eligible to participate in the field study. In this chapter, I report on field data from the PHAST I only, as most of the publications using these data were completed before the completion of PHAST II.

The Marriage of Field- and Lab-Based Protocols

There are well-known advantages and disadvantages to both field-based studies and lab-based studies. In this specific context, field-based studies such as PHAST I allow us to track large numbers of students over time in a relatively efficient manner. The efficiency, however, can sometimes come at the expense of measurement. In the field, we tend to rely on measures that can easily be administered in a timely way. Sometimes, these tools lack the precision that is important for accurate measurement of phenomena such as body composition or physical fitness and physical activity. Moreover, when these tools are administered in field-based settings, especially schools, we often can exert only minimal control over the environment. This can sometimes negatively influence the test results in ways that are difficult to quantify. In this case, we may tolerate greater imprecision to achieve greater numbers of subjects. We have written before about the challenges of doing this kind of research and the compromises that must be made (Cairney, Hay, & Faught, 2009).

Lab-based studies, though they allow for much greater control over the environment and make it possible to perform tests that would be unthinkable in field-based settings (many of which offer greater sensitivity and precision), are often very expensive and time consuming, place limits on the number of participants who can be tested, and often require highly specialized, trained technicians. Often, the cost of greater precision of measurement (and control over environmental confounds) comes at the expense of ecological validity; what we have children do in the lab is so far removed from the real world that we are concerned about what the results may actually mean.

However, under circumstances in which both field and lab can be combined, it becomes possible to obtain the benefits of both methods and minimize the limitations associated with reliance on any one design. By including a nested, prospective case-control study into our school-based prospective cohort study, we were able to do the following: (1) validate or cross-check some of the observations we were making in the field against those obtained under lab conditions and (2) use technology in the lab to pose and test new questions arising from our experiences in the field. In particular, the introduction of a lab-based protocol allowed us to examine measures of cardiovascular risk that could simply not be collected in a school-based setting.

In the sections that follow, I present what we have learned so far from both methods in relation to the following questions: (1) Are children with DCD really less active than other children, and does this change over time? (2) Are children with DCD more likely to be overweight or obese when compared to typically developing children, and does this risk change over time? (3) Are children with DCD more likely than their typically developing peers to show early signs (premorbid clinical signs) of cardiovascular disease?

Before proceeding, I wish to acknowledge that what follows represents the work of a team (colleagues, graduate students, and I) whose members have just begun to analyse the extensive trove of data that has been amassed over the past 7 to 8 years. The focus is on what has been published so far at the time of writing of this chapter.

Participation in Active Play over Time in Children with and without Developmental Coordination Disorder

After the completion of the first phase of PHAST, we examined the question of stability and change in participation in active play, for the first 2.5 years of the study (as the children transitioned from the end of fourth grade to the end of sixth grade). In addition to comparing children with DCD to typically developing children, we also questioned whether gender might also influence the impact of DCD on participation trajectories (Cairney et al., 2010b). There is a well-established finding that boys tend to be more physically active than girls and this gap widens over time, particularly in adolescence, largely because girls withdraw from activity at an accelerated rate through this developmental period (Kimm et al., 2005). There is also a literature suggesting that it may be harder for boys with coordination difficulties to be inactive, as there is much more social pressure placed on them to be active, particularly in sports (Chase & Dummer, 1992). It seemed imperative not to ignore the important role gender could play in influencing activity patterns in children with DCD and those without the condition.

The results of this study are depicted, graphically, in Figures 3.3 and 3.4 (Cairney et al., 2010b).[2] Our measure of participation in active play is based on the work of John Hay, a PHAST co-principal investigator. His participation questionnaire (or PQ) is a self-reported measure

---

2 These graphs are derived from a mixed-effects model, where group (DCD vs no-DCD), gender, and time are taken into account simultaneously. A detailed description of the analysis and the results are provided in the original publication. All graphs reporting change over time in this chapter use this statistical method.

Figure 3.3. Differences in total participation questionnaire (PQ) scores over time for boys and girls with and without DCD.

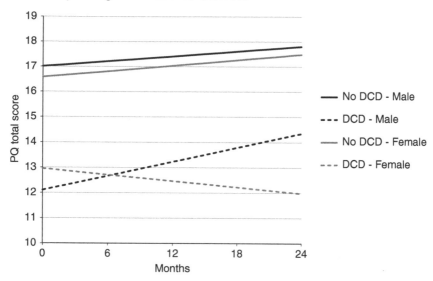

Source: Reprinted from Cairney et al. (2010b).

that captures common active and sedentary pursuits that children and adolescents engage in (Hay, 1992). The scale measures activity (and inactivity) in single units, which represent participation in discrete play activities (e.g., playing on an intramural basketball team, taking swimming lessons). These are further divided into free play, where the child has discretionary control over participation and where the play is unstructured, and organized play such as team sports, where the play is both structured and directed, usually by an adult. Activity units are dependent on recall, subjective reporting of the child over the past year from the time at which the survey was completed.

When we examined total activity (participation in both free play and organized play), we observed important differences between boys and girls with and without DCD. First, regardless of gender, there were differences between groups with regard to participation in active play: Over the duration of the study period typically developing boys and girls had consistently higher activity scores than did boys and girls with DCD. Overall, there was very little difference between typically

Figure 3.4. Differences in participation questionnaire (PQ) free play scores (only) over time for boys and girls with and without DCD.

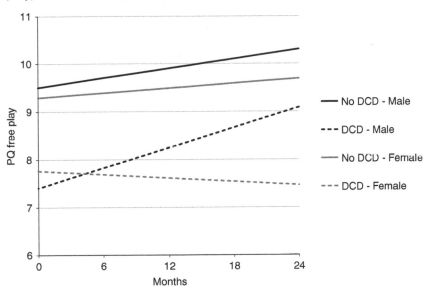

Source: Reprinted from Cairney et al. (2010b).

developing boys and girls. The situation was more complex for boys and girls with DCD. While boys with DCD started out less active than girls with the disorder, after 6 months (~200 days or 6.5 months), boys began to surpass girls with DCD and, by study completion, had significantly narrowed the gap in activity between themselves and typically developing boys and girls. For girls, the pattern of change in activity is best described as a gradual, albeit modest, decline in activity over the course of the study.

We wondered whether this effect was specific to the kinds of activity a child engages in, so we further analysed participation by separating free play from organized activities, using the same independent variables and statistical approach as used in the first analysis. The results are depicted in Figure 3.4.

The pattern of results is identical for free play, but not for organized activities, for which there was no evidence that the association between DCD and participation over time was different for boys than girls. Gender-based influences on participation in children with and without

DCD are true only for activities in which the child has discretionary control over his or her participation.

For girls with DCD, we see evidence for the activity deficit with age hypotheses (Bouffard et al., 1996; Cairney et al., 2006); over time, participation for girls with the disorder remains steady, while typically developing girls' participation increases. The result is a widening gap over time. More difficult to explain is the pattern for boys with DCD. There are two likely explanations for the pattern in play observed here. First, the increase may be an artefact of measurement. Our participation measure is self-reported, so there could be error due to recall, or perhaps bias in reporting owing to social desirability that may affect boys with DCD differently than other children. As we have noted, there is pressure for boys to be physically active, particularly in sports (Chase & Dummer, 1992). Boys with DCD may be reporting what they desire (or are reporting what they think we want them to report), but in actual fact their participation rates have not changed or may even be decreasing. The ultimate test of this will be to use more objective means of assessing activity participation (see the sections below). Second, boys with DCD may really be increasing their participation, but the quality of this participation may be at a level lower than that of their typically developing peers. For example, in many team sports (e.g., soccer, road hockey) boys could participate, but in a way that requires little skill or energy expenditure. For example, in a game of pick-up road hockey, it is not uncommon to see a child "hanging back" on defence, waiting for the play to come to them without much physical exertion, and where size, even excess body fat, can offer some advantages for things like blocking other players. This child is participating but other than gaining social interaction, may be getting little in way of a physical health benefit. The same reason boys with DCD may tell us they are participating when they are not is likely also the explanation for the kind of "minimal" participation just described. The social pressure to be included in active play pushes boys with DCD into participating, even if the level is well below that of their peers.

What Have We Learned about DCD and Physical Activity from Our Lab-Based Studies?

As noted above, the usefulness of self-report measures of participation is limited. Direct assessment of physical activity using heart rate monitoring or accelerometry can provide a more objective measure of energy expenditure (though this is, of course, different from participation). The cost of such technology, however, often prohibits its use in large, field-based studies (such as PHAST). In the lab, we had the opportunity to use accelerometry on a smaller subset of our children (Baerg et al., 2011). In addition, unlike our field study, we assessed symptoms of ADHD in all of the children attending the lab. We wondered whether the presence of symptoms of hyperactivity and inattention might further increase the risk of inactivity in children with DCD, as some research had suggested (Harvey & Reid, 1997; Harvey et al., 2009).

Like the results with participation, we found gender to also be an important factor influencing physical activity patterns in children with and without DCD. We also found differences based on the kinds of physical activity data generated using accelerometry. Step counts (number of steps taken by children) were highest in girls with DCD and ADHD, and lowest in typically developing girls. This suggests that hyperactivity, when present with DCD, may actually increase overall activity levels in girls. A more predictable pattern of results was observed for boys. Typically developing children had the highest step counts, boys with DCD and ADHD were in the middle, and boys with only DCD had the lowest levels of physical activity. The presence of ADHD in the boys with DCD does seem to increase activity, but overall, DCD reduces activity levels relative to children unaffected by the condition.

It is also possible to estimate energy expenditure using an algorithm that considers not only steps but also the velocity or rate of change in motion and duration (measured in 60-second epochs, repeatedly sampled during the total time the device was worn). When this measure is used, the finding for girls is unchanged: Girls with DCD and ADHD report the highest levels of energy expenditure, typically developing girls the lowest. For boys, overall energy expenditure is highest in the DCD group, lowest among those with both DCD and ADHD.

The differences are not easily explained. Girls with DCD (with or without ADHD) are more active than typically developing girls, regardless of how activity is measured. While ADHD may be seen to increase activity in girls, as some research suggests it might (e.g., Dane, Schachar, & Tannock, 2000), it is unclear why girls with DCD only are still more active than typically developing girls. For boys, step counts are lower in those with DCD, but overall energy expenditure appears to be higher. It has been suggested that children with DCD may move less efficiently (Chia, Guelfi, & Licari, 2010; Hands & Larkin, 2002), meaning they may actually expend more energy to move the same distance as a child without the condition. It is possible that what we are observing here is a measure of movement inefficiency.

A more likely explanation, however, is that this result is a product of the measure itself. It is important to note that both step counts and energy expenditure estimates in this study are based on raw counts. Conversion of raw counts into energy expenditure estimates that take into account time and the intensity of the exertion during a specific time interval can be used to more precisely capture physical activity. For example, validation studies of accelerometers have produced algorithms that allow researchers to classify children based on the time spent in moderate, vigorous, and sedentary activity as a percentage of wear time of the motion sensor. These data can then be used to categorize children based on current physical activity guidelines (e.g., 60 minutes of moderate to vigorous physical activity per day, everyday of the week). Categorizing activity this way is very different from step count and raw energy expenditures. This analysis has not yet been done, but it may account for some of the counterintuitive findings noted here.

Direct comparisons between the field results and the lab results for physical activity in PHAST are problematic for a number of reasons. First, as noted earlier, participation is not the same thing as energy expenditure. It is possible to participate in a sport or activity without necessarily expending a lot of energy; conversely, a child can expend a lot of energy in daily activities without participating in a lot of organized or free play games. At best, we are measuring different components of physical activity. Moreover, the introduction of ADHD to further characterize our children with DCD means direct comparison is not possible, as this measure was not collected in our field study. Clearly, the introduction of symptoms of inattention and hyperactivity further complicates the association between DCD and activity. At the very least, the results from both the field and the lab highlight the importance of considering comorbid developmental conditions when examining the impact of DCD on activity. Moreover, the moderating influence of gender is clearly important, as gender differences within and between groups were evident in both studies.

DCD and the Risk of Overweight or Obesity over Time

The second question posed earlier in this chapter asks whether or not children with DCD are at greater risk for overweight or obesity, and whether this risk increases, decreases, or remains stable over time.

Unlike the literature on DCD and physical activity, research on obesity risk in children with DCD is somewhat more mixed: Some studies showed a heightened risk (e.g., Cairney et al., 2005a; Cairney et al., 2010c; Cantell et al., 2008; Faught et al., 2005; Hands & Larkin, 2006; Hands, Larkin, Parker, Straker, & Perry, 2009; Kaufman & Schilling, 2007; O'Beirne, Larkin, & Cable, 1994; Schott et al., 2007; Tsiotra et al., 2009; Wrotniak et al., 2006), while others did not (Hands, 2008; Williams et al., 2008; Wu, Lin, Li, Tsai, & Cairney, 2010). Most of this research was cross-sectional, so the question of change over time was largely unaddressed when we began our work. We wondered if gender would again play a moderating role in the association between DCD and overweight or obesity, as at least one study had shown that increased risk was evident for boys but not girls (Cairney et al., 2005a). Finally, most research in the field had relied upon BMI. While commonly used to identify overweight and obesity, the measure is problematic for developing children. It has been shown, for example, to be less accurate in children because it does not take into account lean tissue mass (Rowland, 1996). Other measures, such as waist-to-hip ratio, waist circumference, or measurement of body fat using skinfold assessment, bioelectrical impedance, or whole body air-displacement plethysmography, can overcome some limitations associated with BMI. With relatively few exceptions (Cairney et al., 2005a), these measures had not been used to assess overweight or obesity in children with DCD.

The results from PHAST I are shown in the Figures 3.5, 3.6, and 3.7 below; these were reported in a previous publication (Cairney et al., 2010c). First, we examined total BMI scores. What is immediately evident, and different from the results for physical activity, is that there are no gender differences within groups. In other words, gender does not influence the association between DCD and BMI in these data. What is clear is that children with DCD had higher average BMI at the beginning of the study, and that this difference in BMI persisted over time. Moreover, these graphs show a slight widening in the gap in BMI between groups, a function of a faster rate of increase in BMI in children with DCD.

Figure 3.6 shows the same association between DCD, gender, and time, this time for waist circumference instead of BMI. The results are very similar: large differences in average waist girth between groups at baseline, with a gap that appears to be increasing due to an accelerated increase in waist circumference in the DCD group.

In both sets of results, the focus is on BMI or waist girth estimates. This does not tell us how many children in each group are overweight or

Figure 3.5. Predicted BMI for boys and girls with and without "possible" DCD.

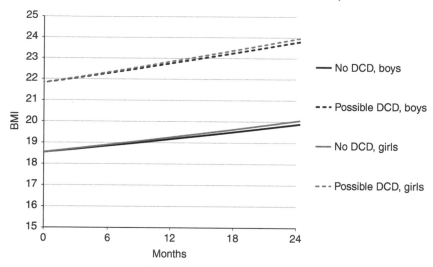

Source: Reprinted from Cairney et al. (2010c).

Figure 3.6. Predicted waist circumference (girth) for boys and girls with and without "possible" DCD.

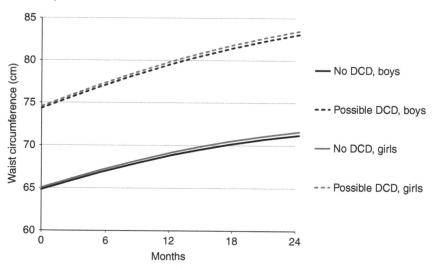

Source: Reprinted from Cairney et al. (2010c).

Figure 3.7. Predicted probability of obesity for children with and without "possible" DCD.

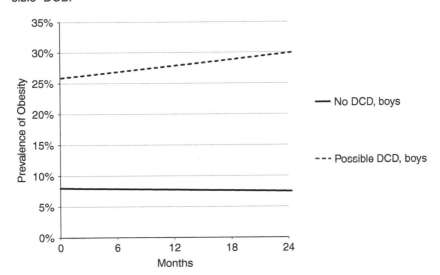

Source: Reprinted from Cairney et al. (2010c).

obese, nor does it show what happens to this number over time. Figure 3.7 shows the prevalence of obesity in children with and without DCD.

The relationship between DCD and obesity is plotted for boys only because the effect for girls is essentially the same. Again, the graph shows that sizeable group differences in prevalence already exist at the beginning of the study (boys with DCD are more than twice as likely to be obese than boys without the disorder), it also shows that while the prevalence of obesity remains essentially flat for typically developing boys, the prevalence increases by almost 5% for children with DCD over the first phase of the study.

What Have We Learned in the Lab?

As noted above, field-based measures of relative body weight like BMI are of limited use in children. While certainly waist circumference is an improvement over BMI, as it is a more direct measure of one kind of adiposity – belly fat – there are more sensitive ways to estimate body mass that take into account both fat and lean tissue mass.

In the lab, we used several different measures of body composition. The one I report here estimates total body composition using whole-body air displacement (Cairney, Hay, Veldhuizen, & Faught, 2011a). This technique allows us to estimate total body mass. To our knowledge, no previous work has actually examined fat-free mass differences between children with and without DCD. This may be important because if differences in muscle mass exist between groups, this would be evidence that children with DCD may be at greater risk for muscle atrophy (wasting) than children without the condition.

The results of the analysis with whole-body air displacement confirm the findings we observed in the field (see Figure 3.8 below). Children with DCD had a higher percentage of body fat and BMI scores; moreover, when we divided children with DCD into groups based on severity (i.e., those below the 6th percentile on the M-ABC-2 vs those who score between the 6th and the 15th percentile), there was evidence of a gradient: the lower the level of overall motor coordination ability, the higher

Figure 3.8. Difference in percentage of body fat and BMI in children with and without DCD. The *y*-axis comprises both percentage of body fat and BMI scores.

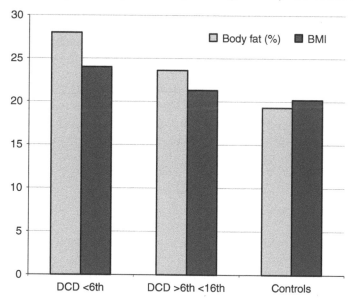

Source: From Cairney et al. (2011a).

the percentage of body fat and BMI. Finally, we did not find any differences in fat-free (lean muscle) mass between groups. Any differences in total body mass, therefore, are due to differences in fat, not muscle mass (Cairney et al., 2011a).

It appears that regardless of how body weight is assessed and whether we are describing weight (total BMI, lean muscle mass versus fat mass) or overweight or obesity based on defined cut points, boys and girls with DCD are at greater risk when compared to typically developing children. Moreover, this risk seems to be increasing over time, suggesting that if unaltered, these trends may have profoundly negative health consequences later in life.

DCD and Cardiorespiratory Fitness over Time

The final question concerns differences in physical fitness over time between children with DCD and those without. Physical fitness is an important determinant of overall health and well-being. One important component of physical fitness, aerobic or cardiorespiratory fitness, is a measure of the efficiency with which the cardiorespiratory system (heart, lungs, and blood vessels) transports oxygen to the muscles to sustain exercise and remove waste products (Rowland, 1996). Aerobic fitness confers many health benefits, including reduced risk of overall mortality and heart disease, stroke, and diabetes (Blair et al., 1989; Church, Kampert, Gibbons, Barlow, & Blair, 2001).

While we already know that children with DCD are at greater risk for physical inactivity and overweight or obesity, it is reasonable to ask, Can we not simply infer that DCD also has a negative affect on physical fitness, including aerobic capacity? It is true that physical inactivity is associated with lower aerobic fitness and that obesity will negatively affect fitness levels, but in fact, fitness is a unique and independent health-related outcome. This is nicely illustrated by a series of studies that show the unique, additive benefits of aerobic fitness on health and mortality. In one study, researchers divided a group of men into tertiles based on the results of an aerobic fitness test. All the men in the study had metabolic syndrome,[3] meaning they had at least three risk factors for cardiovascular disease (e.g., obesity, high blood pressure, elevated blood cholesterol levels) and therefore had a significantly elevated risk for cardiovascular

---

3 Specific criteria for metabolic syndrome are provided later in this chapter.

disease (CVD). For both all-cause mortality and mortality attributable to CVD, men in the highest fitness group had lower rates of death; those in the lowest fitness had a risk of mortality 2.5 to 3.0 times greater than the men in the high fitness group (Katzmarzyk, Church, & Blair, 2004). Being aerobically fit, therefore, can reduce your risk of adverse outcomes even when other risk factors, including obesity, are present. This same research group showed an identical effect for men who were overweight or obese – whether they were obese or not, being fit reduced the overall and CVD-specific risk of mortality (Wei et al., 1999).

We used PHAST I to explore the effects of gender and time on aerobic fitness in children with and without DCD (Cairney, Hay, Veldhuizen, & Faught, 2011b). The main results are depicted in Figure 3.9. As with relative weight and participation, there were noticeable differences in fitness already present when the children were first tested. These differences persisted over time and showed some evidence of widening. The trends are similar across genders, although girls in both groups have lower fitness levels than boys. Overall, girls with DCD show the lowest levels of fitness in this sample.

Figure 3.9. Predicted VO$_2$ max for boys and girls with and without DCD.

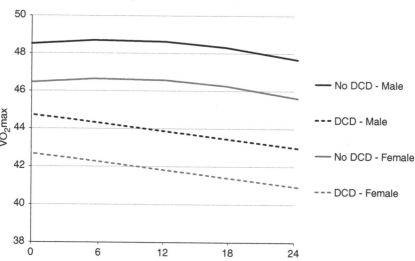

Source: Reprinted from Cairney et al. (2011b).

What Have We Learned in the Lab?

In the field, we assessed aerobic fitness using a test known as the 20-metre shuttle run. In small groups of 5 to 10, boys and girls ran between two lines, spaced 20 metres apart, in time to a beep. The object is to traverse the total distance (there and back) before the sound of the beep. Failing to do so in two consecutive attempts results in removal from the test. The time interval between beeps decreases as the test progresses, making it harder and harder to complete the distance in time.

While, in our experience, children enjoyed doing the test (at least until adolescence) and most seemed to strive to stay in the test for as long as they could, we have concerns with the format of the shuttle run test for children with motor coordination problems. First, there is a competitive element to the test: Children run in small groups, and even though they are racing against a beep, inevitably many end up racing against each other. Children with DCD may not do well in competitive tasks, owing to a history of failure in sport-related competitions. The test was usually conducted in a gym or outside in a playing field. While we tried not to make it feel like being in a physical education class, the environmental cues could have been sending a different message. Children with DCD tend to dislike physical education for the same reasons they dislike other sports-related experiences (Cairney et al., 2007b). Finally, although the test is relatively easy, in the sense that it requires little in the way of motor skill, children with balance and timing problems may find the quick pivots at the line required for turning and running in stride with other children difficult. There is therefore some reason to be concerned that there will be differences in motivation, with children with DCD perhaps more likely to quit before making maximal effort. Our own work has shown that self-efficacy towards physical activity is a significant predictor of shuttle run test performance in typically developing children (Cairney, Hay, Faught, Léger, & Mathers, 2008).

Because we had a subset of children in the lab who had completed aerobic fitness testing using both a cycle ergometer and the 20-metre shuttle run, we had an opportunity to compare results from the two tests (Cairney et al., 2010a). The lab test was conducted one-on-one with a trained research assistant, which eliminated the competitive aspect associated with the shuttle run, as well as the feel of "gym class." Moreover, effort can be assessed in the lab by asking the child about his or her perceived exertion and by paying attention to visible signs of effort (e.g., breathing, facial expression). Moreover, the child can more easily be encouraged in this setting. Finally, more objective measures of effort, captured though heart rate monitoring and the collection of gases (e.g., CO_2) via the mouth, can be used to assess whether the child is truly exercising to exhaustion.

In the lab protocol, children with DCD had lower peak VO_2 than their peers, but there were no significant between-group differences in maximal heart rate (191 bpm in TD compared to 186 bpm in DCD). Similarly, both groups had respiratory exchange ratios (RERs) greater than 1:1 (Silman, Cairney, Hay, Klentrou, & Faught, 2011). RER is an indirect estimate of the ratio of CO_2 produced to O_2 consumed. When the ratio is 1:1 or greater, CO_2 production is the result of lactate buffering and other changes in substrate utilization in muscle, indicative of maximal effort (Rowland, 1996). These results suggest that though overall fitness levels differed, it was not due to differences in effort; both groups were working very hard.

Equally intriguing, the differences between peak VO_2 estimates were remarkably similar, between 8 and 10 points, regardless of the test (lab vs field; Cairney et al., 2010a). While the absolute values differed – as would be expected since they are different tests – the relative difference between groups remained about the same. We concluded on the basis of this that the shuttle run test was a reasonable measure, and that differences in motivation did not account for the poorer performance on the shuttle run test that we and others have observed in children with DCD (e.g., Hands & Larkin, 2006; Mata et al., 2007; Schott et al., 2007). Of course, it should be noted that we were not exactly comparing equivalent tests – one was a running protocol, the other a cycling test. Nevertheless, we were less interested in the precision of the estimate for peak VO_2 than we were in assessing whether group differences were affected by differences in testing protocols. Our data suggest that regardless of the test, children with DCD are less fit than others.

Together, the results of both our field-based studies and our lab-based studies confirm that children with DCD are indeed at greater risk for physical inactivity, overweight, and obesity (although there are important gender differences in these associations) and are less aerobically fit than children without DCD. These differences are evident by 8 years of age and tend to persist through early adolescence. There is also some evidence that differences in relative weight and fitness may widen over time.

Early Signs of Cardiovascular Disease in Children with DCD

Our final question concerns what we might learn about physical health differences between children with DCD and those without the condition.

While inactivity, obesity, and poor fitness are themselves important risk factors for poor cardiovascular health, we wondered if we might be able to observe more sensitive signs of early cardiovascular pathology in children with this condition, given the increased risks we had observed in relation to activity, relative weight, and aerobic fitness. While our work in this regard is ongoing, I report on a few studies that address this question.

When we began PHAST, there were no studies that had explored whether the increased risk of obesity, inactivity, and poor fitness was also associated with early signs of cardiovascular pathology or other CVD risk factors like hypertension or elevated blood cholesterol and triglycerides. Since initiation of our study, however, at least one other group has studied such differences (Cantell et al., 2008). Where appropriate, I will compare our results to theirs.

One important pathological change that can occur to the structure of the heart is increased left ventricular mass (LVM). Essentially, the cardiac muscles that form the wall of the heart begin to hypertrophy as a result of prolonged stress (e.g., pressure overload from hypertension). The result of this is myocardial thickening. The thickening of the walls occurs with no change in the overall size of the heart, so the changes in mass occur at the expense of the cavities, which become smaller. The heart must work harder and harder to pump the same amount of blood through increasingly narrowed cavities. Increased LVM is a marker of this pathological process and has been shown to be an independent risk factor for heart attack, stroke, and cardiovascular mortality (Bluemke et al., 2008).

LVM can be assessed noninvasively using ultrasound imaging technology. When our team, under the leadership of Deborah O'Leary-Myers from Brock University, examined ultrasound images from children in the study, we found no evidence of increased LVM in children with DCD (Chirico et al., 2011). However, children with DCD did show elevated end-diastolic volume, diastolic chamber size, stroke volume, and cardiac output. These differences indicate obesity-related changes in the left ventricle and may represent the early stages of developing left ventricle hypertrophy.

In addition to LVM, we also explored other markers of cardiovascular disease risk. Given the comprehensive battery of assessments performed in the laboratory, we were interested in whether children with DCD exhibited multiple CVD risk factors simultaneously. There is increasing evidence that risk factors for CVD, such as obesity, hypertension, elevated cholesterol, and elevated triglycerides, cluster in individuals.

Table 3.2. International Diabetes Federation Consensus Criteria for Metabolic Syndrome (10–15 years)

> ➤ Metabolic syndrome is diagnosed when a child is:
>   • Obese, defined by waist circumference ≥ 90th for age and sex
> ➤ And at least two of following conditions are met:
>   • Fasting glucose ≥ 100 mg/dl (or Type II diabetes)
>   • Triglycerides ≥ 150 mg/dl
>   • HDL < 40 mg/dl
>   • SBP ≥ 130 or DBP ≥ 85

While the risk for CVD is increased by the presence of any one of these factors, when they occur simultaneously, the risk for heart and cerebrovascular disease is even greater (e.g., McNeill et al., 2005). Metabolic syndrome (MetS) is the term used for the co-occurrence of these risk factors. Table 3.2 outlines the specific criteria for MetS in children and adolescents.

Using these criteria to define MetS, our team investigated whether the risk of metabolic syndrome was greater in children with DCD versus the typically developing children (Wahi et al., 2011). In our sample ($n = 126$) a total of 11 children met the criteria for MetS: 8 (72.3%; prevalence = 6.3%) with DCD and 3 (27.3%; prevalence = 2.4%) controls ($OR = 2.9$, $p = 0.115$). While not statistically significant, the relative proportion of children with DCD meeting criteria relative to controls is worthy of further study. Post hoc power analyses revealed that the study was not powered to detect differences in prevalence of MetS, which is uncommon in this age group. With regard to individual components of MetS, several significant differences were observed. Abdominal obesity was found in 39 (30.9%) children, 29 (46.0%) with DCD and 10 (15.9%) controls ($p < 0.01$). Serum triglycerides were higher in DCD, 91.9 mg/dl (63.1) versus 67.7 mg/dl (33.3) in the control group, $p = 0.001$. Finally, blood pressure (BP) was also significantly higher in the pDCD group, mean systolic BP (110 vs. 105 mmHg, $p = 0.01$) and mean diastolic BP (69 vs. 65 mmHg, $p = 0.01$). Thus, while only a small number of children had MetS, children with DCD may be at greater risk of developing it in the future, given the unhealthy risk profiles documented here.

In sum, while it may be too soon to detect the early signs of CVD in children of this age with DCD, troubling evidence of increased risk is detectable. Along with the patterns of inactivity, higher rates of obesity and poor aerobic fitness we previously observed, there seems little doubt that risk for CVD is higher in children with DCD. However, the only other study to have examined some of these same components failed to find significant differences in heart rate or diastolic or systolic blood pressure in children with and without DCD (Cantell et al., 2008). Further research, preferably with larger samples of children, is required to confirm the associations I have reported here.

PHAST and Future Studies

This chapter, indeed this book, is about secondary consequences arising from DCD. These results suggest that the disorder is a cause of outcomes like inactivity, obesity, and other measures of physical health status. Can we, however, conclude from PHAST, and from other studies that have been conducted, that DCD is truly a cause? Two kinds of study designs, experimental and longitudinal, are most appropriate for understanding cause and effect. While experimental designs are the most powerful, they are not particularly useful in this context: We cannot induce DCD in children and wait to observe its consequences. Longitudinal, observational studies are the most appropriate design.

As I have noted, PHAST is one of only a few studies (e.g., Hands, 2008) that have examined the association between DCD and activity, relative weight, and physical fitness using a prospective design. Nonetheless PHAST is the largest and, in many ways, the most comprehensive. Yet, as is evident throughout this review, when longitudinal results show differences between groups, these differences were already present when the study began. We cannot conclude from these data alone that DCD is a cause of – or even preceded – these outcomes. Where exactly does that leave us?

While our data may be insufficient to demonstrate causation, when considered against other evidence and theory, there is justification for assuming DCD plays an important causal role in relation to physical health. First, we must consider what the presence of baseline differences means for the argument that obesity, poor physical fitness, and inactivity are consequences of DCD. If DCD does not cause these conditions, could the reverse be true? Could inactivity, obesity, and poor fitness lead to poor coordination? Our current understanding of the etiology of DCD (see Chapter 1 in this volume), while incomplete, points to neurological dysfunction that occurs during early fetal brain development as the likely cause of DCD. If this is so, then it is unlikely that inactivity or obesity would occur prior to development of the disorder.[4] While it is true that overweight or obesity can negatively affect motor coordination (e.g., D'Hondt, Deforche, De Bourfeaudhuij, & Lenoir, 2009), and it is certainly plausible that children who are inactive from early childhood may show delayed motor skill development and therefore be at greater risk for obesity, these children should not be diagnosed with DCD. It is important also to consider the difference between motor skill and motor coordination. A skill is a learned motor behaviour, like throwing or catching a ball, whereas motor coordination refers to the underlying neurological and biological apparatus that is necessary for the execution of skill. While it is conceivable that chronic inactivity from early childhood would retard the development of motor skill, it is less clear how this would negatively affect coordination.

Nevertheless, in field-based studies such as PHAST, it is difficult to separate DCD cases from children whose apparent poor coordination is the result of prolonged inactivity and/or obesity. This will continue to be a problem, especially in the absence of a biomarker for the condition. For that matter, separating motor skill from motor coordination with functional assessments like the M-ABC or the BOT is also difficult to do.

Second, the data from PHAST and other studies are at least consistent with the theory that DCD is a cause of poor fitness and obesity. The trends in our PHAST data show not only differences between groups but also different pathways over time: Children with DCD are getting worse over time at a faster rate than their typically developing peers, at least in relation to obesity and fitness. For participation in active play, this is true for girls with DCD but may not be so for boys with the disorder. Moreover, we have also shown a gradational effect between motor ability and percentage of body fat and BMI (Cairney et al., 2011a). Children scoring below the 6th percentile are heavier than children scoring between the 6th and 15th percentiles, who in turn are heavier than children in the typically developing range for motor coordination. These data are consistent with the hypothesis that DCD is a cause of obesity.

Finally, at least one study has shown that motor coordination difficulties present in childhood predicts overweight and obesity in adulthood (Osika & Montgomery, 2008). While this study needs to be replicated, it does provide important data concerning the causal pathway. It also

---

4 It of course does not rule out the possibility that there is a common mechanism that causes DCD and poor physical health.

points to the next generation of studies that will be required to truly test causality. Such studies will also need to explore the independent (or adjusted) association of DCD on outcomes such as obesity, as a large body of research has established the importance of risk factors other than motor coordination, such as socioeconomic status (e.g., Kinra, Nelder, & Lewendon, 2000) and family habits (particularly maternal; e.g., Perez-Pastor et al., 2009), for overweight or obesity in children. The contribution of these factors to obesity needs to be explored, as few studies of children with DCD have incorporated these data (Green et al., 2011).

Given the presence of baseline differences in our data, it seems reasonable to begin to track children at a younger age. Since motor coordination cannot be reliably assessed much earlier than 4 years of age (Geuze, 2007), assembling a large cohort of children at 48 months and following them prospectively, tracking motor coordination, relative weight status (e.g., BMI, waist circumference, percentage of body fat), physical activity (preferably using not only self- or parent-reported data but also using objective measures such as motion sensors), and health-related fitness (e.g., aerobic fitness, as well as other fitness parameters including strength and flexibility) would be the best design to capture causal associations. While it is arguable that this may already be too late, given the increasing prevalence of overweight and obesity in preschool children (de Onis & Blössner, 2000), we researchers are limited by our ability to measure motor coordination. Data on children during this developmental period would certainly help us to understand the associations between these variables over time in early childhood. Moreover, repeated assessments of motor coordination through early childhood would also provide a much needed "natural history" of motor coordination problems early in life and may allow us to separate true cases of DCD from delay. (A more in-depth discussion of the challenges of doing longitudinal studies in this field is offered in Chapter 7).

While such a study would be of scientific interest, I am equally compelled to pursue a different course altogether. Given the theoretical plausibility of a causal link between DCD, inactivity, and poor health, as well as the robustness of these associations over time and across different studies, coupled with the ethical imperative to try to help children with DCD, intervention studies may be as useful, if not more so, than prospective observational studies. First, intervention studies are by design experimental and can therefore be used to address questions of causality. If we can intervene to "compensate" for motoric problems, and this results in an increase in physical activity accompanied by a

STAFF LIBRARY
SINGLETON HOSPITAL
TEL: 01792 205666 EXT: 35281

reduction in the risk of poor health, then we have provided evidence for the hypothesis that these problems are secondary to DCD. Such an intervention could improve the quality of life and reduce the risk for future disease in a group of high-risk children. The challenge, of course, is in designing an intervention that could work. In a previous paper, colleagues and I have outlined some of the issues that should be considered when designing such an intervention (Cairney, Kwan, & King-Dowling, 2011). The core principle of any intervention must be that activities should be matched to the motoric capabilities of the child and should be things that the child enjoys and wants to do. One model for intervention that could be used in this context is provided by Missiuna, Polatajko, and Pollock (Chapter 8 in this volume). What is particularly appealing about the model described by Missiuna and her colleagues is that it targets all children initially and does not rely on one-on-one interventions, but instead it focuses, at least at one level, on environmental accommodation. Creating environments that encourage participation, and which are child centred and therefore matched to motor ability, holds the greatest promise, I believe, for addressing the problem of inactivity and physical health risk in children not only with DCD but also for those whose motor abilities are at the low end of normal functioning.

Conclusion

At the outset of this chapter, I began with the commonly asserted proposition that the child with DCD is more likely to be inactive, and therefore at greater risk for suffering the consequences of inactivity, than the typically developing child. I asked, what is the validity of this claim? There is theoretical plausibility and compelling data to confirm the association between DCD, inactivity, and poor physical health. The body of work that has amassed over the past decade, including the results of the PHAST study, has answered many important questions about these associations (e.g., What is the impact, if any, of gender? Are these associations stable over time?). The answer appears to be that there is indeed validity to this claim. While further research may yet shed more light on the complex associations between these variables, it is also clear that we can no longer wait for more data. The next generation of studies will have to balance the need to understand more about mechanisms against the need to act. Based on what we know about the physical health profiles of children with DCD, it is imperative that we continue this line of research. It would be unethical if we do not seek to intervene.

REFERENCES

Andersen, L.B., Harro, M., Sardinha, L.B., Froberg, K., Ekelund, U., Brage, S., Anderssen, S.A. (2006). Physical activity and clustered cardiovascular risk in children: A cross-sectional study (The European Youth Heart Study). *Lancet, 368*(9532):299–304.

Baerg, S., Cairney, J., Hay, J., Rempel, L., Mahlberg, N., & Faught, B.E. (2011, Jul-Aug). Evaluating physical activity using accelerometry in children at risk of developmental coordination disorder in the presence of attention deficit hyperactivity disorder. *Research in Developmental Disabilities, 32*(4), 1343–1350. http://dx.doi.org/10.1016/j.ridd.2011.02.009 Medline:21420277

Bar-Or, O. (1983). *Pediatric sports medicine for the practitioner.* New York, NY: Springer-Verlag. http://dx.doi.org/10.1007/978-1-4612-5593-2

Berenson, G.S., Srinivasan, S.R., Bao, W., Newman, W.P., III, Tracy, R.E., & Wattigney, W.A. (1998, Jun 4). Association between multiple cardiovascular risk factors and atherosclerosis in children and young adults. The Bogalusa Heart Study. *New England Journal of Medicine, 338*(23), 1650–1656. http://dx.doi.org/10.1056/NEJM199806043382302 Medline:9614255

Blair, S.N., Kohl, H.W., III, Paffenbarger, R.S., Jr., Clark, D.G., Cooper, K.H., & Gibbons, L.W. (1989, Nov 3). Physical fitness and all-cause mortality: A prospective study of healthy men and women. *Journal of the American Medical Association, 262*(17), 2395–2401. http://dx.doi.org/10.1001/jama.1989.03430170057028 Medline:2795824

Bluemke, D.A., Kronmal, R.A., Lima, J.A., Liu, K., Olson, J., Burke, G.L., & Folsom, A.R. (2008, Dec 16). The relationship of left ventricular mass and geometry to incident cardiovascular events: The MESA (Multi-Ethnic Study of Atherosclerosis) study. *Journal of the American College of Cardiology, 52*(25), 2148–2155. http://dx.doi.org/10.1016/j.jacc.2008.09.014 Medline:19095132

Bouffard, M., Watkinson, E.J., Thompson, L.P., Causgrove Dunn, J.L., & Romanow, S.K.E. (1996). A test of the activity deficit hypothesis with children with movement difficulties. *Adapted Physical Activity Quarterly; APAQ, 13*, 61–73.

Bruininks, R.H. (1978). *Bruininks-Oseretsky Test of Motor Proficiency: Examiner's manual.* Circle Pines, MN: American Guidance Service.

Cairney, J., Hay, J.A., & Faught, B.E. (2009). On the finer points of handling googlies: Reflections on hits, near misses and full-blown swings at the air in large, population-based studies involving schools, parents and children. In D.L. Streiner & S. Sidani (Eds.), *When research goes off the rails* (pp. 228–238). New York, NY: Guilford Press.

Cairney, J., Hay, J.A., Faught, B.E., Corna, L., & Flouris, A. (2006). Developmental coordination disorder, age and play: A test of the divergence in activity-deficit with age hypothesis. *Adapted Physical Activity Quarterly; APAQ, 23*(3), 261–276.

Cairney, J., Hay, J.A., Faught, B.E., Flouris, A., & Klentrou, P. (2007a, Feb). Developmental coordination disorder and cardiorespiratory fitness in children. *Pediatric Exercise Science, 19*(1), 20–28. Medline:17554154

Cairney, J., Hay, J.A., Faught, B.E., & Hawes, R. (2005c, Apr). Developmental coordination disorder and overweight and obesity in children aged 9–14 y. *International Journal of Obesity, 29*(4), 369–372. http://dx.doi.org/10.1038/sj.ijo.0802893 Medline:15768042

Cairney, J., Hay, J.A., Faught, B.E., Léger, L., & Mathers, B. (2008, Mar-Apr). Generalized self-efficacy and performance on the 20-metre shuttle run in children. *American Journal of Human Biology, 20*(2), 132–138. http://dx.doi.org/10.1002/ajhb.20690 Medline:17990324

Cairney, J., Hay, J.A., Faught, B.E., Mandigo, J., & Flouris, A. (2005a). Developmental coordination disorder, self-efficacy toward physical activity and participation in free play and organized activities: Does gender matter? *Adapted Physical Activity Quarterly; APAQ, 22*(1), 67–82.

Cairney, J., Hay, J.A., Faught, B.E., Wade, T.J., Corna, L., & Flouris, A. (2005b, Oct). Developmental coordination disorder, generalized self-efficacy toward physical activity, and participation in organized and free play activities. *Journal of Pediatrics, 147*(4), 515–520. http://dx.doi.org/10.1016/j.jpeds.2005.05.013 Medline:16227039

Cairney, J., Hay, J.A., Mandigo, J., Wade, T.J., Faught, B.E., & Flouris, A. (2007b). Developmental coordination disorder and reported enjoyment of physical education in children. *European Physical Education Review, 13*(1), 81–98. http://dx.doi.org/10.1177/1356336X07072678

Cairney, J., Hay, J., Veldhuizen, S., & Faught, B. (2010a, Nov-Dec). Comparison of VO$_2$ maximum obtained from 20 m shuttle run and cycle ergometer in children with and without developmental coordination disorder. *Research in Developmental Disabilities, 31*(6), 1332–1339. http://dx.doi.org/10.1016/j.ridd.2010.07.008 Medline:20702060

Cairney, J., Hay, J.A., Veldhuizen, S., Missiuna, C., Faught, B.E. (2010, Mar). Developmental coordination disorder, sex, and activity deficit over time: A longitudinal analysis of participation trajectories in children with and without coordination difficulties. *Developmental Medicine and Child Neurology, 52*(3):e67-72.

Cairney, J., Hay, J., Veldhuizen, S., & Faught, B. (2011a, Mar-Apr). Assessment of body composition using whole body air-displacement plethysmography in children with and without developmental coordination disorder. *Research in Developmental Disabilities, 32*(2), 830–835. http://dx.doi.org/10.1016/j.ridd.2010.10.011 Medline:21095096

Cairney J, Hay J, Veldhuizen S, Missiuna C, Mahlberg N, Faught B.E. (2010, Aug). Trajectories of relative weight and waist circumference among children with and without developmental coordination disorder. *CMAJ*, 182(11):1167-72. doi: 10.1503/cmaj.091454.

Cairney, J., Hay, J., Veldhuizen, S., & Faught, B.E. (2011b, Dec). Trajectories of cardiorespiratory fitness in children with and without developmental coordination disorder: A longitudinal analysis. *British Journal of Sports Medicine, 45*(15), 1196–1201. http://dx.doi.org/10.1136/bjsm.2009.069880 Medline:20542967

Cairney, J., Kwan, M.Y.W., & King-Dowling, S. (2011). Obesity risk in children with developmental coordination disorder: What do we know and what should we do? *Dyspraxia Foundation Professional Journal, 10*, 21–32.

Cantell, M., Crawford, S.G., & Tish Doyle-Baker, P.K. (2008, Apr). Physical fitness and health indices in children, adolescents and adults with high or low motor competence. *Human Movement Science, 27*(2), 344–362. http://dx.doi.org/10.1016/j.humov.2008.02.007 Medline:18395282

Cantell, M.H., Smyth, M.M., & Ahonen, T.P. (1994). Clumsiness in adolescence: Educational, motor and social outcomes of motor delay detected at 5 years. *Adapted Physical Activity Quarterly; APAQ, 11*, 115–129.

Castelli, D.M., & Valley, J.A. (2007). The relationship of physical fitness and motor competence to physical activity. *Journal of Teaching in Physical Education, 26*, 358–374.

Causgrove Dunn, J., & Dunn, J.G.H. (2006). Psychosocial determinants of physical education behavior in children with movement difficulties. *Adapted Physical Activity Quarterly; APAQ, 23*, 293–309.

Chase, M.A., & Dummer, G.M. (1992, Dec). The role of sports as a social status determinant for children. *Research Quarterly for Exercise and Sport 63*(4), 418–424. http://dx.doi.org/10.1080/02701367.1992.10608764 Medline:1439167

Chia, L.C., Guelfi, K.J., & Licari, M.K. (2010, Mar). A comparison of the oxygen cost of locomotion in children with and without developmental coordination disorder. *Developmental Medicine and Child Neurology, 52*(3), 251–255. http://dx.doi.org/10.1111/j.1469-8749.2009.03392.x Medline:19706141

Chiarelli, F., & Marcovecchio, M.L. (2008, Dec). Insulin resistance and obesity in childhood. *European Journal of Endocrinology, 159*(Suppl 1), S67–S74. http://dx.doi.org/10.1530/EJE-08-0245 Medline:18805916

Chirico, D., O'Leary, D., Cairney, J., Klentrou, P., Haluka, K., Hay, J., & Faught, B. (2011, Jan-Feb). Left ventricular structure and function in children with and without developmental coordination disorder. *Research in Developmental Disabilities, 32*(1), 115–123. http://dx.doi.org/10.1016/j.ridd.2010.09.013 Medline:21035301

Christiansen, A.S. (2000, Jan). Persisting motor control problems in 11- to 12-year-old boys previously diagnosed with deficits in attention, motor control and perception (DAMP). *Developmental Medicine and Child Neurology, 42*(1), 4–7. http://dx.doi.org/10.1017/S0012162200000025 Medline:10665968

Church, T.S., Kampert, J.B., Gibbons, L.W., Barlow, C.E., & Blair, S.N. (2001, Sep 15). Usefulness of cardiorespiratory fitness as a predictor of all-cause and cardiovascular disease mortality in men with systemic hypertension. *American Journal of Cardiology, 88*(6), 651–656. http://dx.doi.org/10.1016/S0002-9149(01)01808-2 Medline:11564389

Conners, C.K., Sitarenios, G., Parker, J.D., & Epstein, J.N. (1998, Aug). The revised Conners' Parent Rating Scale (CPRS-R): Factor structure, reliability, and criterion validity. *Journal of Abnormal Child Psychology, 26*(4), 257–268. http://dx.doi.org/10.1023/A:1022602400621 Medline:9700518

Dane, A.V., Schachar, R.J., & Tannock, R. (2000, Jun). Does actigraphy differentiate ADHD subtypes in a clinical research setting? *Journal of the American Academy of Child and Adolescent Psychiatry, 39*(6), 752–760. http://dx.doi.org/10.1097/00004583-200006000-00014 Medline:10846310

de Onis, M., & Blössner, M. (2000, Oct). Prevalence and trends of overweight among preschool children in developing countries. *American Journal of Clinical Nutrition, 72*(4), 1032–1039. Medline:11010948

D'Hondt, E., Deforche, B., De Bourdeaudhuij, I., & Lenoir, M. (2009, Jan). Relationship between motor skill and body mass index in 5- to 10-year-old children. *Adapted Physical Activity Quarterly; APAQ, 26*(1), 21–37. Medline:19246771

Dietz, W.H. (1998, Mar). Health consequences of obesity in youth: Childhood predictors of adult disease. *Pediatrics, 101*(3 Pt 2), 518–525. Medline:12224658

Faught, B.E., Hay, J.A., Cairney, J., & Flouris, A. (2005, Nov). Increased risk for coronary vascular disease in children with developmental coordination disorder. *Journal of Adolescent Health, 37*(5), 376–380. http://dx.doi.org/10.1016/j.jadohealth.2004.09.021 Medline:16227122

Fisher, A., Reilly, J.J., Kelly, L.A., Montgomery, C., Williamson, A., Paton, J.Y., & Grant, S. (2005, Apr). Fundamental movement skills and habitual physical activity in young children. *Medicine and Science in Sports and Exercise, 37*(4), 684–688. http://dx.doi.org/10.1249/01.MSS.0000159138.48107.7D Medline:15809570

Foulder-Hughes, L.A., & Cooke, R.W. (2003). Developmental co-ordination disorder in preterm children born <32 weeks gestational age. *Dyspraxia Foundation Professional Journal, 2*, 3–13.

Geuze, R.H. (Ed.). (2007). *Developmental Coordination Disorder: A Review of Current Approaches.* Marseille, France: Solal

Gibbs, J., Appleton, J., & Appleton, R. (2007, Jun). Dyspraxia or developmental coordination disorder? Unravelling the enigma. *Archives of Disease in*

Childhood, 92(6), 534–539. http://dx.doi.org/10.1136/adc.2005.088054 Medline:17515623

Green, D., Lingam, R., Mattocks, C., Riddoch, C., Ness, A., & Emond, A. (2011, Jul-Aug). The risk of reduced physical activity in children with probable developmental coordination disorder: A prospective longitudinal study. *Research in Developmental Disabilities, 32*(4), 1332–1342. http://dx.doi.org/10.1016/j.ridd.2011.01.040 Medline:21334850

Haga, M. (2008a). Physical fitness in children with movement difficulties. *Physiotherapy, 94*(3), 253–259. http://dx.doi.org/10.1016/j.physio.2007.04.011

Haga, M. (2008b, May). The relationship between physical fitness and motor competence in children. *Child: Care, Health and Development, 34*(3), 329–334. http://dx.doi.org/10.1111/j.1365-2214.2008.00814.x Medline:18410639

Hands, B. (2008, Apr). Changes in motor skill and fitness measures among children with high and low motor competence: A five-year longitudinal study. *Journal of Sports Science & Medicine, 11*(2), 155–162. http://dx.doi.org/10.1016/j.jsams.2007.02.012 Medline:17567536

Hands, B., & Larkin, D. (2002). Physical fitness and developmental coordination disorder. In S.A. Cermak & D. Larkin (Eds.), *Developmental coordination disorder* (pp. 174–184). Albany, NY: Delmar.

Hands, B., & Larkin, D. (2006). Physical fitness differences in children with and without motor learning difficulties. *European Journal of Special Needs Education, 21*(4), 447–456. http://dx.doi.org/10.1080/08856250600956410

Hands, B., Larkin, D., Parker, H., Straker, L., & Perry, M. (2009, Oct). The relationship among physical activity, motor competence and health-related fitness in 14-year-old adolescents. *Scandinavian Journal of Medicine & Science in Sports, 19*(5), 655–663. http://dx.doi.org/10.1111/j.1600-0838.2008.00847.x Medline:18694431

Harvey, W.J., & Reid, G. (1997). Motor performance of children with attention-deficit hyperactivity disorder: A preliminary investigation. *Adapted Physical Activity Quarterly; APAQ, 14*, 189–202.

Harvey, W.J., Reid, G., Bloom, G.A., Staples, K., Grizenko, N., Mbekou, V., … Joober, R. (2009, Apr). Physical activity experiences of boys with and without ADHD. *Adapted Physical Activity Quarterly, 26*(2), 131–150. Medline:19478346

Hay, J. (1992). Adequacy in and predilection for physical activity in children. *Clinical Journal of Sport Medicine, 2*(3), 192–201. http://dx.doi.org/10.1097/00042752-199207000-00007

Hay, J., & Missiuna, C. (1998). Motor proficiency in children reporting low levels of participation in physical activity. *Canadian Journal of Occupational Therapy, 65*(2), 64–71. http://dx.doi.org/10.1177/000841749806500203

Henderson, S.E., Sugden, D.A., & Barnett, A.L. (2007). *Movement Assessment Battery for Children-2 examiner's manual.* London, England: Harcourt Assessment.

Janssen, I., & LeBlanc, A.G. (2010). Systematic review of the health benefits of physical activity and fitness in school-aged children and youth. *International Journal of Behavioral Nutrition and Physical Activity, 7*(1), 40. http://dx.doi. org/10.1186/1479-5868-7-40 Medline:20459784

Kanioglou, A. (2006). Estimation of physical abilities in children with developmental coordination disorder. *Studies in Physical Culture and Tourism, 13*(2), 25–32.

Katzmarzyk, P.T., Church, T.S., & Blair, S.N. (2004, May 24). Cardiorespiratory fitness attenuates the effects of the metabolic syndrome on all-cause and cardiovascular disease mortality in men. *Archives of Internal Medicine, 164*(10), 1092–1097. http://dx.doi.org/10.1001/archinte.164.10.1092 Medline:15159266

Kaufman, A.S., & Kaufman, N.L. (2004). *Kaufman Brief Intelligence Test* (2nd ed.). Bloomington, MN: Pearson.

Kaufman, L.B., & Schilling, D.L. (2007, Apr). Implementation of a strength training program for a 5-year-old child with poor body awareness and developmental coordination disorder. *Physical Therapy, 87*(4), 455–467. http://dx.doi.org/10.2522/ptj.20060170 Medline:17374632

Kimm, S.Y., Glynn, N.W., Obarzanek, E., Kriska, A.M., Daniels, S.R., Barton, B.A., & Liu, K. (2005, Jul 23–29). Relation between the changes in physical activity and body-mass index during adolescence: A multicentre longitudinal study. *Lancet, 366*(9482), 301–307. http://dx.doi.org/10.1016/S0140-6736(05)66837-7 Medline:16039332

Kinra, S., Nelder, R.P., & Lewendon, G.J. (2000, Jun). Deprivation and childhood obesity: A cross sectional study of 20,973 children in Plymouth, United Kingdom. *Journal of Epidemiology and Community Health, 54*(6), 456–460. http://dx.doi.org/10.1136/jech.54.6.456 Medline:10818122

Léger, L.A., & Lambert, J. (1982). A maximal multistage 20-m shuttle run test to predict $VO_{2\,max}$. *European Journal of Applied Physiology and Occupational Physiology, 49*(1), 1–12. http://dx.doi.org/10.1007/BF00428958 Medline:7201922

Li, Y.C., Wu, S.K., Cairney, J., & Hsieh, C.Y. (2011, Nov-Dec). Motor coordination and health-related physical fitness of children with developmental coordination disorder: A three-year follow-up study. *Research in Developmental Disabilities, 32*(6), 2993–3002. http://dx.doi. org/10.1016/j.ridd.2011.04.009 Medline:21632207

Maggio, A.B.R., Aggoun, Y., Marchand, L.M., Martin, X.E., Herrmann, F., Beghetti, M., & Farpour-Lambert, N.J. (2008, Apr). Associations among obesity, blood pressure, and left ventricular mass. *Journal of Pediatrics, 152*(4), 489–493. http://dx.doi.org/10.1016/j.jpeds.2007.10.042 Medline:18346502

Mandich, A.D., Polatajko, H.J., & Rodger, S. (2003, Nov). Rites of passage: Understanding participation of children with developmental coordination disorder. *Human Movement Science, 22*(4-5), 583–595. http://dx.doi. org/10.1016/j.humov.2003.09.011 Medline:14624835

Marcovecchio, M., Mohn, A., & Chiarelli, F. (2005, Oct). Type 2 diabetes mellitus in children and adolescents. *Journal of Endocrinological Investigation,* *28*(11), 853–863. http://dx.doi.org/10.1007/BF03347581 Medline:16370570

Mata, E., Ruiz, L.M., & Hay, J.A. (2007). Motor competence and aerobic fitness in Spanish secondary school children. *Acta Kinesiologiae Universitatis Tartuensis, 12*(Suppl), 89–90.

McNeill, A.M., Rosamond, W.D., Girman, C.J., Golden, S.H., Schmidt, M.I., East, H.E., ... Heiss, G. (2005, Feb). The metabolic syndrome and 11-year risk of incident cardiovascular disease in the atherosclerosis risk in communities study. *Diabetes Care, 28*(2), 385–390. http://dx.doi.org/10.2337/diacare.28.2.385 Medline:15677797

Nuñez, C., Kovera, A.J., Pietrobelli, A., Heshka, S., Horlick, M., Kehayias, J.J., ... Heymsfield, S.B. (1999, May). Body composition in children and adults by air displacement plethysmography. *European Journal of Clinical Nutrition,* *53*(5), 382–387. http://dx.doi.org/10.1038/sj.ejcn.1600735 Medline:10369494

O'Beirne, C., Larkin, D., & Cable, L. (1994). Coordination problems and anaerobic performance in children. *Adapted Physical Activity Quarterly; APAQ, 11,* 141–149.

Osika, W., Montgomery, S.M., & Longitudinal Birth Cohort Study. (2008, Aug 12). Physical control and coordination in childhood and adult obesity: Longitudinal Birth Cohort Study. *British Medical Journal* (Clinical research ed.), *337*(3), a699. http://dx.doi.org/10.1136/bmj.a699 Medline:18698093

Perez-Pastor, E.M., Metcalf, B.S., Hosking, J., Jeffery, A.N., Voss, L.D., & Wilkin, T.J. (2009, Jul). Assortative weight gain in mother–daughter and father–son pairs: An emerging source of childhood obesity. Longitudinal study of trios (EarlyBird 43). *International Journal of Obesity, 33*(7), 727–735. http://dx.doi.org/10.1038/ijo.2009.76 Medline:19434065

Poulsen, A.A., Ziviani, J.M., & Cuskelly, M. (2006, Dec). General self-concept and life satisfaction for boys with differing levels of physical coordination: The role of goal orientations and leisure participation. *Human Movement Science, 25*(6), 839–860. http://dx.doi.org/10.1016/j.humov.2006.05.003 Medline:16859792

Poulsen, A.A., Ziviani, J.M., & Cuskelly, M. (2007a, Jul). Perceived freedom in leisure and physical co-ordination ability: Impact on out-of-school activity participation and life satisfaction. *Child: Care, Health and Development, 33*(4), 432–440. http://dx.doi.org/10.1111/j.1365-2214.2007.00730.x Medline:17584399

Poulsen, A.A., Ziviani, J.M., & Cuskelly, M. (2008). Leisure time physical activity energy expenditure in boys with developmental coordination disorder: The role of peer relations self-concept perceptions. *Occupational Therapy Journal of Research: Occupation, Participation and Health, 28*(1), 30–41. http://dx.doi.org/10.3928/15394492-20080101-05

Poulsen, A.A., Ziviani, J.M., Cuskelly, M., & Smith, R. (2007b, Jul-Aug). Boys with developmental coordination disorder: Loneliness and team sports participation. *American Journal of Occupational Therapy., 61*(4), 451–462. http://dx.doi.org/10.5014/ajot.61.4.451 Medline:17685178

Powell, L.M., Han, E., & Chaloupka, F.J. (2010, Jun). Economic contextual factors, food consumption, and obesity among U.S. adolescents. *Journal of Nutrition, 140*(6), 1175–1180. http://dx.doi.org/10.3945/jn.109.111526 Medline:20392882

Rivilis, I., Hay, J., Cairney, J., Klentrou, P., Liu, J., & Faught, B.E. (2011, May). Physical activity and fitness in children with developmental coordination disorder: A systematic review. *Research in Developmental Disabilities, 32*(3), 894–910. http://dx.doi.org/10.1016/j.ridd.2011.01.017 Medline:21310588

Rowland, T. (1996). *Developmental exercise physiology*. Champaign, IL: Human Kinetics.

Schott, N., Alof, V., Hultsch, D., & Meermann, D. (2007, Dec). Physical fitness in children with developmental coordination disorder. *Research Quarterly for Exercise and Sport, 78*(5), 438–450. http://dx.doi.org/10.1080/02701367.2007. 10599444 Medline:18274216

Shields, M. (2006, Aug). Overweight and obesity among children and youth. *Health Reports, 17*(3), 27–42. Medline:16981484

Silman, A., Cairney, J., Hay, J., Klentrou, P., & Faught, B.E. (2011, Jun). Role of physical activity and perceived adequacy on peak aerobic power in children with developmental coordination disorder. *Human Movement Science, 30*(3), 672–681. http://dx.doi.org/10.1016/j.humov.2010.08.005 Medline:21414676

Skinner, R.A., & Piek, J.P. (2001, Mar). Psychosocial implications of poor motor coordination in children and adolescents. *Human Movement Science, 20*(1-2), 73–94. http://dx.doi.org/10.1016/S0167-9457(01)00029-X Medline:11471399

Sorof, J., & Daniels, S. (2002, Oct). Obesity hypertension in children: A problem of epidemic proportions. *Hypertension, 40*(4), 441–447. http:// dx.doi.org/10.1161/01.HYP.0000032940.33466.12 Medline:12364344

Stodden, D.F., Goodway, J.D., Langendorfer, S.J., Roberton, M., Rudisill, M.E., Garcia, C., & Garcia, L.E. (2008). A developmental perspective on the role of motor skill competence in physical activity: An emergent relationship. *Quest, 60*(2), 290–306. http://dx.doi.org/10.1080/00336297.2008.10483582

Taylor, S.J., Whincup, P.H., Hindmarsh, P.C., Lampe, F., Odoki, K., & Cook, D.G. (2001, Jan). Performance of a new pubertal self-assessment questionnaire: A preliminary study. *Paediatric and Perinatal Epidemiology, 15*(1), 88–94. http:// dx.doi.org/10.1046/j.1365-3016.2001.00317.x Medline:11237120

Tremblay, M.S., Shields, M., Laviolette, M., Craig, C.L., Janssen, I., & Connor Gorber, S. (2010, Mar). Fitness of Canadian children and youth: Results from the 2007–2009 Canadian Health Measures Survey. *Health Reports, 21*(1), 7–20. Medline:20426223

Tsiotra, G.D., Flouris, A.D., Koutedakis, Y., Faught, B.E., Nevill, A.M., Lane, A.M., & Skenteris, N. (2006, Jul). A comparison of developmental coordination disorder prevalence rates in Canadian and Greek children.

Journal of Adolescent Health, 39(1), 125–127. http://dx.doi.org/10.1016/j.
jadohealth.2005.07.011 Medline:16781974

Tsiotra, G.D., Nevill, A.M., Lane, A.M., & Koutedakis, Y. (2009). Perceptions
of physical competence, motor competence, and participation in organized
sport: Their interrelationships in young children. *Research Quarterly in Sport
and Exercise, 58*(1), 21, 186–195.

Ulrich, B.D. (1987). Perceptions of physical competence, motor competence,
and participation in organized sport: Their interrelationships in young
children. *Research Quarterly for Exercise and Sport, 58*(1), 57–67. http://
dx.doi.org/10.1080/02701367.1987.10605421

Visser, J. (2007). Subtypes and co-morbidities. In R.H. Geuze (Ed.),
Developmental coordination disorder: A review of current approaches
(pp. 83–100). Marseille, France: Solal.

Visser, J., Geuze, R.H., & Kalverboer, A.F. (1998). The relationship between physical growth, level of activity and the development of motor skills in adolescence:
Differences between children with DCD and controls. *Human Movement Science,
17*(4-5), 573–608. http://dx.doi.org/10.1016/S0167-9457(98)00014-1

Wahi, G., LeBlanc, P.J., Hay, J.A., Faught, B.E., O'Leary, D., & Cairney, J. (2011,
Nov-Dec). Metabolic syndrome in children with and without developmental
coordination disorder. *Research in Developmental Disabilities, 32*(6), 2785–2789.
http://dx.doi.org/10.1016/j.ridd.2011.05.030 Medline:21708447

Wall, A.E. (2004). The developmental skill-learning gap hypothesis: Implications
for children with movement difficulties. *Adapted Physical Activity Quarterly;
APAQ, 21*(3), 197–218.

Wei, M., Kampert, J.B., Barlow, C.E., Nichaman, M.Z., Gibbons, L.W.,
Paffenbarger, R.S., Jr., & Blair, S.N. (1999, Oct 27). Relationship between low
cardiorespiratory fitness and mortality in normal-weight, overweight, and
obese men. *Journal of the American Medical Association, 282*(16), 1547–1553.
http://dx.doi.org/10.1001/jama.282.16.1547 Medline:10546694

Williams, H.G., Pfeiffer, K.A., O'Neill, J.R., Dowda, M., McIver, K.L., Brown,
W.H., & Pate, R.R. (2008, Jun). Motor skill performance and physical
activity in preschool children. *Obesity 16*(6), 1421–1426. http://dx.doi.
org/10.1038/oby.2008.214 Medline:18388895

Wrotniak, B.H., Epstein, L.H., Dorn, J.M., Jones, K.E., & Kondilis, V.A. (2006,
Dec). The relationship between motor proficiency and physical activity
in children. *Pediatrics, 118*(6), e1758–e1765. http://dx.doi.org/10.1542/
peds.2006-0742 Medline:17142498

Wu, S.K., Lin, H.H., Li, Y.C., Tsai, C.L., & Cairney, J. (2010, Mar-Apr).
Cardiopulmonary fitness and endurance in children with developmental
coordination disorder. *Research in Developmental Disabilities, 31*(2), 345–349.
http://dx.doi.org/10.1016/j.ridd.2009.09.018 Medline:19913384

4 Psychosocial and Behavioural Difficulties in Children with Developmental Coordination Disorder

JAN P. PIEK AND DANIELA RIGOLI

Introduction

The area of developmental psychopathology has been extensively researched over the last decade, and an area that has been of particular interest has been that of comorbidity or co-occurrence of disorders. Rutter and Sroufe (2000) argued that this was one of the major research challenges of the future. Despite this, there remains one disorder that has lacked the research attention given to other developmental disorders, namely, a disorder characterizing those children who have what has been termed "minor motor deficits," referred to in the DSM-V as developmental coordination disorder (DCD).

Research has now identified social, emotional, and behavioural difficulties often co-occurring with DCD, although these are not defining features. In fact, it has been argued that the deficits of children with DCD are more pervasive than the current definition implies and that the criteria that define DCD do not provide a complete picture of these children's underachievement and, consequently, are misleading (Wisdom, Dyck, Piek, Hay, & Hallmayer, 2007). Gillberg and Kadesjö (2003) have noted that few psychiatrists are aware of the motor and perceptual difficulties that often coexist with childhood neuropsychiatric disorders, and many child neurologists pay little attention to the behavioural and emotional difficulties shown by many of their "clumsy" patients.

Fox and Lent (1996) highlighted how professionals may dismiss motor difficulties as transient and unimportant. It is plausible that these misunderstandings stem partly from the widely held assumption that children would "grow out of" clumsiness, a belief that has been challenged by a number of longitudinal studies showing that these difficulties do in fact persist (e.g., Cantell, Ahonen, & Smyth, 1994; Losse et al., 1991). It is important that studies have now also revealed that motor skill impairment may be a significant risk factor for poor psychosocial outcome such as anxiety in childhood and adolescence (Sigurdsson, Van Os, & Fombonne, 2002; Skinner & Piek, 2001). Even more concerning are our findings suggesting that preschool-age children at risk of DCD demonstrate significantly higher anxious-depressive symptoms compared with their peers who do not have difficulty in the motor domain (Piek et al., 2008). Other studies have also shown the high co-occurrence of other developmental conditions such as attention deficit hyperactivity disorder (ADHD) with motor difficulties (Kaplan, Dewey, Crawford, & Wilson, 2001; Kaplan, Wilson, Dewey, & Crawford, 1998). In the case of developmental disorders (including DCD), it has been argued that co-occurrence is the rule rather than the exception (Kaplan et al., 1998), and that there needs to be a much clearer focus on DCD in child psychiatry and neurology in both research and clinical practice (Gillberg & Kadesjö, 2003).

Self-Worth, Self-Perceptions, and Social Functioning

Links between poor motor coordination and poor social or emotional outcome were identified as early as the 1930s. However, these links were based primarily on intuition and clinical experience rather than systematic research (Shaffer et al., 1985). In the 1990s, researchers identified a relationship between motor competence and children's understanding of themselves. Cratty (1994) suggested that children with motor coordination difficulties are likely to have poor self-perceptions and experience negative social feedback due to difficulties faced in the classroom (e.g., writing) as well as difficulties with playing games, which can subsequently result in lowered self-esteem.

Many terms can be found in the literature to describe the concept of "self," which has been found in the psychological literature for over a century since the work of William James (1908). There is a lack of consistency in defining terms such as *self- concept, self-esteem, self-worth,* and *self-efficacy* (Byrne, 1996). Self-esteem is often used interchangeably with self-worth and self-respect and is considered a value judgment of attributes and limitations (Gallahue & Ozmun, 1998). An awareness of one's attributes and limitations without placing a value on these is generally referred to as self-concept, self-perception, or self-awareness (Hattie, 1992).

Children with poor coordination have been found to rate both their general self-worth and their perceptions of their own abilities, especially concerning their athletic competence, as lower than their peers' (Losse et al., 1991). More disturbing is the evidence that children with DCD also rate their perceptions in such areas as academic achievement, physical appearance, and social acceptance as lower than their peers' (Cantell et al., 1994; O'Dwyer, 1987; Rose, Larkin, & Berger, 1997; Skinner & Piek, 2001). That is, although these children were considered as having "only a minor motor disability," many aspects of their academic and social life appear to be affected. We (Miyahara & Piek, 2006) carried out a meta-analysis on studies that measured the self-esteem or self-worth of children and adolescents with major and minor motor disability, such as, DCD, cerebral palsy (CP), spina bifida. Our findings were quite surprising in that the self-worth of children with major physical disabilities such as CP or spina bifida was identified as higher than for children with minor physical disability such as DCD. We suggested that because many of these children did not have a clinical diagnosis, their disability was not understood or accepted, and may be misinterpreted as something else, such as an intellectual or behavioural problem.

Chen and Cohn (2003) note how the self-systems (i.e., self-perceptions, self-worth) of children with DCD are important in understanding their participation in physical or social activities. For example, Engel-Yeger and Hanna Kasis (2010) noted relationships among DCD, perceived self-efficacy, and participation preference, not only in physical activities but also in other recreational, skill-based, and self-improvement activities. As noted in an earlier study, in Western society sporting competence and the ability to play games with friends is highly regarded (Piek, Dworcan, Barrett, & Coleman, 2000). As a result, competence in such areas is important for social status and peer acceptance (Cratty, 1994; Mandich, Polatajko, & Rodger, 2003). Using Harter's (1987) competence motivation theory, we highlighted how children with DCD may often try to avoid participation in such activities for fear of failure and/or peer criticism (Skinner & Piek, 2001). This is supported by the findings of Poulsen, Ziviani, and Cuskelly (2006) that children with DCD are less likely to participate in team sports or physical play with others. Poulsen and colleagues (Poulsen, Johnson, & Ziviani, 2011; Poulsen, Ziviani, & Cuskelly, 2006) assessed participation using a 7-day diary and a 12-month leisure survey, which measured structured versus unstructured, individual versus social, and physical activity versus non-physical activity participation. Children with DCD were less likely to participate in structured as well as unstructured social physical activities, but they were more likely to participate in structured nonphysical social activities compared with the non-DCD group (Poulsen et al., 2006). (The issue of participation is described more fully in Chapter 2 in this volume.)

By avoiding participation, children therefore limit their opportunity to practise skills and to participate in a social environment (Cermak, Gubbay, & Larkin, 2002; Skinner & Piek, 2001; Smyth & Anderson, 2000). A number of studies have linked poor coordination to social concerns, such as difficulties with peer relations (Losse et al., 1991). We found that children and adolescents with DCD perceived less social support compared to children without motor deficits (Skinner & Piek, 2001).

Social interaction requires accurate detection, coding, and processing of perceptual information in order for the child to understand the emotional information provided by other children (Piek & Dyck, 2004). If children with DCD have poor visuospatial organization, this may affect their ability to accurately perceive their peers' emotional cues such as facial expressions and body language and may therefore affect their social performance. Limited research has investigated this relationship. However, we assessed whether children with motor coordination difficulties have problems across a range of empathic abilities and demonstrated that children with motor coordination difficulties are less competent than typically developing peers in their ability to respond to facial emotion cues (Cummins, Piek, & Dyck, 2005). This delay was specific to recognizing facial expressions of emotions and not the ability to recognize vocal cues or understand emotions (i.e., auditory perception and tasks with larger verbal component). Our results provide important information when considered in the context of the child's social functioning (e.g., poor peer relations).

Regardless of the causes of these social skills deficits, by avoiding participation, children limit their opportunity to practise skills and to participate in a social environment, creating a vicious circle (Skinner & Piek, 2001). This highlights the importance of motor skill competency and its relationship to a child's self-perceptions, social functioning, and ultimately, emotional adjustment.

Mental Health Outcomes

A child's evaluation of him -or herself is closely linked with mental health outcomes such as anxiety and depression (Harter, 1987), the most common mental health concerns found in Australian children and adolescents (Prior, Sanson, Smart, & Oberklaid, 1999), and significant problems worldwide (Boyd, Kostanski, Gullone, Ollendick, & Shek, 2000). Cole and colleagues (Cole, 1991; Cole, Martin, & Powers, 1997) developed a competency-based model of depression in young people arguing that low self-perceived competence may be a risk factor for a number of problems including depression. In a longitudinal study of children 8–12 years of age, Burt, Obradović, Long, and Masten (2008) found that social competence in childhood was inversely related to internalizing symptoms in adolescence suggesting a causal relationship between the two. Given the significant negative self-perceptions and social difficulties experienced by those with coordination difficulties, emotional outcomes such as anxiety and depression seem likely.

DCD and Anxiety

Accumulating evidence suggests a strong association between poor coordination and anxiety difficulties in children (Schoemaker & Kalverboer, 1994; Sigurdsson et al., 2002; Skinner & Piek, 2001). We investigated perceived competence, social support, self-worth, and anxiety in children and adolescents with and without DCD (Skinner & Piek, 2001) and found that DCD groups (children ages 8–10 years and adolescents ages 12–14 years) perceived themselves as less competent in various domains and had less social support than those without DCD. The two DCD groups also demonstrated lower global self-worth and higher anxiety compared with the controls. We suggested that negative self-concept and social support may mediate the relationship between motor skill difficulties and anxiety.

Recently, research not only compared the levels of anxiety between children with a clinical diagnosis of DCD and those from a typically developing sample but also examined the profile of anxiety in children with DCD (Pratt & Hill, 2011). Children with DCD were found to experience higher levels of anxiety overall, as well as increased difficulties in the areas of panic or agoraphobia, social phobia, and obsessive compulsive disorder compared to the typically developing group. In terms of panic-related symptoms, it was hypothesized that if a child struggles on a daily basis to undertake tasks that appear to be relatively easy for peers (e.g., participating in team games), he or she may become anxious for current and future situations, feel a sense of panic when such tasks need to be attempted, and possibly avoid the situations. This avoidance may subsequently hinder the child from developing the appropriate strategies needed when tasks are challenging. Approximately 30% of the DCD sample experienced social phobia at a clinical level, and similarly, it was suggested that reduced participation in activities may negatively affect the development of social skills, resulting in a lack of social skills and the perception of poor quality friendships. It was also noted that rather than having social deficits per se, children with DCD may also experience social exclusion due to their difficulties, thus possibly resulting in social anxiety in these cases. Ultimately, Pratt and Hill (2011) argued, it is easy to visualize how having a motor disorder may lead to anxiety-related difficulties, although the mechanism for this link is yet unknown.

Extending on our earlier findings of an association between poor motor ability and anxiety symptoms in school-age children, we revealed a concerning finding that preschool children (as young as 3 and 4 years of age) at risk of DCD demonstrate significantly higher anxious-depressed scores compared with children who perform better in the motor domain (Piek, Bradbury, Elsley, & Tate, 2008). Therefore, it appears that motor difficulties also place a child at risk for increased depressive symptoms, which is not surprising given the high overlap between depressive disorders and anxiety disorders (Angold, Costello, & Erkanli, 1999).

DCD and Depression

Concerns are growing in the Australian community regarding the increase in depression prevalence rates, particularly in children and adolescents (Lancaster, 2003).

Before the 1970s, depression in young people was believed to be extremely rare (Klein, Dougherty, & Olino, 2005). However, it is now recognized that depressive symptoms and depressive disorders represent significant mental health concerns in the child and adolescent population (Compas, Connor-Smith, & Jaser, 2004; Roberts, 1999). In an Australia-wide survey, 3% of children and adolescents between the ages of 4 and 17 years met the criteria for depressive disorder (Sawyer et al., 2001). Furthermore, only a small number of these were reported to have received professional help.

These data are concerning because child and youth depression is associated with significant impairment in psychosocial functioning such as with family and peer relationships and in academic performance (Dumas, 1998; Hammen, Rudolph, Weisz, Rao, & Burge, 1999; Sheeber,

Hops, & Davis, 2001). Evidence also indicates continued impairment and a high risk of reoccurrence after the recovery of a depressive episode (Weissman et al., 1999). Depression is also a leading risk factor for youth suicide and may also be a risk factor for the development of other disorders such as substance abuse (Stanard, 2000). Ultimately, the increase in depression prevalence rates in children and adolescents highlights the importance of intervening with preventative efforts. This requires a comprehensive understanding of the associated risk factors.

Little research has examined the relationship between DCD and depression. However, given the considerable physical, social, and emotional effects of DCD, as well as Cole and colleagues' (Cole, 1991; Cole, Martin, & Powers, 1997) model of depression, which argues that low self-perceived competence may be a risk factor for a number of difficulties, including depression, one could assume that depression is a possible outcome for children with DCD. Several studies have identified a relationship between poor motor ability and increased depressive symptomatology (e.g., Francis & Piek, 2003; Piek et al., 2008; Piek et al., 2007a). Using Harter's model of the relationship between self-worth and depression, these studies investigated the unique impact of self-perceived competencies and perceived social support on the level of self-worth and depressive symptoms in children (ages 7 to 11 years) with and without DCD (Francis & Piek, 2003). Children with DCD perceived significantly higher levels of depressive symptomatology compared to children without coordination difficulties. Furthermore, although self-worth did not act as a mediator for depression for the children with DCD, perceived athletic competence was shown to have a direct impact on depression, emphasizing the importance of motor ability on emotional functioning. This sheds some light on the possible causal mechanisms associated with poor motor coordination and co-occurring internalizing disorders.

Causal Factors

It is evident from the preceding sections that internalizing problems and motor skill difficulties co-occur, although the causal links remain unclear (Cairney, Veldhuizen, & Szatmari, 2010). Kristensen and Torgersen (2008) found that children with social anxiety disorder (SAD) demonstrated overall poorer performance on a standardized motor test compared to a control group but were no different when compared to children with ADHD. The SAD group also demonstrated poorer performance on the static and dynamic balance subscale compared to the "other disorder" group comprising mostly children with other anxiety disorders. Similarly, maternal report revealed increased gross motor skill difficulties in children with SAD compared with the control and "other disorder" group, but not when compared to the ADHD group. Consequently, given that fear of scrutiny by others is characteristic of SAD, Kristensen and Torgersen (2008) suggest that the genuine skill deficits experienced by these children may contribute to their increased anxiety and stress, although it is important to note that the cross-sectional nature of such studies cannot establish causality. For example, it is also possible that social anxiety leads to motor difficulties. However, in their study, Kristensen and Torgersen (2008) found only a modest relationship ($r = .23$) between state anxiety and balance, which occurred only in boys with SAD.

Are motor and internalizing difficulties both a result of the same etiology? For example, past research has associated cerebellar dysfunction with DCD (e.g., Lundy-Ekman, Ivry, Keele, & Woollacott, 1991; Piek & Skinner, 1999), and a recent study using transcranial magnetic stimulation has also linked the cerebellum with emotion regulation (Schutter & van Honk, 2009). Also, given that recent evidence has implicated birth complications such as oxygen perfusion difficulties as a possible cause of DCD (Pearsall-Jones et al., 2008; Pearsall-Jones et al., 2009), is it possible that this can affect both motor function and emotional function? Studies suggesting a specific relationship between balance dysfunction and anxiety disorders have also proposed a possible neurological underpinning; furthermore, the neurological hypothesis predicts that either of the disorders may benefit from treatment of the other. For example, Bart and colleagues (2009) found that young children with balance difficulties reported increased anxiety compared with control children. In addition, children with balance difficulties demonstrated reduced anxiety following a 12-week balance treatment compared to the waiting list group. However, this study did not appear to assess other motor skill areas such as fine motor skills. Therefore, it is unclear whether a specific relationship exists. It is also possible that other factors, such as the positive attitude of the therapists, played a role in the balance treatment effects on anxiety (Bart et al., 2009).

Cairney and colleagues (2010) suggested that such a neurodevelopmental explanation is conceivable in some cases, but it is equally possible that motor coordination difficulties themselves cause internalizing problems. They named the environmental stress hypothesis as an alternative explanation for the relationship between motor skill deficits (primary stressor) and internalizing difficulties. Specifically, as children with coordination difficulties are exposed to the cascade of negative psychosocial consequences described earlier (secondary stressors), they develop negative self-appraisals, which may then lead to anxiety and/or depression. If this is the case, then negative self-perceptions may play an important role in the relationship between coordination deficits and the associated emotional difficulties. Evidence is emerging that environmental explanations are indeed a plausible alternative.

Recent studies using a monozygotic (MZ) differences design found that child and adolescent MZ twins with DCD demonstrated significantly higher levels of anxious (Pearsall-Jones et al., 2011) and depressive (Piek et al., 2007) symptomatology compared to their co-twins without DCD. We argued that the MZ differences design allows the effects of genes and shared environmental factors to be controlled, and thus the finding of a significant difference in the level of anxious and depressive symptomatology between the twins may be attributed to the effects of unique environmental factors often associated with children with motor coordination difficulties.

We have also recently used structural equation modelling to investigate possible pathways linking motor ability and emotional status (Wilson, Piek, & Kane, 2013). We examined the mediating role of social skills on the relationship between motor ability and internalizing symptoms in a sample of 475 young children between 4 and 7 years of age. Using the Bruininks-Oseretsky Test of Motor Proficiency (second edition, short form) to measure motor ability (Bruininks & Bruininks, 2005), the Social Skills Rating System Teacher Report version to measure social skills (Gresham & Elliott, 1990), and the Strengths and Difficulties Questionnaire Teacher Report (Goodman, 1997) to measure internalizing symptoms, we found that the best model fit was the mediation model, with social skills mediating the relationship between motor ability and internalizing symptoms, and without a direct pathway between motor ability and internalizing symptoms. However, given that this model accounted for only 5% of the variance in internalizing symptoms, clearly many other factors are important in this relationship.

We have found a much stronger model accounting for 45% of the variance in a sample of 93 adolescents from 12 to 16 years of age (Rigoli, Piek, & Kane, 2012). This model argued that self-perceptions mediate the relationship between motor ability and internalizing symptoms. The Movement Assessment Battery for Children-Second Edition (MABC-2; Henderson, Sugden, & Barnett, 2007) provided two indicators of motor skills: specifically, Aiming and Catching, and Balance; Manual Dexterity was not correlated with the outcome measures. The Mood and Feelings Questionnaire (Costello & Angold, 1988), measuring depressive symptomatology, and the Spence Children's Anxiety Scale (Spence, 1997) assessing anxiety symptoms, provided two indicators of emotional functioning; the Self-Description Questionnaire-II (Marsh, 1992) provided six indicators for self-perceived competence. Structural equation modelling revealed that the relationship between motor skills and emotional functioning in adolescents from a normal population may be understood in terms of a mechanism in which motor skills have an indirect impact on emotional outcomes through various self-perception domains.

Neither of these studies, however, was longitudinal. Longitudinal designs for assessment of temporal associations, along with correlation, are the necessary conditions to establish causality. Several longitudinal studies have identified the relationship between early motor difficulties and later anxiety and depressive symptoms at school age and adolescence (Piek, Barrett, Smith, Rigoli, & Gasson, 2010; Shaffer et al., 1985; Sigurdsson et al., 2002). For example, Shaffer et al. found that the relationship between motor skills at 7 years of age and anxiety difficulties at age 17 remained even when anxiety had not been present at the earlier age. Consequently, it is plausible that motor skill and emotional difficulties do not necessarily coexist and thus may be better explained through environmental rather than biological factors. However, stronger evidence is needed to further elucidate whether a causal relationship exists (Piek et al., 2010).

Summary

Despite the ongoing debate on causality, research highlighting the relationship between motor deficits and emotional difficulties has important implications for the provision of services for these children, regardless of whether these difficulties are seen as primary (i.e., coexisting) or secondary and possibly consequential (Green, Baird, & Sugden, 2006). However, Missiuna (2003), in her commentary response to Sigurdsson, Van Os, and Fombonne (2002), noted that although the large-scale longitudinal study reinforced the findings of other studies demonstrating that having impaired motor skills is a risk factor for later anxiety difficulties, these studies are open to the potential criticism that learning or attentional difficulties may have contributed to the results.

In fact, Missiuna, Moll, King, King, and Law (2006), in another paper, argued that the recognition of DCD appears to be complicated by the fact that it often coexists with other disorders such as ADHD. Furthermore, although DCD and ADHD have a high rate of co-occurrence, it is noted that DCD is frequently mistaken for ADHD because children appear disruptive as they knock things over, drop and bump into things, have trouble sitting still due to difficulty maintaining a stable posture, and avoid work by seeking attention from the teacher and interfering with other children (Missiuna, Moll, King, King, & Law, 2006). It is important to distinguish which specific disorders are likely to affect psychosocial functioning, as this would have important implications for therapeutic approaches.

Behavioural Difficulties in DCD and Co-occurring Disorders

As with other developmental disorders, DCD is a heterogeneous disorder, and children with DCD display difficulties across a variety of domains. Extensive research in this area over the last decade has identified links between DCD and behavioural disorders such as ADHD (e.g., Dewey, Kaplan, Crawford, & Wilson, 2002; Lingam et al., 2010; Pitcher et al., 2003), oppositional defiant disorder (e.g., Kooistra, Crawford, Dewey, Cantell, & Kaplan, 2005; Martin, Piek, Baynam, Levy, & Hay, 2010), and autism spectrum disorders (e.g., Dyck, Piek, Hay, & Hallmayer, 2007; Reiersen, Constantino, & Todd, 2008). Cognitive deficits such as reading and spelling deficits (e.g., Dewey et al., 2002; Lingam et al., 2010; Martin et al., 2010) and executive functioning deficits (e.g., Alloway & Temple, 2007; Michel, Roethlisberger, Neuenschwander, & Roebers, 2011; Piek, Dyck, Francis, & Conwell, 2007) have also been identified in children with DCD. (Neurocognitive deficits are discussed more fully in Chapter 5 in this volume.)

In reviewing the literature on co-occurring difficulties with DCD it is worth considering McConaughy and Achenbach's (1994) comments in relation to the differences associated with the use of clinical versus community samples. They discussed "Berkson's bias" (Berkson, 1946, in McConaughy & Achenbach, 1994), which describes how comorbidity rates are generally higher when using a clinic sample rather than a non-referred or general population. McConaughy and Achenbach argued that in order to get valid estimates of comorbidity "it is necessary to assess large samples that are representative of the general population, unaffected by referral bias" (p. 1143). Given that the referral rate for

DCD is generally very low, most studies investigating comorbidity have been based on samples from the general population.

DCD and Attention Deficit Hyperactivity Disorder

ADHD is one of the most commonly diagnosed childhood psychiatric disorders and is characterized by inattention, impulsivity, and increased levels of motor activity termed "hyperactivity" (Treuting & Hinshaw, 2001). These symptoms must be persistent, developmentally inappropriate, and maladaptive (American Psychiatric Association, 2000). According to the DSM-IV, there are two distinct clusters of symptoms, inattention and hyperactivity-impulsivity, and either of these must be present to meet a diagnosis of ADHD. On the basis of these symptoms the DSM-IV has identified three subtypes of ADHD: ADHD-Predominantly Inattentive type, ADHD-Predominantly Hyperactive-Impulsive type, and ADHD-Combined type, which has both inattentive and hyperactive-impulsive symptoms (APA, 2000).

Although findings have been inconsistent, research has linked ADHD with poor self-esteem and low self-perceptions (Dumas & Pelletier, 1999; Slomkowski, Klein, & Mannuzza, 1995). However, other studies have found inflated self-esteem despite the academic, behaviour, and social difficulties children with ADHD experience (Hoza, Pelham, Milich, Pillow, & McBride, 1993). Studies involving clinic-based samples have found that children and adolescents with ADHD are more likely to be diagnosed with mood disorders, including depression and anxiety, compared with other children (Angold & Costello, 1993; Biederman, Newcorn, & Sprich, 1991). Studies employing community-based samples have also linked ADHD, like DCD, with elevated depressive symptomatology if not a diagnosis of depression per se (Jensen, Shervette, Xenakis, & Richters, 1993; Kitchens, Rosen, & Braaten, 1999; LeBlanc & Morin, 2004). It should be noted, however, that these studies did not control for possible comorbid motor difficulties, which as we have shown are also associated with psychosocial and emotional difficulties.

As with DCD, the relationship between ADHD and depression in children is unclear. It has been noted that there are two most likely possibilities (Cytryn & McKnew, 1996). First, a biological explanation argues that ADHD and depression share a parallel etiology and coexist in the same child as autonomous entities (Cytryn & McKnew, 1996). This view is supported by genetic studies showing common familial vulnerabilities when examining the relationship between ADHD and mood disorders (Faraone & Biederman, 1997). An alternative environmental explanation argues that depression is a secondary disorder in response to the difficulties these children face, for example, family conflict, school failure, and lack of friends (Cytryn & McKnew, 1996). It has been suggested that the difficulties associated with ADHD, such as repeated failure at school and inadequate social support, increase a child's vulnerability to depression. Schmidt, Stark, Carlson, and Anthony (1998) suggested that given the behavioural, social, and academic difficulties characteristic of ADHD, depression represents a "logical secondary disorder to a primary manifestation of ADHD" (Schmidt et al., p. 677).

The latter explanation has been supported in one of our recent studies using an MZ differences design (Piek et al., 2007b), as child and adolescent MZ twins with ADHD were found to have significantly higher levels of depressive symptomatology when compared with their identical twin without ADHD. This suggests that the unique environmental factors described above for children with ADHD may account for their increased depressive symptomatology. The other important finding in this study was that when each of the disorders was controlled (i.e., no children with ADHD had DCD and vice versa), the subjects each displayed significantly higher levels of depressive symptoms compared with their identical twins without the disorder. This finding demonstrates that the unique features of each disorder are responsible for the depressive symptoms, and one cannot explain the other.

Our research has found a strong link between ADHD and motor difficulties, where approximately 50% of children with ADHD also experience motor difficulties severe enough to be diagnosed as DCD (Piek, Pitcher, & Hay, 1999; Pitcher, Piek, & Hay, 2003). Studies employing community samples have shown that diagnoses of ADHD and DCD often co-occur (Kadesjö & Gillberg, 1999), and children diagnosed with DCD often have attentional difficulties (Kaplan et al., 1998; Lingam et al., 2010).

Kaplan and colleagues (1998; 2001) suggested that the increased overlap between ADHD, DCD, and other developmental difficulties may be explained by a generalized heterogeneous, neurodevelopmental condition (viz., atypical brain development) resulting from a disruption to the early development of the brain (Kaplan et al., 1998). Consequently, comorbidities are the rule rather than the exception due to the proposed diffuse nature and extent of the underlying neurological abnormality (Kaplan et al., 1998). However, we have challenged this idea by stating that a general neurodevelopmental delay does not explain the way in which developmental disorders mostly appear as recognizable syndromes and also tend to be comorbid with particular disorders (Piek et al., 2004). For example, ADHD has been associated with conduct disorder and oppositional defiant disorder (Biederman et al., 1991; Jensen, Martin, & Cantwell, 1997), yet we have found that DCD is associated with oppositional defiant disorder but not conduct disorder (Martin et al., 2010). Furthermore, our studies using an MZ co-twin control design have suggested different etiologies for DCD and ADHD, with evidence suggesting that birth difficulties resulting in oxygen perfusion problems may be an explanation for DCD but not necessarily for ADHD (Pearsall-Jones et al., 2008; Pearsall-Jones et al., 2009).

Gillberg (1995) described the overlap between coordination and attention difficulties as deficits in attention, motor control, and perception, commonly referred to as DAMP, and provided indirect evidence that the combination of DCD and ADHD has an interactive negative effect on various measures, among them academic outcome (Gillberg, 1983; Kadesjö & Gillberg, 1999). Follow-up studies involving children with DAMP ages 6 to 7, 10, 13, 16, and 22 years have demonstrated that children with both DCD and ADHD are at greater risk for poorer long-term outcomes such as neurodevelopmental problems, psychiatric difficulties, personality disorders, school dysfunction, and reading, writing, and language difficulties compared to a comparison group without ADHD or DCD (e.g., Hellgren, Gillberg, Bågenholm, & Gillberg, 1994). Other studies have also revealed a worse outcome in individuals with comorbid ADHD and DCD compared to ADHD-only and DCD-only groups (Kadesjö & Gillberg, 1999, 2001).

According to Gillberg (1995) the main psychiatric difficulties experienced by children with DAMP are depression, conduct disorder, and autistic features. This view was supported by our findings (Piek et al., 2007b), as we noted that children and adolescents with a diagnosis of both ADHD and DCD (equivalent to DAMP) had higher levels of depressive symptoms compared with children who had only ADHD or DCD. Furthermore, Reiersen, Constantino, and Todd (2008) found that children and adolescents with ADHD who also had parent-reported motor difficulties were more likely to have autistic symptoms. Our results also revealed that children with DCD were not clearly differentiated from those with autistic disorder (AD), as each group performed poorly on motor ability, emotional understanding, and theory-of-mind tasks (Wisdom et al., 2007). Children in the AD group, however, had more severe difficulties in these areas. When a more able AD group was compared to the DCD group, no significant differences in these scores were found. This suggests that the AD and DCD groups differed more in severity than in kind and highlights the need for further research to determine whether DCD is part of the autistic spectrum.

DCD and Autism Spectrum Disorders

While the DSM-IV (APA, 2000) ruled out a diagnosis of DCD if the child has a pervasive developmental disorder such as AD or Asperger's syndrome, we found that children with AD could perform in the normal range of motor ability, a finding that suggests that poor motor ability is not a necessary impairment in AD (Dyck et al., 2007). Furthermore, poor motor ability was associated with greater qualitative impairments in social interaction in children with AD. What appeared to be a buffer to autism symptoms was a better Performance IQ score, which includes the measure of visuospatial organization. It was when both motor ability and Performance IQ scores were low that the symptoms were most severe. We argued that this correlation indicated that these children were more likely to have DCD as well as AD (Piek & Dyck, 2004) because poor visuospatial organization as measured by Performance IQ is a key deficit in DCD (e.g., Wilson & McKenzie, 1998).

The possibility that children can be diagnosed with both DCD and a pervasive developmental disorder has been raised by others. For example, Sugden, Chambers, and Utley (2006) in the Leeds Consensus Statement argued that children with autistic spectrum disorder should not be excluded from a DCD diagnosis if they meet the other criteria for this disorder. This view was adopted by Lingam, Hunt, Golding, Jongmans, and Emond (2009) in their examination of the prevalence of DCD in the United Kingdom. Furthermore, the advisory subgroup examining the DCD criteria for the Neurodevelopmental Disorder Work Group of the American Psychiatric Association recommended that a diagnosis of pervasive developmental disorders be removed as an exclusion criterion for criterion C on the DSM-V, a recommendation that has since been accepted (American Psychiatric Association, 2013). This will create a new challenge for researchers in terms of identifying which social and emotional deficits are associated with the autism symptoms and which with the motor deficits in these children.

Treatment

Research examining the associated psychological and behavioural implications of DCD has highlighted the importance of early identification and intervention. For example, our finding that adolescents with DCD demonstrated lower self-esteem, self-perceptions, and higher anxiety not only when compared to their coordinated peers but also in comparison to younger children with DCD emphasizes the need for early intervention in order to deter the later detrimental outcomes (Skinner & Piek, 2001).

Given the emotional and behavioural difficulties that have been found in children with DCD, it is crucial that these possible outcomes be carefully considered in the assessment and intervention phase of children referred for their motor difficulties. Furthermore, coordination difficulties should be assessed for those children referred for behavioural difficulties such as ADHD or emotional difficulties such as anxiety, and appropriate interventions should be determined. This is particularly important when one considers the poorer outcomes identified in children with combined motor and behavioural difficulties than in those with only motor or behavioural difficulties (e.g., Hellgren et al., 1994; Piek et al., 2007b). Furthermore, it is also likely that these children will have different responses to treatment.

Engel-Yeger and Hanna Kasis (2010) argue that it is important to move beyond impairment-based interventions focusing solely on improving motor abilities. Given the evidence that self-perceptions and social skills may affect a child's emotional well-being, it is crucial to focus on these aspects of development in children with DCD and through ecological interventions encourage the children's participation in school, home, and community (Engel-Yeger & Hanna Kasis, 2010). One suggestion is to incorporate a leisure counseling component that guides the child with DCD towards activities that are likely to enhance a sense of competency (Hay & Missiuna, 1998). In fact, Dewey and Wilson (2001) state that the training of motor skills makes sense only when it also involves an increase in self-esteem and motivation to participate in physical activities of daily living. Given the strong link between self-perceived competence and symptoms of depression and anxiety, particularly social anxiety (e.g., Smári, Pétursdóttir, & Porsteinsdóttir, 2001), an intervention aimed at improving a sense of competency may prove vital in preventing and treating possible emotional difficulties in children with DCD.

Since both motor competence and self-concept of children are deemed two important components of their overall well-being, a recent study investigated the effectiveness of motor intervention, a self-concept-enhancing intervention, versus psychomotor intervention in improving motor competency and self-concept in children with DCD ages 7 to 9 years (Peens, Pienaar, & Nienaber, 2008). The motor-based intervention contributed to the biggest change in children's motor ability; however, for this group neither the children's self-concept nor anxiety significantly improved. The self-concept of the psychologically based treatment group improved significantly after intervention, as did their levels of anxiety, but with no significant improvement in their motor proficiency. On the other hand, the psychomotor group, integrating both the motor and psychological programs, demonstrated the biggest improvement in total self-concept, an improvement in anxiety (although nonsignificant) as well as a significant improvement in motor proficiency. The control group in this study demonstrated the same self-concept after the intervention period but reported a nonsignificant increase in anxiety. Consequently, it is argued that both motor skills and self-concept should be addressed in treatment in order achieve optimal benefits for children with DCD (Peens et al., 2008). However, further research is needed, particularly since the authors of this study reported a confounding result in terms of the contribution of the motor-based program, because an improvement in the motor proficiency of the control group was found. A small sample size, the influence of maturity, and possible exposure to the program (as it was sometimes conducted during school break times in non-secluded areas) were given by the authors as plausible explanations for this (Peens et al., 2008).

It is also evident that the social functioning of children with DCD is of great concern, given the research findings revealing increased withdrawal, isolation, and peer rejection in these children. Chen and Cohn (2003) argued that a primary goal of intervention should involve increasing the social participation of children with DCD. They suggested that when evaluating and formulating interventions for the child, clinicians should take a "top-down" approach, whereby participation in activities at home, community, and school needs to be examined, as do cultural and gender factors and the impact of values, perceptions, and attitudes of the child and significant others. Finally, clinicians should also assess the underlying motor, cognitive, social, and communication skills influencing participation within these contexts.

Poulsen, Ziviani, and Cuskelly (2008) highlighted the importance of considering self-perceptions when planning intervention. In their study, self-perceptions of peer relationships were found to mediate the relationship between physical coordination ability and low energy expenditure patterns in boys. Furthermore, the researchers note the value of a client-centred approach that includes children's perceptions of their own abilities. This approach, it is argued, may not only result in better therapeutic results but also enhance the emotional and physical well-being of these children (Engel-Yeger & Hanna Kasis, 2010).

Activity preference is also an important consideration related to interventions for increasing social participation. Given that children with DCD may value and seek different activities compared to children without DCD, this may affect their social participation and should be considered when setting goals during intervention (Chen & Cohn, 2003). Chen and Cohn (2003) note that an investigation into the child's daily activities will help researchers understand their patterns of social participation and may also provide a picture of the social participation options for the child, thus guiding intervention.

Throughout intervention, professionals may provide activity counseling to develop well-organized schedules that facilitate social participation (Chen & Cohn, 2003). Poulsen et al. (2008) recommended that therapists also encourage social interactions in clubs involving individual or dyadic physical activities that de-emphasize social evaluation and social comparisons and also provide a socially supportive framework. For example, structured leisure activities such as choir or band may provide protective advantages for those with DCD. Their research identified a meaningful group of boys with motor difficulties who participated in group activities such as band, choir, or chess club and did not demonstrate low self-concept perceptions in any domain. Conversely, a group of boys were identified with motor difficulties and low levels of participation in unstructured group physical activities (e.g., ball games on the street) who demonstrated low peer relations self-concept. Low participation in such informal activities may not buffer low perceived social competence for some children with DCD.

It may also be important not to disregard the value of team sports for some children with DCD. For example, it has been suggested that boys with DCD who remain active in team sports may experience lower feelings of loneliness, with increased feelings of social satisfaction, regardless of their level of coordination ability (Poulsen, Ziviani, Cuskelly, & Smith, 2007). Consequently, team sports may provide psychosocial benefits for some children. Therefore, the child, parents, and professionals should identify the best fit for the child by considering the child's characteristics, the team sport's characteristics, and the environments that will best support the child's mental health (Poulsen et al., 2007). Furthermore, social skills training has been recommend for nonphysical social activities (e.g., talking to classmates at school), as it may encourage a child's participation in these situations (Chen & Cohn, 2003).

Finally, given the increasing findings suggesting possible depression and anxiety in children with DCD, it is noted that some children will require a treatment component focusing directly on these symptoms. For example, panic-related anxiety has been reported in some children with DCD (Pratt & Hill, 2011), and thus these children may benefit from psychological treatment focusing on the panic symptoms.

Future Work

Despite increasing interest in motor difficulties such as DCD, research investigating the social and emotional consequences for children with DCD remains quite sparse. Recent studies using complex modelling have started to shed some light on the relationships between motor difficulties and psychosocial factors such as self-perceptions, social skills, and internalizing disorders such as anxiety and depression (e.g., Rigoli et al., 2012; Wilson et al., 2012). Other techniques such as behavioural analyses using twin studies (e.g., Pearsall-Jones et al., 2011; Piek et al., 2007b) and, more recently, brain-imaging techniques (e.g., Schutter & van Honk, 2009) have also assisted researchers in understanding these relationships. However, few longitudinal studies have been carried out, and these are needed to enhance researchers' understanding of the etiology of DCD and its link with disorders such as anxiety and depression. This research will assist professionals in understanding when and how to address these difficulties. Evidence to date suggests that psychosocial difficulties are present in children with DCD as early as 3 and 4 years of age. If this is the case then early intervention and treatment is clearly needed.

This leads to the other area in need of research. Methodologically sound studies examining different interventions for children with DCD are needed. We are gaining a much clearer understanding of the difficulties faced by these children, but how to address these remains a key issue for future research.

Conclusion

Children with DCD face many challenges as a result of their poor motor ability. However, if children are mentally healthy, they have a much better chance of functioning normally through appropriate social interactions. It is clear from the evidence presented that many children with DCD may experience negative psychosocial outcomes, and this is a major concern, particularly if children are being affected at an early age. Therefore, as researchers and clinicians in the field of DCD we must be aware that the child's physical health and mental health must both be considered if he or she is to lead a healthy and happy life.

REFERENCES

Alloway, T.P., & Temple, K.J. (2007). A comparison of working memory skills and learning in children with developmental coordination disorder and moderate learning difficulties. *Applied Cognitive Psychology, 21*(4), 473–487. http://dx.doi.org/10.1002/acp.1284

American Psychiatric Association. (2000). *Diagnostic and statistical manual of mental disorders* (4th ed.). Washington, DC: Author.

American Psychiatric Association. (2013). *Diagnostic and statistical manual of mental disorders* (5th ed.). Arlington, VA: American Psychiatric Publishing.

Angold, A., & Costello, E.J. (1993, Dec). Depressive comorbidity in children and adolescents: Empirical, theoretical, and methodological issues. *American Journal of Psychiatry, 150*(12), 1779–1791. Medline:8238631

Angold, A., Costello, E.J., & Erkanli, A. (1999, Jan). Comorbidity. *Journal of Child Psychology and Psychiatry, and Allied Disciplines, 40*(1), 57–87. http://dx.doi.org/10.1111/1469-7610.00424 Medline:10102726

Bart, O., Bar-Haim, Y., Weizman, E., Levin, M., Sadeh, A., & Mintz, M. (2009, May-Jun). Balance treatment ameliorates anxiety and increases self-esteem in children with comorbid anxiety and balance disorder. *Research in Developmental Disabilities, 30*(3), 486–495. http://dx.doi.org/10.1016/j.ridd.2008.07.008 Medline:18775641

Biederman, J., Newcorn, J., & Sprich, S. (1991, May). Comorbidity of attention deficit hyperactivity disorder with conduct, depressive, anxiety, and other disorders. *American Journal of Psychiatry, 148*(5), 564–577. Medline:2018156

Boyd, C.P., Kostanski, M., Gullone, E., Ollendick, T.H., & Shek, D.T. (2000, Dec). Prevalence of anxiety and depression in Australian adolescents: Comparisons with worldwide data. *Journal of Genetic Psychology, 161*(4), 479–492. http://dx.doi.org/10.1080/00221320009596726 Medline:11117103

Bruininks, R., & Bruininks, B. (2005). *Bruininks-Oseretsky Test of Motor Proficiency* [Manual](2nd ed.). Minneapolis, MN: NCS Pearson.

Burt, K.B., Obradović, J., Long, J.D., & Masten, A.S. (2008, Mar-Apr). The interplay of social competence and psychopathology over 20 years: Testing transactional and cascade models. *Child Development,*

79(2), 359–374. http://dx.doi.org/10.1111/j.1467-8624.2007.01130.x
Medline:18366428

Byrne, B.M. (1996). *Measuring self-concept across the life span: Issues and instrumentation*. Washington, DC: American Psychological Association.

Cairney, J., Veldhuizen, S., & Szatmari, P. (2010, Jul). Motor coordination and emotional-behavioral problems in children. *Current Opinion in Psychiatry, 23*(4), 324–329. http://dx.doi.org/10.1097/YCO.0b013e32833aa0aa Medline:20520549

Cantell, M.H., Ahonen, T.P., & Smyth, M.M. (1994). Clumsiness in adolescence: Education, motor, and social outcomes of motor delay detected at 5 years. *Adapted Physical Activity Quarterly; APAQ, 11*, 115–129.

Cermak, S.A., Gubbay, S.S., & Larkin, D. (2002). What is developmental coordination disorder? In S.A. Cermak (Ed.), *Developmental coordination disorder* (pp. 2–22). New York, NY: Delmar Thomson Learning.

Chen, H.F., & Cohn, E.S. (2003). Social participation for children with developmental coordination disorder: Conceptual, evaluation and intervention considerations. *Physical & Occupational Therapy in Pediatrics, 23*(4), 61–78. Medline:14750309

Cole, D.A. (1991, May). Preliminary support for a competency-based model of depression in children. *Journal of Abnormal Psychology, 100*(2), 181–190. http://dx.doi.org/10.1037/0021-843X.100.2.181 Medline:2040769

Cole, D.A., Martin, J.M., & Powers, B. (1997, Jul). A competency-based model of child depression: A longitudinal study of peer, parent, teacher, and self-evaluations. *Journal of Child Psychology and Psychiatry, and Allied Disciplines, 38*(5), 505–514. http://dx.doi.org/10.1111/j.1469-7610.1997.tb01537.x Medline:9255694

Compas, B.E., Connor-Smith, J., & Jaser, S.S. (2004, Mar). Temperament, stress reactivity, and coping: Implications for depression in childhood and adolescence. *Journal of Clinical Child and Adolescent Psychology, 33*(1), 21–31. http://dx.doi.org/10.1207/S15374424JCCP3301_3 Medline:15028538

Costello, E.J., & Angold, A. (1988, Nov). Scales to assess child and adolescent depression: Checklists, screens, and nets. *Journal of the American Academy of Child and Adolescent Psychiatry, 27*(6), 726–737. http://dx.doi.org/10.1097/00004583-198811000-00011 Medline:3058677

Cratty, B.J. (1994). *Clumsy child syndromes: Descriptions, evaluation, and remediation*. Philadelphia, PA: Harwood Academic Publishers.

Cummins, A., Piek, J.P., & Dyck, M.J. (2005, Jul). Motor coordination, empathy, and social behaviour in school-aged children. *Developmental Medicine and Child Neurology, 47*(7), 437–442. http://dx.doi.org/10.1017/S001216220500085X Medline:15991862

Cytryn, L., & McKnew, D.H. (1996). *Growing up sad: Childhood depression and its treatment*. New York, NY: W.W. Norton.

Dewey, D., Kaplan, B.J., Crawford, S.G., & Wilson, B.N. (2002, Dec). Developmental coordination disorder: Associated problems in attention, learning, and psychosocial adjustment. *Human Movement Science, 21*(5-6), 905–918. http://dx.doi.org/10.1016/S0167-9457(02)00163-X Medline:12620725

Dewey, D., & Wilson, B.N. (2001). Developmental coordination disorder: What is it? *Physical & Occupational Therapy in Pediatrics, 20*(2-3), 5–27. http://dx.doi.org/10.1080/J006v20n02_02 Medline:11345511

Dumas, M.C. (1998). The risk of social intervention problems among adolescents with ADHD. *Education & Treatment of Children, 21*, 447–460.

Dumas, D., & Pelletier, L. (1999, Jan-Feb). A study of self-perception in hyperactive children. *American Journal of Maternal Child Nursing, 24*(1), 12–19. http://dx.doi.org/10.1097/00005721-199901000-00004 Medline:10036902

Dyck, M.J., Piek, J.P., Hay, D.A., & Hallmayer, J.F. (2007). The relationship between symptoms and abilities in autism. *Journal of Developmental and Physical Disabilities, 19*(3), 251–261. http://dx.doi.org/10.1007/s10882-007-9055-7

Engel-Yeger, B., & Hanna Kasis, A. (2010, Sep). The relationship between developmental co-ordination disorders, child's perceived self-efficacy and preference to participate in daily activities. *Child: Care, Health and Development, 36*(5), 670–677. http://dx.doi.org/10.1111/j.1365-2214.2010.01073.x Medline:20412146

Faraone, S.V., & Biederman, J. (1997, Sep). Do attention deficit hyperactivity disorder and major depression share familial risk factors? *Journal of Nervous and Mental Disease, 185*(9), 533–541. http://dx.doi.org/10.1097/00005053-199709000-00001 Medline:9307614

Fox, A.M., & Lent, B. (1996, Oct). Clumsy children: Primer on developmental coordination disorder. *Canadian Family Physician Médecin de Famille Canadien, 42*, 1965–1971. Medline:8894243

Francis, M., & Piek, J. (2003). The effects of perceived social support and self-worth on depressive symptomatology in children with and without developmental coordination disorder (DCD). Proceedings of the 38th APS Annual Conference, Melbourne The Australian Psychological Society, 70–74. 2–5 October 2003.

Gallahue, D.L., & Ozmun, J.C. (1998). *Understanding motor development: Infants, children, adolescents, adults* (4th ed.). Boston, MA: McGraw Hill.

Gillberg, C. (1983, Jul). Perceptual, motor and attentional deficits in Swedish primary school children: Some child psychiatric aspects. *Journal of Child Psychology and Psychiatry, and Allied Disciplines, 24*(3), 377–403. http://dx.doi.org/10.1111/j.1469-7610.1983.tb00116.x Medline:6874784

130   Jan P. Piek and Daniela Rigoli

Gillberg, C. (1995). Deficits in attention, motor control and perception, and other syndromes attributed to minimal brain dysfunction. In C. Gillberg (Ed.), *Clinical child neuropsychiatry* (pp. 138–172). New York, NY: Cambridge University Press. http://dx.doi.org/10.1017/CBO9780511570094.009

Gillberg, C., & Kadesjö, B. (2003). Why bother about clumsiness? The implications of having developmental coordination disorder (DCD). *Neural Plasticity, 10*(1-2), 59–68. http://dx.doi.org/10.1155/NP.2003.59 Medline:14640308

Goodman, R. (1997, Jul). The Strengths and Difficulties Questionnaire: A research note. *Journal of Child Psychology and Psychiatry, and Allied Disciplines, 38*(5), 581–586. http://dx.doi.org/10.1111/j.1469-7610.1997.tb01545.x Medline:9255702

Green, D., Baird, G., & Sugden, D. (2006, Nov). A pilot study of psychopathology in developmental coordination disorder. *Child: Care, Health and Development, 32*(6), 741–750. http://dx.doi.org/10.1111/j.1365-2214.2006.00684.x Medline:17018049

Gresham, F.M., & Elliott, S.N. (1990). *Social Skills Rating System manual.* Circle Pines, MN: American Guidance Service.

Hammen, C., Rudolph, K., Weisz, J., Rao, U., & Burge, D. (1999, Jan). The context of depression in clinic-referred youth: Neglected areas in treatment. *Journal of the American Academy of Child and Adolescent Psychiatry, 38*(1), 64–71. http://dx.doi.org/10.1097/00004583-199901000-00021 Medline:9893418

Harter, S. (1987). The determinants and mediational role of global self-worth in children. In N. Eisenberg (Ed.), *Contemporary topics in developmental psychology* (pp. 219–242). New York, NY: John Wiley & Sons.

Hattie, J.A. (1992). *Self-Concept.* Hillsdale, New Jersey: Laurence Erlbaum.

Hay, J., & Missiuna, C. (1998). Motor proficiency in children reporting low levels of participation in physical activity. *Canadian Journal of Occupational Therapy, 65*(2), 64–71. http://dx.doi.org/10.1177/000841749806500203

Hellgren, L., Gillberg, I.C., Bågenholm, A., & Gillberg, C. (1994, Oct). Children with deficits in attention, motor control and perception (DAMP) almost grown up: Psychiatric and personality disorders at age 16 years. *Journal of Child Psychology and Psychiatry, and Allied Disciplines, 35*(7), 1255–1271. http://dx.doi.org/10.1111/j.1469-7610.1994.tb01233.x Medline:7806609

Henderson, S.E., Sugden, D.A., & Barnett, A. (2007). *Movement Assessment Battery for Children* (2nd ed.). London, England: Psychological Corporation.

Hoza, B., Pelham, W.E., Milich, R., Pillow, D., & McBride, K. (1993, Jun). The self-perceptions and attributions of attention deficit hyperactivity disordered and nonreferred boys. *Journal of Abnormal Child Psychology, 21*(3), 271–286. http://dx.doi.org/10.1007/BF00917535 Medline:8335764

James, W. (1908). *Textbook of psychology.* London, England: MacMillan.

Jensen, P.S., Martin, D., & Cantwell, D.P. (1997, Aug). Comorbidity in ADHD: Implications for research, practice, and DSM-V. *Journal of the American Academy of Child and Adolescent Psychiatry, 36*(8), 1065–1079. http://dx.doi. org/10.1097/00004583-199708000-00014 Medline:9256586

Jensen, P.S., Shervette, R.E., III, Xenakis, S.N., & Richters, J. (1993, Aug). Anxiety and depressive disorders in attention deficit disorder with hyperactivity: New findings. *American Journal of Psychiatry, 150*(8), 1203–1209. Medline:8328565

Kadesjö, B., & Gillberg, C. (1999, Jul). Developmental coordination disorder in Swedish 7-year-old children. *Journal of the American Academy of Child and Adolescent Psychiatry, 38*(7), 820–828. http://dx.doi.org/10.1097/00004583-199907000-00011 Medline:10405499

Kadesjö, B., & Gillberg, C. (2001, May). The comorbidity of ADHD in the general population of Swedish school-age children. *Journal of Child Psychology and Psychiatry, and Allied Disciplines, 42*(4), 487–492. http:// dx.doi.org/10.1111/1469-7610.00742 Medline:11383964

Kaplan, B.J., Dewey, D.M., Crawford, S.G., & Wilson, B.N. (2001, Nov-Dec). The term comorbidity is of questionable value in reference to developmental disorders: Data and theory. *Journal of Learning Disabilities, 34*(6), 555–565. http://dx.doi.org/10.1177/002221940103400608 Medline:15503570

Kaplan, B.J., Wilson, B.N., Dewey, D., & Crawford, S.G. (1998). DCD may not be a discrete disorder. *Human Movement Science, 17*(4-5), 471–490. http:// dx.doi.org/10.1016/S0167-9457(98)00010-4

Kitchens, S.A., Rosen, L.A., & Braaten, E.B. (1999). Differences in anger, aggression, depression, and anxiety between ADHD and non-ADHD children. *Journal of Attention Disorders, 3*(2), 77–83. http://dx.doi. org/10.1177/108705479900300201

Klein, D.N., Dougherty, L.R., & Olino, T.M. (2005, Sep). Toward guidelines for evidence-based assessment of depression in children and adolescents. *Journal of Clinical Child and Adolescent Psychology, 34*(3), 412–432. http:// dx.doi.org/10.1207/s15374424jccp3403_3 Medline:16026212

Kooistra, L., Crawford, S., Dewey, D., Cantell, M., & Kaplan, B.J. (2005, May-Jun). Motor correlates of ADHD: Contribution of reading disability and oppositional defiant disorder. *Journal of Learning Disabilities, 38*(3), 195–206. http://dx.doi.org/10.1177/00222194050380030201 Medline:15940958

Kristensen, H., & Torgersen, S. (2008, Mar). Is social anxiety disorder in childhood associated with developmental deficit/delay? *European Child & Adolescent Psychiatry, 17*(2), 99–107. http://dx.doi.org/10.1007/s00787-007-0642-z Medline:17849080

Lancaster, S. (Ed.). (2003). *Psychologists working with depression across the lifecycle.* Sydney, Australia: Australian Academic Press.

LeBlanc, N., & Morin, D. (2004, Apr-Jun). Depressive symptoms and associated factors in children with attention deficit hyperactivity disorder. *Journal of Child and Adolescent Psychiatric Nursing, 17*(2), 49–55. http://dx.doi.org/10.1111/j.1744-6171.2004.00049.x Medline:15366311

Lingam, R., Golding, J., Jongmans, M.J., Hunt, L.P., Ellis, M., & Emond, A. (2010, Nov). The association between developmental coordination disorder and other developmental traits. *Pediatrics, 126*(5), e1109–e1118. http://dx.doi.org/10.1542/peds.2009-2789 Medline:20956425

Lingam, R., Hunt, L., Golding, J., Jongmans, M., & Emond, A. (2009, Apr). Prevalence of developmental coordination disorder using the DSM-IV at 7 years of age: A UK population-based study. *Pediatrics, 123*(4), e693–e700. http://dx.doi.org/10.1542/peds.2008-1770 Medline:19336359

Losse, A., Henderson, S.E., Elliman, D., Hall, D., Knight, E., & Jongmans, M. (1991, Jan). Clumsiness in children – Do they grow out of it? A 10-year follow-up study. *Developmental Medicine and Child Neurology, 33*(1), 55–68. http://dx.doi.org/10.1111/j.1469-8749.1991.tb14785.x Medline:1704864

Lundy-Ekman, L., Ivry, R., Keele, S., & Woollacott, M. (1991, Fall). Timing and force control deficits in clumsy children. *Journal of Cognitive Neuroscience, 3*(4), 367–376. http://dx.doi.org/10.1162/jocn.1991.3.4.367 Medline:23967817

Mandich, A.D., Polatajko, H.J., & Rodger, S. (2003, Nov). Rites of passage: Understanding participation of children with developmental coordination disorder. *Human Movement Science, 22*(4-5), 583–595. http://dx.doi.org/10.1016/j.humov.2003.09.011 Medline:14624835

Marsh, H.W. (1992). *Self-Description Questionnaire II: Manual.* Sydney, Australia: University of Western Sydney, SELF Research Centre.

Martin, N.C., Piek, J., Baynam, G., Levy, F., & Hay, D. (2010, Oct). An examination of the relationship between movement problems and four common developmental disorders. *Human Movement Science, 29*(5), 799–808. http://dx.doi.org/10.1016/j.humov.2009.09.005 Medline:19944472

McConaughy, S.H., & Achenbach, T.M. (1994, Sep). Comorbidity of empirically based syndromes in matched general population and clinical samples. *Journal of Child Psychology and Psychiatry, and Allied Disciplines, 35*(6), 1141–1157. http://dx.doi.org/10.1111/j.1469-7610.1994.tb01814.x Medline:7995848

Michel, E., Roethlisberger, M., Neuenschwander, R., & Roebers, C.M. (2011). Development of cognitive skills in children with motor coordination impairments at 12-month follow-up. *Child Neuropsychology, 17*(2), 151–172. http://dx.doi.org/10.1080/09297049.2010.525501 Medline:21271412

Missiuna, C. (2003, Feb). Childhood motor impairment is associated with male anxiety at 11 and 16 years. *Evidence-Based Mental Health, 6*(1), 18. http://dx.doi.org/10.1136/ebmh.6.1.18 Medline:12588824

Missiuna, C., Moll, S., King, G., King, S., & Law, M. (2006). "Missed and misunderstood": Children with coordination difficulties in the school system. *International Journal of Special Education, 21*(1), 53–67.

Miyahara, M., & Piek, J. (2006). Self-esteem of children and adolescents with physical disabilities: Quantitative evidence from meta-analysis. *Journal of Developmental and Physical Disabilities, 18*(3), 219–234. http://dx.doi. org/10.1007/s10882-006-9014-8

O'Dwyer, S. (1987). Characteristics of highly and poorly co-ordinated children. *Irish Journal of Psychology, 8*(1), 1–8. http://dx.doi.org/10.1080/03033910.198 7.10557687

Pearsall-Jones, J.G., Piek, J.P., Martin, N.C., Rigoli, D., Levy, F., & Hay, D.A. (2008). A monozygotic twin design to investigate etiological factors for DCD and ADHD. *Journal of Pediatric Neurology, 6*(3), 209–219.

Pearsall-Jones, J.G., Piek, J.P., Rigoli, D., Martin, N.C., & Levy, F. (2009, Aug). An investigation into etiological pathways of DCD and ADHD using a monozygotic twin design. *Twin Research and Human Genetics, 12*(4), 381–391. http://dx.doi.org/10.1375/twin.12.4.381 Medline:19653839

Pearsall-Jones, J.G., Piek, J.P., Rigoli, D., Neilson, C., Martin, N.C., & Levy, F. (2011). Motor disorder and anxious and depressive symptomatology: A monozygotic co-twin control approach. *Research in Developmental Disabilities.* http://dx.doi.org/10.1016/j.ridd.2011.01.042

Peens, A., Pienaar, A.E., & Nienaber, A.W. (2008, May). The effect of different intervention programmes on the self-concept and motor proficiency of 7- to 9-year-old children with DCD. *Child: Care, Health and Development, 34*(3), 316–328. http://dx.doi.org/10.1111/j.1365-2214.2007.00803.x Medline:18294260

Piek, J.P., Barrett, N.C., Smith, L.M., Rigoli, D., & Gasson, N. (2010, Oct). Do motor skills in infancy and early childhood predict anxious and depressive symptomatology at school age? *Human Movement Science, 29*(5), 777–786. http://dx.doi.org/10.1016/j.humov.2010.03.006 Medline:20650535

Piek, J.P., Bradbury, G.S., Elsley, S.C., & Tate, L. (2008). Motor coordination and social-emotional behaviour in preschool-aged children. *International Journal of Disability Development and Education, 55*(2), 143–151. http://dx.doi. org/10.1080/10349120802033592

Piek, J.P., Dworcan, M., Barrett, N.C., & Coleman, R. (2000). Determinants of self-worth in children with and without developmental coordination disorder. *International Journal of Disability Development and Education, 47*(3), 259–272. http://dx.doi.org/10.1080/713671115

Piek, J.P., & Dyck, M.J. (2004, Oct). Sensory-motor deficits in children with developmental coordination disorder, attention deficit hyperactivity disorder and autistic disorder. *Human Movement Science, 23*(3-4), 475–488. http://dx.doi.org/10.1016/j.humov.2004.08.019 Medline:15541530

Piek, J.P., Dyck, M.J., Francis, M., & Conwell, A. (2007a, Sep). Working memory, processing speed, and set-shifting in children with developmental coordination disorder and attention-deficit-hyperactivity disorder. *Developmental Medicine and Child Neurology, 49*(9), 678–683. http://dx.doi.org/10.1111/j.1469-8749.2007.00678.x Medline:17718824

Piek, J.P., Dyck, M.J., Nieman, A., Anderson, M., Hay, D., Smith, L.M., . . ., & Hallmayer, J. (2004, Dec). The relationship between motor coordination, executive functioning and attention in school aged children. *Archives of Clinical Neuropsychology, 19*(8), 1063–1076. http://dx.doi.org/10.1016/j.acn.2003.12.007 Medline:15533697

Piek, J.P., Pitcher, T.M., & Hay, D.A. (1999, Mar). Motor coordination and kinaesthesis in boys with attention deficit-hyperactivity disorder. *Developmental Medicine and Child Neurology, 41*(3), 159–165. http://dx.doi.org/10.1017/S0012162299000341 Medline:10210248

Piek, J.P., Rigoli, D., Pearsall-Jones, J.G., Martin, N.C., Hay, D.A., Bennett, K.S., & Levy, F. (2007b, Aug). Depressive symptomatology in child and adolescent twins with attention-deficit hyperactivity disorder and/or developmental coordination disorder. *Twin Research and Human Genetics, 10*(4), 587–596. http://dx.doi.org/10.1375/twin.10.4.587 Medline:17708700

Piek, J.P., & Skinner, R.A. (1999, May). Timing and force control during a sequential tapping task in children with and without motor coordination problems. *Journal of the International Neuropsychological Society, 5*(4), 320–329. http://dx.doi.org/10.1017/S1355617799544032 Medline:10349295

Pitcher, T.M., Piek, J.P., & Hay, D.A. (2003, Aug). Fine and gross motor ability in males with ADHD. *Developmental Medicine and Child Neurology, 45*(8), 525–535. http://dx.doi.org/10.1111/j.1469-8749.2003.tb00952.x Medline:12882531

Poulsen, A.A., Johnson, H., & Ziviani, J.M. (2011, Apr). Participation, self-concept and motor performance of boys with developmental coordination disorder: A classification and regression tree analysis approach. *Australian Occupational Therapy Journal, 58*(2), 95–102. http://dx.doi.org/10.1111/j.1440-1630.2010.00880.x Medline:21418232

Poulsen, A.A., Ziviani, J.M., & Cuskelly, M. (2006, Dec). General self-concept and life satisfaction for boys with differing levels of physical coordination: The role of goal orientations and leisure participation. *Human Movement Science, 25*(6), 839–860. http://dx.doi.org/10.1016/j.humov.2006.05.003 Medline:16859792

Poulsen, A.A., Ziviani, J.M., & Cuskelly, M. (2008). Leisure time physical activity energy expenditure in boys with developmental coordination disorder: The role of peer relations self-concept perceptions. *OTJR: Occupation, Participation and Health, 28*(1), 30–39. http://dx.doi.org/10.3928/15394492-20080101-05

Poulsen, A.A., Ziviani, J.M., Cuskelly, M., & Smith, R. (2007, Jul-Aug). Boys with developmental coordination disorder: Loneliness and team sports participation. *American Journal of Occupational Therapy., 61*(4), 451–462. http://dx.doi.org/10.5014/ajot.61.4.451 Medline:17685178

Pratt, M.L., & Hill, E.L. (2011, Jul-Aug). Anxiety profiles in children with and without developmental coordination disorder. *Research in Developmental Disabilities, 32*(4), 1253–1259. http://dx.doi.org/10.1016/j.ridd.2011.02.006 Medline:21377831

Prior, M., Sanson, A., Smart, D., & Oberklaid, F. (1999, May). Psychological disorders and their correlates in an Australian community sample of preadolescent children. *Journal of Child Psychology and Psychiatry, and Allied Disciplines, 40*(4), 563–580. http://dx.doi.org/10.1111/1469-7610.00474 Medline:10357163

Reiersen, A.M., Constantino, J.N., & Todd, R.D. (2008, Jun). Co-occurrence of motor problems and autistic symptoms in attention-deficit/hyperactivity disorder. *Journal of the American Academy of Child and Adolescent Psychiatry, 47*(6), 662–672. http://dx.doi.org/10.1097/CHI.0b013e31816bff88 Medline:18434922

Rigoli, D., Piek, J.P., & Kane, R. (2012, Apr). Motor coordination and psychosocial correlates in a normative adolescent sample. *Pediatrics, 129*(4), e892–e900. http://dx.doi.org/10.1542/peds.2011-1237 Medline:22451714

Roberts, C.M. (1999). The prevention of depression in children and adolescents. *Australian Psychologist, 34*(1), 49–57. http://dx.doi.org/10.1080/00050069908257425

Rose, B., Larkin, D., & Berger, B.G. (1997). Coordination and gender influences on the perceived competence of children. *Adapted Physical Activity Quarterly; APAQ, 14*, 210–221.

Rutter, M., & Sroufe, L.A. (2000, Summer). Developmental psychopathology: Concepts and challenges. *Development and Psychopathology, 12*(3), 265–296. http://dx.doi.org/10.1017/S0954579400003023 Medline:11014739

Sawyer, M.G., Arney, F.M., Baghurst, P.A., Clark, J.J., Graetz, B.W., Kosky, R.J., … Zubrick, S.R. (2001, Dec). The mental health of young people in Australia: Key findings from the child and adolescent component of the national survey of mental health and well-being. *Australian and New Zealand Journal of Psychiatry, 35*(6), 806–814. http://dx.doi.org/10.1046/j.1440-1614.2001.00964.x Medline:11990891

Schmidt, K.L., Stark, K.D., Carlson, C.L., & Anthony, B.J. (1998, Aug). Cognitive factors differentiating attention deficit-hyperactivity disorder

STAFF LIBRARY
SINGLETON HOSPITAL
TEL: 01792 205666 EXT: 35281

with and without a comorbid mood disorder. *Journal of Consulting and Clinical Psychology*, 66(4), 673–679. http://dx.doi.org/10.1037/0022-006X.66.4.673 Medline:9735585

Schoemaker, M., & Kalverboer, A. (1994). Social and affective problems of children who are clumsy: How early do they begin? *Adapted Physical Activity Quarterly; APAQ*, 11, 130–140.

Schutter, D.J.L.G., & van Honk, J. (2009, Mar). The cerebellum in emotion regulation: A repetitive transcranial magnetic stimulation study. *Cerebellum (London, England)*, 8(1), 28–34. http://dx.doi.org/10.1007/s12311-008-0056-6 Medline:18855096

Shaffer, D., Schonfeld, I., O'Connor, P.A., Stokman, C., Trautman, P., Shafer, S., & Ng, S. (1985, Apr). Neurological soft signs: Their relationship to psychiatric disorder and intelligence in childhood and adolescence. *Archives of General Psychiatry*, 42(4), 342–351. http://dx.doi.org/10.1001/archpsyc.1985.01790270028003 Medline:3977551

Sheeber, L., Hops, H., & Davis, B. (2001, Mar). Family processes in adolescent depression. *Clinical Child and Family Psychology Review*, 4(1), 19–35. http://dx.doi.org/10.1023/A:1009524626436 Medline:11388562

Sigurdsson, E., Van Os, J., & Fombonne, E. (2002, Jun). Are impaired childhood motor skills a risk factor for adolescent anxiety? Results from the 1958 U.K. birth cohort and the National Child Development Study. *American Journal of Psychiatry*, 159(6), 1044–1046. http://dx.doi.org/10.1176/appi.ajp.159.6.1044 Medline:12042195

Skinner, R.A., & Piek, J.P. (2001, Mar). Psychosocial implications of poor motor coordination in children and adolescents. *Human Movement Science*, 20(1-2), 73–94. http://dx.doi.org/10.1016/S0167-9457(01)00029-X Medline:11471399

Slomkowski, C., Klein, R.G., & Mannuzza, S. (1995, Jun). Is self-esteem an important outcome in hyperactive children? *Journal of Abnormal Child Psychology*, 23(3), 303–315. http://dx.doi.org/10.1007/BF01447559 Medline:7642839

Smári, J., Pétursdóttir, G., & Porsteinsdóttir, V. (2001, Apr). Social anxiety and depression in adolescents in relation to perceived competence and situational appraisal. *Journal of Adolescence*, 24(2), 199–207. http://dx.doi.org/10.1006/jado.2000.0338 Medline:11437480

Smyth, M.M., & Anderson, H.I. (2000). Coping with clumsiness in the school playground: Social and physical play in children with coordination impairments. *British Journal of Developmental Psychology*, 18(3), 389–413. http://dx.doi.org/10.1348/026151000165760

Spence, S.H. (1997, May). Structure of anxiety symptoms among children: A confirmatory factor-analytic study. *Journal of Abnormal Psychology*, 106(2), 280–297. http://dx.doi.org/10.1037/0021-843X.106.2.280 Medline:9131848

Stanard, R.P. (2000). Assessment and treatment of adolescent depression and suicidality. *Journal of Mental Health Counseling, 22,* 204–217.

Sugden, D.A., Chambers, M., & Utley, A. (2006). Leeds Consensus Statement. Retrieved 1 April 2011 from www.dcd-uk.org/consensus.html

Treuting, J.J., & Hinshaw, S.P. (2001, Feb). Depression and self-esteem in boys with attention-deficit/hyperactivity disorder: Associations with comorbid aggression and explanatory attributional mechanisms. *Journal of Abnormal Child Psychology, 29*(1), 23–39. http://dx.doi.org/10.1023/A:1005247412221 Medline:11316333

Weissman, M.M., Wolk, S., Goldstein, R.B., Moreau, D., Adams, P., Greenwald, S., ... Wickramaratne, P. (1999, May 12). Depressed adolescents grown up. *Journal of the American Medical Association, 281*(18), 1707–1713. http://dx.doi.org/10.1001/jama.281.18.1707 Medline:10328070

Wilson, A., Piek, J.P., & Kane, R. (2013). An investigation of the relationship between motor ability and internalising symptoms in pre-primary children: The mediating role of social skills. *Infant and Child Development, 22*(2), 151–164. http://dx.doi.org/10.1002/icd.1773

Wilson, P.H., & McKenzie, B.E. (1998, Sep). Information processing deficits associated with developmental coordination disorder: A meta-analysis of research findings. *Journal of Child Psychology and Psychiatry, and Allied Disciplines, 39*(6), 829–840. http://dx.doi.org/10.1017/S0021963098002765 Medline:9758192

Wisdom, S.N., Dyck, M.J., Piek, J.P., Hay, D., & Hallmayer, J. (2007, Apr). Can autism, language and coordination disorders be differentiated based on ability profiles? *European Child & Adolescent Psychiatry, 16*(3), 178–186. http://dx.doi.org/10.1007/s00787-006-0586-8 Medline:17136301

5 Neurocognitive Processing Deficits in Children with Developmental Coordination Disorder

PETER H. WILSON

This chapter examines the neurocognitive processing deficits that are common in children with developmental coordination disorder (DCD), focusing on issues of motor control and executive function. Taking an embodied approach, it is argued that the development of motor behaviour is constrained by maturational and experiential factors. Movement skills and underlying control processes emerge over a relatively protracted period of development and are viewed as being embedded within a broader neurocognitive system. One prominent account of DCD that is a focus of this chapter is the *internal modelling deficit* (IMD) account, perhaps better termed a deficit of predictive control. The chapter will trace the main lines of evidence that support this model and will then give particular focus to the development of online control in children. A mature system of online control can orchestrate movement corrections in-flight with minimal time lag (in many cases responding to visual and other perturbations in less than 100 ms). This remarkable feat can be achieved only to the extent that feedforward (or predictive) control is well developed and integrated seamlessly with real-time sensory feedback. This refined level of control is supported by maturation of neurocognitive networks involving fronto-parietal and parieto-cerebellar loops. More importantly, it is argued that the process of motor prediction must be constantly updated with maturation and experience as individual biomechanics change during physical growth and as other brain systems emerge. Of the latter, the chapter will describe trends in the development of spatial and executive control systems in children with and without DCD. The increasing level of neural coupling that occurs between anterior (viz., executive) and posterior (perceptual-motor) systems over childhood has important implications for learning and skill development. As the capacity of working memory, inhibitory control, and spatial attention expands, the child is able to organize more sophisticated actions over longer spatial and temporal scales. These changes, along with physical maturation, necessitate a reorganization of predictive control. Middle childhood marks a crucial period during which this occurs. Hence, the main objectives of this chapter are as follows: (1) to outline an embodied approach to the study of motor development and dysfunction in children; (2) to explain the importance of online control in the context of motor development, and the process of predictive control as a driver of developmental sophistication in movement; (3) to impress the view that impairments to predictive control may explain many of the motor skill issues we see in DCD; (4) to explore how the development of executive function (EF) may interact with motor control processes and examine the strong co-occurrence of impaired EF and predictive control in DCD; and (5) to highlight some fruitful areas for future investigation in this regard.

An Embodied Approach to the Development of Motor Control and Skill

Whereas traditional accounts of child development tend to break down different aspects of function (motor, cognitive, social, and affective) as though they were independent, few theorists today would question the view that behavioural development is multidetermined and its domains interactive (Deutsch & Newell, 2005). From an embodied perspective, cognitive control and motor control emerge from common biological bases and are sculpted by experience. Interactions among developing neural systems will, therefore, give rise to periodic alterations in the very nature of control.

It is not surprising that the development of motor control in children is not linear in progression. Rather, the nature of control appears to alter with the changing constraints of maturation and environment. In the case of reaching, young children between 4 and 6 years of age can freely initiate preplanned movements (i.e., a feedforward mode of control); this is shown by relatively smooth acceleration phases for reaching and late use of sensory feedback in the movement cycle (Chicoine, Lassonde, & Proteau, 1992). Most intriguing, this changes to earlier and greater use of sensory feedback in 7–8-year-olds (e.g., Chicoine et al., 1992) while functional skills continue to unfold. Later, at around 9–10 years, feedback and feedforward control become better integrated, with a resultant smoothing of reach trajectories and reduced end-point error (Bard, Hay, &

Fleury, 1990). This pattern of change has been described in numerous studies of reaching, but its neurocognitive basis is only now becoming apparent.

In the following sections, I describe key aspects of motor control in children with and without DCD, trends in the development of executive functions, and the changing relationship between motor and cognitive systems. First, using a computational model, I examine the neurocognitive basis of *rapid online control* (ROC), a system that uses predictive estimates of limb position to organize movement corrections in-flight, with minimal time lag. Second, I discuss trends in the development of ROC and describe converging data that suggest that a basic neurocognitive deficit in predictive control may explain many of the performance issues we see in children with DCD–also known as the IMD hypothesis mentioned above. Third, I examine associated neurocognitive deficits of executive function in DCD and consider the broader consequences of these impairments for development.

This review will raise some interesting hypotheses about possible interactions between developing motor and executive systems, shaping different modes of motor control and skill acquisition with age. A working assumption here is that with cortical maturation there is reciprocal development of motor, spatial, and executive systems that support goal-directed behaviour. A key transition occurs in middle childhood (around 7–8 years of age) when frontal executive systems begin to exert more top-down (or voluntary) control, modulating the activity of posterior attentional and motor systems (Johnson, 2005). With the unfolding of frontal control, the child's sense and experience of time and space is extended. As the control and capacity of attentional orienting, working memory, and response inhibition expand, the older child is more able to plan actions over longer time scales and into extrapersonal space. For children with DCD, executive control deficits may place further constraints on motor learning, particularly of more sophisticated motor skills during middle and later childhood.

I argue that this pattern of change in executive function, along with physical maturation, would necessitate change at the level of motor control. We see how, in typically developing children, the predominant mode of motor control shifts temporarily to a more feedback-based system during middle childhood, which coincides with the unfolding of (frontal) cognitive control. At the same time, the child must learn to compensate for physical changes to his or her body with maturation. These changes present a problem of control at a neurocomputational level: With physical and neural maturation, how does the motor system learn or update the systematic relationship between motor command signals and the effect of these signals on body dynamics? Only with such "knowledge" can predictive control be implemented seamlessly (Desmurget & Grafton, 2003) and, with it, the rapid online adjustments we come to associate with mature reaching. For the child with DCD, a putative delay in cortical maturation (particularly at the level of parietal cortex) will further constrain this transition to mature reaching during middle childhood. This broad hypothesis will be shown to provide a parsimonious account of the neurocognitive processes that support typical motor development and their disruption in DCD. This model has a number of intriguing implications for our understanding of DCD and the longer-term consequences of the disorder for child development. I finish with a brief discussion of the implications of neurocognitive modelling in DCD for intervention.

Online Control as Fundamental to the Development of Movement Skill

Rapid Online Control Requires Seamless Integration of Feedforward and Feedback Processing.

Predictive control (viz., forward internal modelling) is based on the idea that the motor system learns to estimate its own behaviour. The ability to estimate the sensory consequences of an action is particularly important for fast manual actions, especially when they undergo some perturbation, either visual or mechanical. Whereas traditional models of reaching suggest independent feedforward and feedback (or "homing-in") phases, neurocomputational models now view reaching as being controlled by a hybrid system. In the case of *rapid online control* (labelled here as ROC), a fast internal feedback system is used to correct movements in-flight, with minimal time lag (e.g., Desmurget & Grafton, 2003). ROC is viable to the extent that the nervous system can predict the future location of the moving limb using a forward *internal model* that integrates efferent and afferent signals (Desmurget & Grafton, 2003; Jeannerod, 2006; Wolpert, 1997). This type of control circumvents delays associated with processing sensory feedback because the position of the moving hand has changed appreciably by the time sensory feedback can be used to alter the motor command as it unfolds. For instance, using a visual perturbation task where targets jump by up to 10 deg at movement onset, trajectories can be altered smoothly and early, evident in as little as 70–80 ms after liftoff (e.g., Desmurget & Grafton, 2003), and not with two distinct movements (a la earlier dual-process models). Moreover, these corrections can occur in the absence of any nonvisual sensory information (e.g., Bard, Hay, & Fleury, 1990), as seen in deafferented patients, and without vision of the moving hand. Forward models are thought to contribute to movement control by anticipating the sensory consequences of movement, which enables the detection of discrepancies between predicted movement and that indicated by actual sensory inflow; error signals are thus generated to correct the ongoing motor command at the level of motor cortex (Wolpert, Ghahramani, & Flanagan, 2001).

The neural network that supports predictive control is becoming clearer to researchers and provides some explanation of the patterns of performance evident over childhood as these structures mature with age. Forward models generated by frontal motor areas, including supplementary motor area (SMA), are used to cancel reafferent signals processed in the parietal cortex (Haggard & Whitford, 2004). Haggard argued that this suppression of neural activity is a type of "attention for action," as it involves deselection of predicted sensory inputs. Parietal cortex is thought to be intimately involved in generating a predictive forward model for an intended movement (Sirigu et al., 2004). The original motor intention appears to emanate from the frontal motor areas; however, with it, the parietal lobe forms part of a reciprocal cortico-cortical sensorimotor loop that subserves the forward planning process. Internal models generated by the parietal lobe would thus play a role in monitoring intentions and motor plans at high levels of representation, verifying whether actions match their intended goals. Posterior parietal cortex (PPC) is also well positioned, topographically, to generate and/or monitor forward models of expected changes in the visual flux that would occur with self-movement. It has been suggested that feedforward information from downstream motor areas could be compared with (local) visual-spatial representations in parietal cortex that specify the current state of the visual environment (Desmurget & Grafton, 2003; Heide, Blankenburg, Zimmermann, & Kömpf, 1995). Any mismatch between expected and actual visual flow would generate error signals that are conveyed to (premotor) action controllers, which in turn specify the motor commands necessary to achieve a desired outcome (Blakemore Frith, & Wolpert, 2001). Hence, a reciprocal network of cortical structures works to update motor commands in real time.

In cases where the environment is changing in the course of movement or where the limb itself is perturbed, this type of network is vitally important in stabilizing the movement.

The changing nature of predictive control during childhood is seen in studies of movement kinetics and kinematics. In the case of force control in healthy adults, grip force is modulated seamlessly in the early stages of lifting according to anticipated changes in the inertial properties of objects. In lifting experiments, basic predictive strategies are seen in children as young as 4 years of age; however, the energetic cost of lifting (or grip-to-load force ratio) shows continued improvement over childhood (e.g., Forssberg et al., 1992). It is interesting that the correlation between peak acceleration and peak grip force also increases up to around 9 years of age (Paré & Dugas, 1999). By around age 10–11 years, children begin to approximate adult levels of performance for single-arm movements or lifting (e.g., Blank et al., 2001).

Visual perturbation studies also show that older children implement online changes earlier in the reach trajectory in response to target jumps than do younger children (Van Braeckel, Butcher, Geuze, Stremmelaar, & Bouma, 2007). In Van Braeckel et al. (2007), target jumps occurred on two thirds of trials and, unlike most studies using this paradigm, jumps did not coincide with movement onset: The initial target was extinguished at 100 ms after children lifted their finger from a home base, reappearing 120 ms later at a different location. Of note in the study by Van Braeckel and colleagues was a change in strategy over the 7–10-year-old period: While 8-year-olds were able to correct movements in response to a target jump more quickly than 7-year-olds, they still spent the same amount of time in deceleration, which indicated that the ability to implement the correction was still immature. Only in the 9–10-year-old group were children able to both update the movement "program" using visual information and implement the corrective movement towards the new target location. Unfortunately, deviations from the standard paradigm limit what can be said about the upper reaches of ROC in these children. However, there is enough here to suggest that older children are able to integrate a forward estimate of limb position with sensory inflow with only marginal time lag. In developmental terms, as children learn the correlation between their own motor output signals and resultant effects on the moving limbs, they are better able to predict the visuo-perceptual and somatic consequences of their own movement (i.e., form internal models). We know that this internal "knowledge" of one's own movement dynamics can support rapid online adjustments by 9–10 years of age. One issue, however, is that most studies that have examined reaching have done so using targets in near space. It is likely that a system of predictive control would need to be updated as action targets in extrapersonal space become more compelling for children as they develop and as their physical system matures.

Internal Modelling Is Impaired in Children with DCD.

Earlier work has suggested that DCD might be explained by neuro-cognitive impairment to systems involved in generating or monitoring internal models for action. My colleagues and I have termed this the IMD hypothesis (Hyde & Wilson, 2011a, 2011b; Williams, Thomas, Maruff, & Wilson, 2008; Wilson, Maruff, Williams, Lum, & Thomas, 2004), although I now favour the idea that the deficit is one of predictive control (or forward modelling). We have argued that this deficit places limits on the speed and efficiency of online control (Desmurget & Grafton, 2003; Hyde & Wilson, 2011a, 2011b). The consequence of this impairment would be an overreliance on slower, feedback-based control, and movements that are less responsive to real-time changes in the environment. The IMD model is based on converging data, which are outlined below.

First, children with DCD show selective impairments in the voluntary control of covert attention (Tsai, Pan, Cherng, Hsu, & Chiu, 2009; Wilson & Maruff, 1999; Wilson, Maruff, & McKenzie, 1997). Work here is based on the spatial pre-cuing task of Posner, Inhoff, Friedrich, and Cohen (1987), the *covert orienting of visual spatial attention task* (COVAT). We found that attentional shifts were normal when initiated by pre-cues presented at peripheral locations, enlisting a more reflexive shift of covert attention. However, when initiated by central symbolic cues that enlist voluntary attention, children with DCD had difficulty disengaging attention from incorrectly cued locations (Wilson et al., 1997). This deficit occurred even when more time was allowed for processing spatial pre-cues (Wilson & Maruff, 1999). A similar pattern of results was shown more recently by Tsai et al. (2009), who attributed the difficulty to one of movement inhibition. As important, covert attention is thought equivalent to mentally simulating a "reaching" movement with the eyes (Rizzolatti, Riggio, Dascola, & Umiltá, 1987). Imaging studies reveal that it is subserved by the same network of structures as motor imagery (e.g., Nobre et al., 1997). Taken together, these results for DCD suggest an underlying impairment in generating or monitoring internal models of oculomotor plans.

Second, a neurocognitive deficit in the ability to use movement imagery has been shown in a number of studies. Behavioural data show high correlations between the speed of actual movements and imagined movements (Maruff, Wilson, Trebilcock, & Currie, 1999) and reveal that the biomechanical and environmental limitations on actual movements also operate when the same movements are imagined (Maruff et al., 1999). On this basis it has been argued persuasively that motor imagery represents an internal model of a movement with force-timing parameters coded according to the inertial properties of the effector and the structure of the environment. The motor representation comes to consciousness only because the actual movement has been inhibited (see Jeannerod, 2006). Impairments in motor imagery were found in DCD for the imagination of sequential movements – *visually guided pointing task* (VGPT) – complex gestures, and mental rotation of limbs, but not for object-based transformations (e.g., Williams, Thomas, Maruff, Butson, & Wilson, 2006; Wilson et al., 2004; Wilson, Thomas, & Maruff, 2005). Most intriguing, we showed that children with DCD were particularly disadvantaged when more complex (whole body) mental rotation was required, and they benefited little from explicit instruction on these tasks (Williams, Thomas, Maruff, Butson, & Wilson, 2006). It is important to note that these deficits in movement imagery appeared to be more pronounced in children with severe DCD (Williams et al., 2008). Taken together, results suggest difficulties performing imagined transformations from an egocentric (or body-centred) perspective, consistent with the IMD hypothesis.

The IMD hypothesis was also challenged by evaluating an imagery training protocol (randomized controlled trial) designed to train the ability to generate predictive (internal) models for action. The protocol, delivered by interactive DVD, was equally effective as physical therapy in skill development (Wilson, Thomas, & Maruff, 2002), a finding replicated in children with more severe DCD (Wilson et al., 2005). Clearly the type of instruction is important. We used a combination of peer modelling and progressive mental simulation, starting initially with movements reproduced from an external or third-person perspective and extending to an egocentric or first-person perspective. Using this staged approach, we showed that children with more severe DCD improved their motor performance most.

Third, others have also inferred deficits in predictive control on the basis of impaired grip force modulation in DCD (e.g., Hill & Wing, 1999).

In Hill and Wing's (1999) manual lifting study, increases in grip force occurred earlier in a child with DCD. As well, when the lifted object (a force transducer) was perturbed by adding an unexpected increase in load, the child was slower to accommodate the altered inertia of the object. The pattern of deficits was said to indicate poor predictive control, likely involving the cerebellar-parietal axis (see also Nowak, Topka, Timmann, Boecker, & Hermsdörfer, 2007). Similar results were also shown by Pereira, Landgren, Gillberg, and Forssberg (2001) in children with comorbid ADHD and DCD (or deficits in attention, motor control, and perception, DAMP). A high ratio of grip force to load force during lifting movements suggested poor anticipatory control.

Fourth, more recently, goal-directed reaching in DCD has been examined using a (visual) step perturbation task, a paradigm used to great effect to investigate mechanisms of rapid online control and internal modelling (e.g., Castiello, Bennett, Bonfiglioli, Lim, & Peppard, 1999; Pisella, Gréa, Vighetto, Desmurget, Rode, Boisson, & Rossetti, 2000). It was used by Plumb, Wilson, Mulroue, Brockman, Williams, & Mon-Williams (2008) to explore two alternative accounts for why children with DCD have difficulties making corrections while moving: the first a core deficit in detecting errors and making corrections online, and the second a central deficit in movement execution. They used a variation on this approach when they compared the performance of children with DCD and controls. Here, children were required to stand and complete the task using a hand-held stylus. Although the performance of children with DCD was slower than that of controls, both groups were equally disadvantaged on perturbation trials. The authors suggested that these results indicated a generalized deficit in producing movements rather than a specific online control deficit. However, children with DCD in this study had difficulty completing the task, which saw the paradigm being modified for them only: Due to difficulties standing unassisted while performing, they were seated, and because they had difficulty holding the stylus, a much thicker one was used. By the authors' own admission, these modifications simplified the postural and grasp demands of the task for the DCD group. It is well documented that children with DCD have particular difficulty completing complex movements (Sugden & Chambers, 2005). By simplifying the task, it can be argued, the complexity of "perturbed" trials may have been reduced for children with DCD. Thus, valid comparison between groups is limited.

To address these issues, colleagues and I evaluated double-step performance while controlling for task complexity (Hyde & Wilson, 2011a).

Participants were 11 children with DCD and 29 without, between 6 and 12 years of age. The task display consisted of a green circle centred at the bottom of a large LCD touchscreen, which served as a home base, and three potential target locations (2 cm in diameter) arranged in an arc across the top of the screen, spaced 20° apart. After a random delay, the central target location was illuminated. For 80 per cent of the trials, the central location remained lit for the duration of the movement (non-jump trials). For the remaining trials (20%), the central target was initially illuminated, but at the point of lift-off from the home base it was turned off and one of the two lateral targets was illuminated (jump trials). Analysis of MT data showed that the jump condition constrained the performance of the DCD group to a significantly greater extent than controls. Children with DCD also committed significantly more response errors on jump trials. Overall, the pattern of responding was similar to that seen in parietal patients (Pisella et al., 2000) and suggests a selective impairment in children with DCD of the ability to efficiently adapt their movements online, consistent with the IMD hypothesis.

Neural Basis of Impaired Predictive Control in DCD

Recent studies using functional magnetic resonance imaging (fMRI) have shown that children with DCD display abnormal PPC activation patterns during motor learning tasks. Kashiwagi, Iwaki, Narumi, Tamai, and Suzuki (2009) asked children to use a joystick to track a moving target on a monitor. Comparison of activation maps showed suppressed activity in the left posterior parietal cortex (PPC) and the post-central (or somatosensory) cortex in children with DCD. Left PPC is involved in the internal representation of one's body schema (Ogawa & Inui, 2007), hand control, and motor imagery (Gerardin et al., 2000), while right PPC supports more generic aspects of visuospatial processing. These same areas have been implicated in the predictive modelling of movement commands.

The cluster of deficits isolated in DCD also occur in people with ideomotor apraxia (e.g., Buxbaum, Johnson-Frey, & Bartlett-Williams, 2005), who manifest dysfunction at the level of the PPC (Sirigu et al., 1996). Ideomotor apraxia is characterized by difficulty planning movements in body-centred coordinates; movements are clumsy and the individual is unlikely to make corrective movements should an action be perturbed in any way, by an external force, for example (Buxbaum Sirigu, Schwartz, & Klatzky, 2003). It is my view that parieto-cerebellar dysfunction may well underlie the issues with predictive control that have been observed in DCD. Whether the dysfunction reflects developmental delay or deviance is an issue on ongoing debate. The deviance hypothesis suggests that the underlying processing issue is specific to the disorder and represents some departure from a normal developmental trajectory. By comparison, the delay hypothesis suggests some immaturity to the unfolding brain systems that support motor control and learning; the implication here is that children may catch up to their peers with adequate support. The important point here is that efficient ROC occurs only to the extent that feedback and feedforward processes are fully integrated with development. The control system that uses a predictive model to streamline error processing during the course of movement has strong links to the posterior parietal cortex and cerebellum (Desmurget & Grafton, 2003).

Caveats on the IMD Account and Its Neurocognitive Basis

It is important to note that most of the performance tasks described above involve movement in near (or peripersonal) space, whether real or imagined. From a neurocomputational perspective, the development of predictive control is relatively specific to a set of task constraints, the ambient workspace, and the structural integrity of the individual motor system (Wolpert et al., 2001). In other words, motor control develops to support the children's ability to coordinate movements that enable them to interact with their particular physical and social environment. The mode and fidelity of control must be updated as both the demands of the environment and the maturational constraints of the motor system change over time.

Neurocomputational models posit complementary processes for motor control and learning (e.g., Shadmehr, Smith, & Krakauer, 2010; Wolpert et al., 2001). In the case of predictive control, forward estimates of limb kinematics permit real-time, error-based corrections, commensurate with control, and these same error signals help train internal models per se. Motor learning, in part, is the process by which control mechanisms are trained through the medium of repeated, goal-directed activity. More specifically, control and coordination emerge from dynamic interaction of the individual child, a task configuration or problem, and the scale and structure of the environment (Deutsch & Newell, 2005). Learned over time, with repeated practice, is the crucial relationship between motor output signals and the effects of these signals on the body. It is likely that this relationship is encoded by the motor system according to the task and environmental constraints under which the learning occurred. For example, if practice involves small-scale movements, mostly in near space, then "knowledge" of the system's internal dynamics will develop within a narrower set of constraints. This then raises an important question: What developmental factors help determine the scale of this "movement space" in the first place?

The types of exploratory activity that characterize children of different ages are shaped by the child's attentional capacities and perception of what the environment might afford for action (Gibson, 1988). Researchers know that different modes of visuospatial attention exist and unfold along different timelines (Johnson & Munakata, 2005); for example, more reflexive modes unfold early, followed by more voluntary, top-down control. Moreover, perception of object affordances and visuospatial attention go hand in hand. Visuospatial attention appears to use a combination of location- and feature-based selection (Maunsell & Treue, 2006). In the case of infants and younger children, attentional bias tends to be proximal, which then sets in play a set of planned actions that occur for the most part within peripersonal space. Mechanisms of motor control are "trained" to enable dexterity and a degree of flexibility within the boundaries of this workspace.

Changes in the inertia of the moving limb through physical maturation also alter the relationship between the motor signals issued by motor cortices and their effects on arm position (Flanagan, Vetter, Johansson, & Wolpert, 2003; Wolpert et al., 2001). This presents a problem for control. Predictive models need to be constantly updated, especially during periods of rapid physical growth. This process appears to be error driven. Forward estimates of limb position need to be compared with some representation of actual limb position, the best indicator of which is sensory feedback (Desmurget & Grafton, 2003). Any discrepancy between the predicted state and the actual state of the system would indicate some problem with the predictive model itself; the resultant error signal is then used to train the forward model (Wolpert et al., 2001). In short, a system of control based on forward estimates would support both real-time modifications to limb trajectory and learning over longer time scales (Braun, Mehring, & Wolpert, 2010). Moreover, the system can adapt with experience to changing constraints, both internal (e.g., maturational changes in brain systems and biomechanics) and external (e.g., changing task demands with age). Put another way, the learning outputs of the control system are sensitive to context but also permit extraction of common features of different environments to support new learning. Particular modes of exploratory behaviour in particular environments will train prediction within that action space (Braun et al., 2010). In developmental terms, experience in self-produced movement appears to provide just the type of input needed to refine internal models over time, provided the maturational bases of control are sufficiently developed. This form of adaptive control provides a nice explanatory model for the process of both typical and atypical motor skill development.

In the following section I describe developmental changes to key neurocognitive systems that support and bias motor behaviour in children. I also present evidence to show that these systems are compromised in many children with DCD. These deficits have important consequences for the ongoing development of movement skill.

Systems of Spatial and Executive Function: Developmental Trends and Dysfunction in DCD

Spatial Systems and Attentional Orienting

Supporting goal-directed action, there appear to be two main systems for representing space which are both ecologically and developmentally plausible (Previc, 1998): First, a *peripersonal* system supports exploratory manual activity within the immediate boundary for reaching, up to around 1 m from the body (Butler, Eskes, & Vandorpe, 2004; Higuchi, Imanaka, & Patla, 2006), and is biased towards the lower visual field; and, second, an *extrapersonal* system that is concerned with person–environment interactions that extend beyond "reaching space," biased towards the upper visual field. These two spatial systems are defined by separable networks of attention that link goal representations with action.

During early infancy, action in peripersonal space is largely stimulus driven, but gradually more voluntary (attentional) control is exerted with experience-dependent maturation of the forebrain and associated perceptual-motor loops. This is evident in the pattern of visuospatial orienting that we see over the course of infancy and to some extent during early childhood. Attentional orienting in older infants and young children is relatively efficient when triggered by strong external cues in near space (Johnson, Posner, & Rothbart, 1991; Ristic & Kingstone, 2009). But the ability to orient attention using an endogenous mode of control is less well developed in younger children (Brodeur & Enns, 1997), especially when the attentional focus is drawn into extrapersonal space. This mode of control is enlisted when the performer has to weigh up stimulus-response probabilities and/or the symbolic content of task cues (e.g., arrow-shaped pre-cues presented at a central fixation point that indicate the location of an upcoming target location with high probability). Issues in attentional orienting among younger children is shown by a reduced ability to initiate rapid shifts of voluntary attention, ignore cues that are irrelevant to goal completion (so-called invalid cues), and rapidly disengage attention from these cues (Ristic & Kingstone, 2009).

The patterns of response evident in older children with DCD overlap to some extent with those seen in younger, typically developing children. But the selective impairment in disengaging attention from invalid cues looks more like the pattern shown by patients with parietal lobe damage. Children with DCD show an attentional cost for invalid cues regardless of the time interval between cue and target, or stimulus-onset asynchrony (SOA). Indeed, the magnitude of the invalid cue effect (or difference in response time to valid and invalid trials) is similar to that seen in parietal dysfunction, which is in excess of 50 ms at short and long SOAs (Wilson & Maruff, 1999). Neuroimaging work also suggests a strong posterior parietal involvement in the disengage process (Nobre et al., 1997).

The Development of Executive Function in Typically Developing Children and in DCD

Middle childhood marks a period of neurocognitive reorganization as the scope of goal-directed behaviour expands. During this time, there is a progressive coupling of frontal executive functions to more posterior motor control centres (Johnson, 2005). If we track the pattern of neural growth – myelination and synaptic connectivity – over this period, we see maximal levels of synaptic density in the forebrain of children at around 5–6 years of age; this is followed by a period of selective pruning and consolidation through childhood (Casey, Galvan & Hare, 2005). It is during this period that executive systems become more specialized, exerting more control on action systems (Dyck, Piek, Kane, & Patrick, 2009).

The neural basis of executive control. Current models of cognitive control, or executive function (EF), suggest that EF comprises a set of dissociable components including inhibition, working memory, and executive attention (Bennetto & Pennington, 2003; Diamond, 2006). Development of these components serves to enable more adaptive and flexible responses to novel situations and to environments that are information laden and changeable (Diamond, 2006). More important, maturation of prefrontal and parietal cortex connectivity has been shown to support gains in working memory and inhibitory function, processes that help extend the spatiotemporal boundaries of cognition and behaviour (Casey, Galvan & Hare, 2005). Diffusion tensor imaging, for example, shows more focal activation of these networks during task performance with age, whereas diffuse activation (associated with poor inhibition of distractors, for instance) is a characteristic of an immature cognitive system.

There is now good evidence to show that basic sensorimotor processes mature first, but they are then subject to more top-down control as the association cortex (e.g., prefrontal cortex, or PFC) starts to mature, exerting a level of control that extends increasingly from front to back in cortical terms. The net effect of these maturational processes is an increasing ability among older children to modulate more automatic processing (Gogtay et al., 2004). In terms of movement preparation, a limiting factor in children younger than 8 years of age appears to be how volitional control is used to modulate more primitive reflexive processes (Ristic & Kingstone, 2009). For instance, older children and those with better cognitive control, especially inhibition, tend to recruit posterior parietal regions more efficiently than do younger children, particularly on tasks with high cognitive demand (Bunge, Hazeltine, Scanlon, Rosen, & Gabrieli, 2002). This permits greater flexibility of control in the face of task complexity and distractor processing.

Perhaps the most significant watershed in the development of EF occurs between the ages of 4 and 8 years, when cognitive flexibility emerges concomitant to the proliferation of neural connectivity within the PFC and its reciprocal connections downstream (PMC, PPC, cingulate cortex, and midline structures). Maturation of the dorsolateral prefrontal cortex (DL-PFC), in particular, is defined by two major changes: (1) increased concentration of dopamine receptors over the course of infancy and childhood, and (2) the progressive myelination of neural pathways in a posterior-to-anterior direction (Benes, 2001; Diamond, 2006; Mareschal, Johnson, & Grayson, 2004). During this period we see a distinct rise in working memory capacity, inhibitory control (e.g., initiation of anti-saccades), and attentional flexibility in middle childhood (Johnson, 2005).

Working memory. Working memory, as part of the executive system, provides the capacity to temporarily maintain information, or representations, in conscious awareness when this information is not physically present, to manipulate such information, and to use it in directing behaviour (Postle, 2006). Its developmental trajectory is also strongly linked to maturation of the DL-PFC (Benes, 2001; Diamond, 2006); virtually all neurophysiological studies of working memory report delay-period activity of the PFC (Postle, 2006). It is intriguing that this activity may reflect not necessarily storage per se in PFC but rather other aspects of processing associated with goal-directed performance such as minimizing interference from sensory processing areas during delay periods and in channelling executive attention. (For more on the *emergent view* of working memory, see Postle, 2006). In developmental terms, maturation of PFC and its connections to parietal cortex affords smooth and sustained operation of motor planning systems in the face of interference and task complexity.

Working memory impairments have been widely reported in children with DCD. In a series of studies, Alloway and colleagues (Alloway, 2007; Alloway & Archibald, 2008; Alloway & Temple, 2007; Alloway, Rajendran, & Archibald, 2009) showed that children with DCD performed poorly on most measures of visuo-spatial working memory (VSWM) relative to children with specific language impairment, moderate learning difficulties, ADHD, Asperger's syndrome, and typically developing controls. On the Automated Working Memory Assessment (AWMA), deficits were greatest on visuospatial measures, including short-term memory of a tapping sequence, a maze path, and dot location. Piek, Dyck, Francis, and Conwell (2007) have also shown VSWM, processing speed, and executive attention deficits in DCD of the same magnitude as the motor impairments. Moreover, in a recent meta-analysis of DCD–Control studies (Wilson, Ruddock, Smits-Engelsman, Polataiko, & Blank, 2013), we have found that effect sizes on working memory tasks are high regardless of the sensory modality used.

Inhibition and movement skill. It is important that recent data also suggest a strong link between inhibitory function and movement skill in children – for example, Stroop performance and initiation of anti-saccades and movement skill, both in young children (Livesey, Keen, Rouse, & White, 2006) and those who were older (Piek et al., 2007). Deficits of inhibition are particularly common in children with DCD and those with comorbid DCD and ADHD. Piek et al. (2007), for example, found that children with DCD were poorer on EF tasks that measured response inhibition, working memory, and set shifting: They were significantly slower and more variable. It is interesting that this pattern of performance has been linked with deficits in planning associated with cerebellar functioning. One possibility is that the ability to modulate action planning by inhibitory control might be reduced in these children, placing limits on motor learning (see also Barkley, 1997). Under circumstances where task demands are high (e.g., spatial or temporal load), this performance issue is likely to be exacerbated.

New Directions in Thinking about Neurocognitive Development in Children with and without DCD

Does the Development of Predictive Control Mirror Age-Related Changes in Spatial and Executive Networks?

The temporary reorganization of motor control that occurs during middle childhood coincides with the expansion of executive control. The larger neural dynamic may be one of coupling anterior and posterior systems. For children with DCD, who have well documented deficits in both predictive control and executive function, this process of coupling may be particularly challenging, with important long-term consequences for development of skilled action (Piek et al., 2007).

The major changes in PFC during early and middle childhood bestow a processing capability that takes time and experience to fully harness, at least into later childhood and adolescence (Diamond & Kirkham, 2005). Put another way, "Fine-tuning of cortical systems occurs with protracted refinement of association cortex (e.g. prefrontal cortex) relative to sensorimotor cortex" (Casey, Galvan & Hare, 2005, p.108). The "protracted refinement" that Casey speaks of is really getting at the heart of experience-dependent plasticity. For example, in comparison to older children, young children are less able to coordinate advanced skills that enlist working memory and executive attention, despite rapid increases in PFC volume during this period of development (Diamond, 2006). Repeated experience and guided discovery are needed to sculpt the neural networks that support these more advanced skills.

Dorsal (or *how to*) and ventral (*what*) streams also appear to acquire specialization under different timeframes, reflecting regional differences in cortical maturation. Recent developmental research shows that perceptual processing of objects has acquired a high degree of sophistication by early childhood, whereas body-centred representation lags behind (Dilks, Hoffman, & Landau, 2008). In other words, the ability to represent an object per se precedes the child's understanding and ability to interact with the object. The latter involves mapping a body schema onto a 3-D representation of space, a coding that is intrinsically ego or body centred. Moreover, the setting of movement parameters must also take into account the known physical characteristics of the object itself: its given shape, weight, proximity, and inertial characteristics.

There appears to be an important relationship between attentional orienting and the development of body schema. Voluntary reaching during early development is thought to help calibrate an egocentric frame of reference in infancy; this body schema later forms the platform for exploratory activity with locomotion. In other words, attention for action develops within a peripersonal frame in early development and later extends outward into extrapersonal space as voluntary attentional control continues to unfold. Indeed, the extrapersonal system appears to work synergistically with frontal executive control to expand goal-directed action into topographically defined space (Previc, 1998). It follows that the maturational timeline of frontal cortex may act as a rate-limiting factor in the development of skilled movement into extrapersonal space. Similarly, other executive control functions associated with frontal maturation are also working synergistically with motor centres.

Taken together, it is highly plausible that action planning and its supporting control processes must undergo a period of readjustment to accommodate an expansion in action space. Indeed, for actions directed into extrapersonal space, movement is even more reliant on prospective control (Higuchi et al., 2006). Internal models must be learned dynamically as various constraints change with development: the perceived workspace, neurocognitive bases, individual biomechanics, and specific task demands (Wolpert, Ghahramani, & Flanagan, 2001). Emerging functional loops between PMC, PPC, and cerebellum are integral to this process (see also Spratling & Johnson, 2004). In short, I argue that mechanisms of rapid online control undergo a period of reorganization as action potentialities extend beyond peripersonal space as a result of cortical development. Fortunately, we have a number of powerful methods available to examine this broad hypothesis. This is discussed in the next section.

Key questions for research. These theoretical arguments about the interdependence of motor and cognitive systems in children are consistent with the results of descriptive, longitudinal studies of DCD and DAMP. As the level of motor impairment and associated executive difficulties increases (e.g., attentional control), the worse the long-term outcome is for children with DCD. What researchers need to establish is exactly how deficits at the level of motor control might interact with executive processing deficits to disrupt different types of skilled action in children. Indeed, for children with DCD, an already compromised ability to enlist predictive control will be exacerbated when movement tasks also demand high levels of executive control (e.g., inhibitory load). We might expect the performance profile for DCD in middle childhood to resemble that of younger children; the executive skills of the younger child are still emerging, and the process of coupling these to sensorimotor cortex rudimentary.

It is also important to establish how these interactive effects might change with age and to determine the sorts of therapy that best equip children with DCD to learn new skills. For instance, it is possible that a multimodal treatment that combines methods to train predictive control (e.g., movement imagery) with a more top-down approach (like Cognitive Orientation to daily Occupational Performance, or CO-OP) may help overcome some of the challenges to motor planning that are imposed by impaired executive control.

Longitudinal data will provide by far the most rigorous test of these intriguing questions. Cross-sequential longitudinal designs, as well as *growth curve modelling* (GCM; Bryk & Raudenbush, 1992), are particularly useful in measuring change over time at both an individual level and a population level, which is entirely consistent with developmental theory. The moderating effect of movement experience or exposure to learning on the development of ROC and functional skill can also be factored into these models. Ironically, this approach also gets at the notion of biological vulnerability. It is likely that a certain proportion of children develop adequate levels of online control and functional skills in the face of low levels of participation. This suggests a level of neurocognitive plasticity that children with DCD, for example, may not have. Alternatively, for children who fail to develop sound motor skills despite high levels of participation or exposure, a delayed or deviant pattern of neural maturation would be indicated; the theory presented here suggests that the locus of this disruption is likely to be PPC and possibly its reciprocal connections to the cerebellum. Clustering techniques and paradigms based on strong neurocognitive models will enable researchers to answer these questions.

Finally, new techniques in neuroimaging promise to shed light on the emerging neurocognitive mechanisms of motor control and learning.

One exciting new development has been the use of structural MRI (sMRI), in tandem with fMRI. Anatomical changes reported in longitudinal sMRI studies show a particularly tight correlation with cognitive growth, a point that has tended to drive functional investigations (Casey, Galvan & Hare, 2005). Structural tractography, for example, can reveal subtle differences between groups and patterns of individual change with careful use of repeated assessment. Of particular interest will be the ability to track cortical changes in individuals over time as a consequence of not only maturation but also learning. One prediction would be that in children with persistent DCD, reduced connectivity may be revealed between PPC and prefrontal cortex or, indeed, a reduced cortical terrain in regions of PPC, the intraparietal cortex (IPC) being one prime candidate. IPC is strongly linked to visual-motor coordinate transformation and predictive control (e.g., Desmurget & Grafton, 2003). More specifically, while the exact site(s) of internal modelling is a topic of vigorous exploration, the error correction process on visual perturbation tasks has been linked to parietal activity, especially of the lateral intraparietal cortex (LIP). This region is thought to be involved in computing a dynamic movement error signal by comparing the updated location of the target with a predicted estimate of the movement endpoint (e.g., Desmurget et al., 2001).

General Conclusion

DCD is no longer the poor cousin in the study of child development (Piek, Dawson, Smith, & Gasson, 2008; Sommerville & Decety, 2006; Wilson, 2005). Understanding the neurocognitive deficits associated with the disorder has important implications for developing a unifying account of motor development per se, for mapping causal mechanisms of the disorder, and for intervention. Given the extended period of neural maturation over childhood, and variations in the growth trajectories of different neural systems, the motor system is subject to changing internal constraints. The development of predictive control is a prime example of this, contributing to a mature system of rapid online control (e.g., Desmurget et al., 2001; Desmurget & Grafton, 2003). In children with DCD, neurocognitive mechanisms of predictive control appear to be compromised. In addition, the presence of executive control deficits places these children at a significant disadvantage, in developmental terms. I propose that with physical maturation and as spatial and temporal scale of action expand over childhood, predictive models for action need to be recalibrated; this is necessary to support the development of more sophisticated and flexible movement skills. This process may be compromised in DCD, particularly in children with a constellation of motor control and executive deficits.

REFERENCES

Alloway, T.P. (2007, Jan). Working memory, reading, and mathematical skills in children with developmental coordination disorder. *Journal of Experimental Child Psychology*, *96*(1), 20–36. http://dx.doi.org/10.1016/j.jecp.2006.07.002 Medline:17010988

Alloway, T.P., & Archibald, L. (2008, May-Jun). Working memory and learning in children with developmental coordination disorder and specific language impairment. *Journal of Learning Disabilities*, *41*(3), 251–262. http://dx.doi.org/10.1177/0022219408315815 Medline:18434291

Alloway, T.P., Rajendran, G., & Archibald, L.M.D. (2009, Jul-Aug). Working memory in children with developmental disorders. *Journal of Learning Disabilities*, *42*(4), 372–382. http://dx.doi.org/10.1177/0022219409335214 Medline:19380495

Alloway, T.P., & Temple, K.J. (2007). A comparison of working memory skills and learning in children with developmental coordination disorder and moderate learning difficulties. *Applied Cognitive Psychology*, *21*(4), 473–487. http://dx.doi.org/10.1002/acp.1284

Bard, C., Hay, L., & Fleury, M. (1990, Aug). Timing and accuracy of visually directed movements in children: Control of direction and amplitude components. *Journal of Experimental Child Psychology*, *50*(1), 102–118. http://dx.doi.org/10.1016/0022-0965(90)90034-6 Medline:2398328

Barkley, R.A. (1997, Jan). Behavioral inhibition, sustained attention, and executive functions: Constructing a unifying theory of ADHD. *Psychological Bulletin*, *121*(1), 65–94. http://dx.doi.org/10.1037/0033-2909.121.1.65 Medline:9000892

Benes, F.M. (2001). The development of prefrontal cortex: The maturation of neurotransmitter systems and their interactions. In C. Nelson & M. Luciana (Eds.), *Handbook of developmental cognitive neuroscience* (pp. 79–92). Cambridge, MA: Massachusetts Institute of Technology Press.

Bennetto, L., & Pennington, B. (2003). Executive functioning in normal and abnormal development. In S. Segalowitz & I. Rapin (Eds.), *Handbook of neuropsychology*. (2nd ed., Vol. 8, pp. 785–802). Amsterdam, the Netherlands: Elsevier.

Blakemore, S.-J., Frith, C.D., & Wolpert, D.M. (2001, Jul 3). The cerebellum is involved in predicting the sensory consequences of action. *Neuroreport*, 12(9), 1879–1884. http://dx.doi.org/10.1097/00001756-200107030-00023 Medline:11435916

Blank, R., Breitenbach, A., Nitschke, M., Heizer, W., Letzgus, S., & Hermsdörfer, J. (2001, May). Human development of grip force modulation relating to cyclic movement-induced inertial loads. *Experimental Brain Research*, 138(2), 193–199. http://dx.doi.org/10.1007/s002210000622 Medline:11417460

Braun, D.A., Mehring, C., & Wolpert, D.M. (2010, Jan 20). Structure learning in action. *Behavioural Brain Research*, 206(2), 157–165. http://dx.doi.org/10.1016/j.bbr.2009.08.031 Medline:19720086

Brodeur, D.A., & Enns, J.T. (1997, Mar). Covert visual orienting across the lifespan. *Canadian Journal of Experimental Psychology*, 51(1), 20–35. http://dx.doi.org/10.1037/1196-1961.51.1.20 Medline:9206322

Bryk, A., & Raudenbush, S. (1992). *Hierarchical linear models*. Newbury Park, CA: Sage.

Bunge, S.A., Hazeltine, E., Scanlon, M.D., Rosen, A.C., & Gabrieli, J.D.E. (2002, Nov). Dissociable contributions of prefrontal and parietal cortices to response selection. *NeuroImage*, 17(3), 1562–1571. http://dx.doi.org/10.1006/nimg.2002.1252 Medline:12414294

Butler, B.C., Eskes, G.A., & Vandorpe, R.A. (2004). Gradients of detection in neglect: Comparison of peripersonal and extrapersonal space. *Neuropsychologia*, 42(3), 346–358. http://dx.doi.org/10.1016/j.neuropsychologia.2003.08.008 Medline:14670573

Buxbaum, L.J., Johnson-Frey, S.H., & Bartlett-Williams, M. (2005). Deficient internal models for planning hand-object interactions in apraxia. *Neuropsychologia*, 43(6), 917–929. http://dx.doi.org/10.1016/j.neuropsychologia.2004.09.006 Medline:15716162

Buxbaum, L.J., Sirigu, A., Schwartz, M.F., & Klatzky, R. (2003). Cognitive representations of hand posture in ideomotor apraxia. *Neuropsychologia*, 41(8), 1091–1113. http://dx.doi.org/10.1016/S0028-3932(02)00314-7 Medline:12667544

Casey, B.J., Galvan, A., Hare, T.A. (2005). Changes in cerebral functional organization during cognitive development. *Current Opinion in Neurobiology*, 15, 239–244.

Castiello, U., Bennett, K., Bonfiglioli, C., Lim, S., & Peppard, R.F. (1999). The reach-to-grasp movement in Parkinson's disease: Response to a simultaneous perturbation of object position and object size. *Experimental Brain Research*, 125(4), 453–462.

Chicoine, A.J., Lassonde, M., & Proteau, L. (1992). Developmental aspects of sensorimotor integration. *Developmental Neuropsychology, 8*(4), 381–394. http://dx.doi.org/10.1080/87565649209540533

Desmurget, M., & Grafton, S. (2003). Feedback or forward control: End of a dichotomy. In S. Johnson-Frey (Ed.), *Taking action: Cognitive neuroscience perspectives on intentional action* (pp. 289–338). Cambridge, MA: Massachusetts Institute of Technology Press.

Desmurget, M., Gréa, H., Grethe, J.S., Prablanc, C., Alexander, G.E., & Grafton, S.T. (2001, Apr 15). Functional anatomy of nonvisual feedback loops during reaching: a positron emission tomography study. *Journal of Neuroscience, 21*(8), 2919–2928. Medline:11306644

Deutsch, K.M., & Newell, K.M. (2005). Noise, variability, and the development of children's perceptual-motor skills. *Developmental Review, 25*(2), 155–180. http://dx.doi.org/10.1016/j.dr.2004.09.001

Diamond, A. (2006). The early development of executive functions. In E. Bialystok (Ed.), *Lifespan cognition* (pp. 70–95). Oxford, England: Oxford University Press. http://dx.doi.org/10.1093/acprof:o so/9780195169539.003.0006

Diamond, A., & Kirkham, N. (2005, Apr). Not quite as grown-up as we like to think: Parallels between cognition in childhood and adulthood. *Psychological Science, 16*(4), 291–297. http://dx.doi.org/10.1111/j.0956-7976.2005.01530.x Medline:15828976

Dilks, D.D., Hoffman, J.E., & Landau, B. (2008, Jul). Vision for perception and vision for action: Normal and unusual development. *Developmental Science, 11*(4), 474–486. http://dx.doi.org/10.1111/j.1467-7687.2008.00693.x Medline:18576955

Dyck, M.J., Piek, J.P., Kane, R., & Patrick, J. (2009). How uniform is the structure of ability across childhood? *European Journal of Developmental Psychology, 6*(4), 432–454. http://dx.doi.org/10.1080/17405620701439820

Flanagan, J.R., Vetter, P., Johansson, R.S., & Wolpert, D.M. (2003, Jan 21). Prediction precedes control in motor learning. *Current Biology, 13*(2), 146–150. http://dx.doi.org/10.1016/S0960-9822(03)00007-1 Medline:12546789

Forssberg, H., Kinoshita, H., Eliasson, A.C., Johansson, R.S., Westling, G., & Gordon, A.M. (1992). Development of human precision grip: II, Anticipatory control of isometric forces targeted for object's weight. *Experimental Brain Research, 90*(2), 393–398. Medline:1397153

Gerardin, E., Sirigu, A., Lehéricy, S., Poline, J.B., Gaymard, B., Marsault, C., ... Le Bihan, D. (2000, Nov). Partially overlapping neural networks for real and imagined hand movements. *Cerebral Cortex, 10*(11), 1093–1104. http://dx.doi.org/10.1093/cercor/10.11.1093 Medline:11053230

Gibson, E.J. (1988). Exploratory behavior in the development of perceiving, acting, and the acquiring of knowledge. *Annual Review of Psychology, 39*(1), 1–42. http://dx.doi.org/10.1146/annurev.ps.39.020188.000245

Gogtay, N., Giedd, J.N., Lusk, L., Hayashi, K.M., Greenstein, D., Vaituzis, A.C., ... Thompson, P.M. (2004, May 25). Dynamic mapping of human cortical development during childhood through early adulthood. *Proceedings of the National Academy of Sciences of the United States of America, 101*(21), 8174–8179. http://dx.doi.org/10.1073/pnas.0402680101 Medline:15148381

Haggard, P., & Whitford, B. (2004, Mar). Supplementary motor area provides an efferent signal for sensory suppression. *Brain Research. Cognitive Brain Research, 19*(1), 52–58. http://dx.doi.org/10.1016/j.cogbrainres.2003.10.018 Medline:14972358

Heide, W., Blankenburg, M., Zimmermann, E., & Kömpf, D. (1995, Nov). Cortical control of double-step saccades: Implications for spatial orientation. *Annals of Neurology, 38*(5), 739–748. http://dx.doi.org/10.1002/ana.410380508 Medline:7486865

Higuchi, T., Imanaka, K., & Patla, A.E. (2006). Action-oriented representation of peripersonal and extrapersonal space: Insights from manual and locomotor actions. *Japanese Psychological Research, 48*(3), 126–140. http://dx.doi.org/10.1111/j.1468-5884.2006.00314.x

Hill, E.l., & Wing, A. M. (1999). Coordination of grip force and load force in developmental coordination disorder: A case study. *Neurocase, 5*(6), 537–544.

Hyde, C., & Wilson, P.H. (2011a, Apr). Dissecting online control in developmental coordination disorder: A kinematic analysis of double-step reaching. *Brain and Cognition, 75*(3), 232–241. http://dx.doi.org/10.1016/j.bandc.2010.12.004 Medline:21256656

Hyde, C., & Wilson, P. (2011b, Jan). Online motor control in children with developmental coordination disorder: Chronometric analysis of double-step reaching performance. *Child: Care, Health and Development, 37*(1), 111–122. http://dx.doi.org/10.1111/j.1365-2214.2010.01131.x Medline:20637020

Jeannerod, M. (2006). *Motor cognition.* Oxford, England: Oxford University Press. http://dx.doi.org/10.1093/acprof:oso/9780198569657.001.0001

Johnson, M.A. (2005). *Developmental cognitive neuroscience* (2nd ed.). Wiley-Blackwell.

Johnson, M.H., & Munakata, Y. (2005, Mar). Processes of change in brain and cognitive development. *Trends in Cognitive Sciences, 9*(3), 152–158. http://dx.doi.org/10.1016/j.tics.2005.01.009 Medline:15737824

Johnson, M.H., Posner, M.I., & Rothbart, M.K. (1991, Fall). Components of visual orienting in early infancy: Contingency learning, anticipatory looking, and disengaging. *Journal of Cognitive Neuroscience, 3*(4), 335–344. http://dx.doi.org/10.1162/jocn.1991.3.4.335 Medline:23967813

Kashiwagi, M., Iwaki, S., Narumi, Y., Tamai, H., & Suzuki, S. (2009, Oct 7). Parietal dysfunction in developmental coordination disorder: A functional MRI study. *Neuroreport, 20*(15), 1319–1324. http://dx.doi.org/10.1097/WNR.0b013e32832f4d87 Medline:19730138

Livesey, D., Keen, J., Rouse, J., & White, F. (2006, Feb). The relationship between measures of executive function, motor performance and externalising behaviour in 5- and 6-year-old children. *Human Movement Science, 25*(1), 50–64. http://dx.doi.org/10.1016/j.humov.2005.10.008 Medline:16442172

Mareschal, D., Johnson, M.H., & Grayson, A. (2004). Brain and cognitive development. In J. Oates & A. Grayson (Eds.), *Cognitive and language development in children* (pp. 113–162). Wiley-Blackwell.

Maruff, P., Wilson, P., Trebilcock, M., & Currie, J. (1999, Oct). Abnormalities of imaged motor sequences in children with developmental coordination disorder. *Neuropsychologia, 37*(11), 1317–1324. http://dx.doi.org/10.1016/S0028-3932(99)00016-0 Medline:10530731

Maunsell, J.H.R., & Treue, S. (2006, Jun). Feature-based attention in visual cortex. *Trends in Neurosciences, 29*(6), 317–322. http://dx.doi.org/10.1016/j.tins.2006.04.001 Medline:16697058

Nobre, A.C., Sebestyen, G.N., Gitelman, D.R., Mesulam, M.M., Frackowiak, R.S., & Frith, C.D. (1997, Mar). Functional localization of the system for visuospatial attention using positron emission tomography. *Brain, 120*(3), 515–533. http://dx.doi.org/10.1093/brain/120.3.515 Medline:9126062

Nowak, D.A., Topka, H., Timmann, D., Boecker, H., & Hermsdörfer, J. (2007). The role of the cerebellum for predictive control of grasping. *Cerebellum 6*(1), 7–17. http://dx.doi.org/10.1080/14734220600776379 Medline:17366262

Ogawa, K., & Inui, T. (2007, Nov). Lateralization of the posterior parietal cortex for internal monitoring of self- versus externally generated movements. *Journal of Cognitive Neuroscience, 19*(11), 1827–1835. http://dx.doi.org/10.1162/jocn.2007.19.11.1827 Medline:17958485

Paré, M., & Dugas, C. (1999, Apr). Developmental changes in prehension during childhood. *Experimental Brain Research, 125*(3), 239–247. http://dx.doi.org/10.1007/s002210050679 Medline:10229014

Pereira, H.S., Landgren, M., Gillberg, C., & Forssberg, H. (2001). Parametric control of fingertip forces during precision grip lifts in children with DCD (developmental coordination disorder) and DAMP (deficits in attention motor control and perception). *Neuropsychologia, 39*(5), 478–488. http://dx.doi.org/10.1016/S0028-3932(00)00132-9 Medline:11254930

Piek, J.P., Dawson, L., Smith, L.M., & Gasson, N. (2008, Oct). The role of early fine and gross motor development on later motor and cognitive ability. *Human Movement Science, 27*(5), 668–681. http://dx.doi.org/10.1016/j.humov.2007.11.002 Medline:18242747

Piek, J., Dyck, M.J., Francis, M., & Conwell, A. (2007). Working memory, processing speed and set-shifting in children with developmental coordination disorder and attention-deficit-hyperactivity disorder. *Developmental Medicine and Child Neurology, 49*, 678–683. http://dx.doi.org/10.1111/j.1469-8749.2007.00678.x Medline:17718824

Pisella, L., Gréa, H., Tilikete, C., Vighetto, A., Desmurget, M., Rode, G., Boisson, D., Rossetti, Y. (2000, Jul). An "automatic pilot" for the hand in human posterior parietal cortex: Toward reinterpreting optic ataxia. *Nature Neuroscience, 3*(7), 729–736. http://dx.doi.org/10.1038/76694 Medline:10862707

Plumb, M.S., Wilson, A.D., Mulroue, A., Brockman, A., Williams, J.H., & Mon-Williams, M. (2008, Oct). Online corrections in children with and without DCD. *Human Movement Science, 27*(5):695-704. http://dx.doi.org/10.1016/j.humov.2007.11.004.

Posner, M.I., Inhoff, A.W., Friedrich, F.J., & Cohen, A. (1987). Isolating attentional systems: A cognitive-anatomical analysis. *Psychobiology, 15*, 107–121.

Postle, B.R. (2006, Apr 28). Working memory as an emergent property of the mind and brain. *Neuroscience, 139*(1), 23–38. http://dx.doi.org/10.1016/j.neuroscience.2005.06.005 Medline:16324795

Previc, F.H. (1998, Sep). The neuropsychology of 3-D space. *Psychological Bulletin, 124*(2), 123–164. http://dx.doi.org/10.1037/0033-2909.124.2.123 Medline:9747184

Ristic, J., & Kingstone, A. (2009, Mar). Rethinking attentional development: Reflexive and volitional orienting in children and adults. *Developmental Science, 12*(2), 289–296. http://dx.doi.org/10.1111/j.1467-7687.2008.00756.x Medline:19143801

Rizzolatti, G., Riggio, L., Dascola, I., & Umiltá, C. (1987). Reorienting attention across the horizontal and vertical meridians: Evidence in favor of a premotor theory of attention. *Neuropsychologia, 25*(1 Suppl. 1A), 31–40. http://dx.doi.org/10.1016/0028-3932(87)90041-8 Medline:3574648

Shadmehr, R., Smith, M.A., & Krakauer, J.W. (2010). Error correction, sensory prediction, and adaptation in motor control. *Annual Review of Neuroscience, 33*(1), 89–108. http://dx.doi.org/10.1146/annurev-neuro-060909-153135 Medline:20367317

Sirigu, A., Daprati, E., Ciancia, S., Giraux, P., Nighoghossian, N., Posada, A., & Haggard, P. (2004, Jan). Altered awareness of voluntary action after damage to the parietal cortex. *Nature Neuroscience, 7*(1), 80–84. http://dx.doi.org/10.1038/nn1160 Medline:14647290

Sirigu, A., Duhamel, J.R., Cohen, L., Pillon, B., Dubois, B., & Agid, Y. (1996, Sep 13). The mental representation of hand movements after parietal cortex damage. *Science, 273*(5281), 1564–1568. http://dx.doi.org/10.1126/science.273.5281.1564 Medline:8703221

Sommerville, J.A., & Decety, J. (2006, Apr). Weaving the fabric of social interaction: Articulating developmental psychology and cognitive neuroscience in the domain of motor cognition. *Psychonomic Bulletin & Review, 13*(2), 179–200. http://dx.doi.org/10.3758/BF03193831 Medline:16892982

Spratling, M.W., & Johnson, M.H. (2004). Neural coding strategies and mechanisms of competition. *Cognitive Systems Research, 5*(2), 93–117. http://dx.doi.org/10.1016/j.cogsys.2003.11.002

Sugden, D.A. & Chambers, M.E. (Eds.). (2005). *Children with developmental coordination disorder*. London, England: Whurr Publishers.

Tsai, C.L., Pan, C.Y., Cherng, R.J., Hsu, Y.W., & Chiu, H.H. (2009, Dec). Mechanisms of deficit of visuospatial attention shift in children with developmental coordination disorder: A neurophysiological measure of the endogenous Posner paradigm. *Brain and Cognition, 71*(3), 246–258. http://dx.doi.org/10.1016/j.bandc.2009.08.006 Medline:19751962

Van Braeckel, K., Butcher, P.R., Geuze, R.H., Stremmelaar, E.F., & Bouma, A. (2007, Dec). Movement adaptations in 7- to 10-year-old typically developing children: Evidence for a transition in feedback-based motor control. *Human Movement Science, 26*(6), 927–942. http://dx.doi.org/10.1016/j.humov.2007.07.010 Medline:17904673

Williams, J., Thomas, P.R., Maruff, P., Butson, M., & Wilson, P.H. (2006). Motor, visual and egocentric transformations in children with Developmental Coordination Disorder. *Child: Care, Health and Development, 32*, 633–648. http://dx.doi.org/10.1111/j.1365-2214.2006.00688.x Medline:17018040

Williams, J., Thomas, P.R., Maruff, P., & Wilson, P.H. (2008). The link between motor impairment level and motor imagery ability in children with developmental coordination disorder. *Human Movement Science, 27*, 270–285. http://dx.doi.org/10.1016/j.humov.2008.02.008 Medline:18384899

Wilson, P.H. (2005, Aug). Practitioner review: Approaches to assessment and treatment of children with DCD. An evaluative review. *Journal of Child Psychology and Psychiatry, and Allied Disciplines, 46*(8), 806–823. http://dx.doi.org/10.1111/j.1469-7610.2005.01409.x Medline:16033630

Wilson, P.H., Ruddock, S., Smits-Engelsman, B., Polatajko, H., & Blank, R. (2013, Mar). Understanding performance deficits in developmental coordination disorder: A meta-analysis of recent research. *Developmental*

Medicine and Child Neurology, 55(3), 217–228. http://dx.doi.org/10.1111/
j.1469-8749.2012.04436.x Medline:23106668

Wilson, P.H., & Maruff, P. (1999). Deficits in the endogenous control of
covert visuospatial attention in children with developmental coordination
disorder. *Human Movement Science, 18*, 421–442. http://dx.doi.org/10.1016/
S0167-9457(99)00017-2

Wilson, P.H., Maruff, P., & McKenzie, B.E. (1997). Covert orienting
of attention in children with developmental coordination disorder.
Developmental Medicine and Child Neurology, 39, 736–745. http://dx.doi.
org/10.1111/j.1469-8749.1997.tb07375.x Medline:9393887

Wilson, P.H., Maruff, P., Williams, J., Lum, J.A., & Thomas, P.R. (2004).
Impairments in the internal representation of movement in children with
developmental coordination disorder: Evidence from a mental rotation
task. *Developmental Medicine and Child Neurology, 46*, 754–759. http://dx.doi.
org/10.1111/j.1469-8749.2004.tb00995.x Medline:15540636

Wilson, P.H., Thomas, P.R., & Maruff, P. (2002, Jul). Motor imagery training
ameliorates motor clumsiness in children. *Journal of Child Neurology, 17*(7),
491–498. http://dx.doi.org/10.1177/088307380201700704 Medline:12269727

Wilson, P.H., Thomas, P.R., & Maruff, P. (2005). *Motor imagery training
ameliorates motor clumsiness in children: A replication study.* Paper presented
at the 7th Motor Control and Human Skill Conference, Fremantle, Australia
3–6 February 2005.

Wolpert, D.M. (1997, Sep). Computational approaches to motor control.
Trends in Cognitive Sciences, 1(6), 209–216. http://dx.doi.org/10.1016/S1364-
6613(97)01070-X Medline:21223909

Wolpert, D.M., Ghahramani, Z., & Flanagan, J.R. (2001, Nov 1). Perspectives
and problems in motor learning. *Trends in Cognitive Sciences, 5*(11), 487–494.
http://dx.doi.org/10.1016/S1364-6613(00)01773-3 Medline:11684481

SECTION THREE

Identification and Methodological Challenges

6 Screening for Developmental Coordination Disorder in School-Age Children

MARINA M. SCHOEMAKER AND BRENDA N. WILSON

Considering the nature of the primary motor problems of children with developmental coordination disorder (DCD) and the consequences of these problems for daily life functioning, it is beyond doubt that early identification of these children is important in order to provide timely intervention. Indeed, as many chapters in this edited collection highlight, the potential secondary consequences, in regard to physical, emotional, and social well-being are pervasive and troubling (see Chapters 2, 3, and 4 in particular). However, although the prevalence of 5% to 6% for DCD reported in the DSM-IV-TR (APA, 2000) implies the presence of at least one child with DCD in every classroom, DCD is still relatively unrecognized. Lack of awareness of the disorder interferes with identification and intervention (Missiuna, Gaines, & Soucie, 2006a; Wilson, Neil, Kamps, & Babcock, 2013). In addition, if parents seek help for the motor impairments of their child, they are often told that the child will grow out of them (Stephenson & Chesson, 2008). In order to provide children with DCD with the timely help they need, early identification is recommended.

The Importance of Screening for DCD

Screening for DCD is usually an important first step in identification of the disorder. Screening involves sorting those children who *probably have* DCD from those who *probably do not*. Then, those positively screened should be referred for further assessment to confirm the diagnosis, preferably with a "gold standard" test. From a cost-efficient health care perspective, the initial screening should be as accurate as possible to avoid referring children without the disorder or to avoid missing children with the disorder, who consequently may develop more severe deficits or comorbid impairments. Recently, several measurement instruments in the form of questionnaires that focus on identification of DCD have been developed and can be used as screening tools. In this chapter, an overview will be given of these measurement instruments and of their accuracy for identifying children with DCD. In addition, some methodological problems surrounding screening of motor coordination problems will be discussed.

Measuring Instruments Developed for Screening

In order to classify a child as DCD, the four diagnostic criteria outlined in the DSM-IV-TR have to be met. The first two inclusion criteria stress that performance in daily life activities that requires motor coordination should be affected (Criterion A) and that the disorder should significantly interfere with academic achievement or activities of daily living (ADL; Criterion B). To ascertain whether criterion A has been met, the administration of a standardized motor test is recommended in both the Leeds Consensus Statement (Sugden, Chambers, & Utley, 2006) and in the European Guideline for DCD (Blank, Smits-Engelsman, Polatajko, & Wilson, 2012). However, the administration of a motor test is time consuming, often costly, and not suitable for screening large numbers of children. As a consequence, questionnaires have been proposed as a first step in the identification process for children with DCD, as they are relatively inexpensive, fast, and easy to administer. Furthermore, questionnaires offer valuable information about the performance of motor skills within the child's daily environment, an important factor given that problems with performance of ADL are central to both criteria. In addition, questionnaires have the advantage of taking into account performance across a longer period of time.

A disadvantage of questionnaires, however, is that they are more subjective. The rating on a questionnaire depends to a large extent on the ability of the observer to judge differences in motor performance between children, which in turn is dependent on the rater's knowledge of motor skills and the child, as well as personal characteristics, such as socioeconomic status or personal well-being. Several questionnaires, outlined here, have been developed that take into account the perception of the teacher, or the parent, or the child and that can been used to screen for DCD. Although work is being done to develop screening tools for preschool children who are at risk of being diagnosed as DCD at school age (Rihtman, Wilson, & Parush, 2011) only those questionnaires that can be used from 5 years of age onward will be discussed, as it is recommended not to diagnose DCD before that age (Blank et al., 2012). There are also new self-report questionnaires being developed for adolescents and young adults (Kirby, Edwards, Sugden, & Rosenblum, 2010; Saban, Ornoy, Grotto, & Parush, 2012), but this chapter will focus on those for children between the ages of 5 and 16 years.

Teachers have a unique opportunity to observe and compare children of different ages during school breaks and academic activities. Yet Larkin and Rose (2005) report that the results regarding the accuracy of teacher's perceptions of motor ability have led to mixed results (Gubbay, 1975; Henderson & Hall, 1982; Morris & Whiting, 1971; Revie & Larkin, 1993). The ability of teachers to accurately identify children with DCD seems to be enhanced when they are provided with relevant information about the disorder (Henderson & Hall, 1982). Recently, four teacher-based questionnaires have been developed specifically for, or are being used for, identification of school-age children with DCD: (1) Checklist of the Movement Assessment Battery for Children-Second Edition (MABC-2; Henderson & Sugden, 1992; Henderson, Sugden, & Barnett, 2007), (2) Teacher Estimation of Activity Form (TEAF; Faught & et al., 2008), (3) Children Activity Scales for Teachers (ChAS-T; Rosenblum; 2006), and (4) Motor Observation Questionnaire for Teacher (MOQ-T; Schoemaker, Flapper, Reinders-Messelink, & de Kloet, 2008).

The MABC Checklist provides an assessment of how a child performs everyday movement tasks at home or at school. The original MABC Checklist consisted of 48 items, divided over four sections. Recently, it has been revised and reduced to 30 items, divided over two sections (Henderson et al, 2007). The content of some of the items has been changed and includes skills related to self-care, classroom and physical education activities, and ball skill and recreation (Henderson et al., 2007). For each item, teachers have to rate the motor competence of a child on a four-point scale (0 = *very well*, 3 = *not close*).

The ChAS-T was developed in Israel to identify children at risk for DCD in the 4–8-year-old age range. The questionnaire contains 21 items relating to functional gross and fine motor skills, children's organization in time and space during the performance of ADL and self-care, mobility, ball skills, play activities, and academic activities (Rosenblum, 2006). Teachers rate the functional performance of the children on a five-point, adjectival scale (1 = *very well*, 5 = *less adequately*).

With the TEAF, developed in Canada (Hay, 1992), teachers assess their student's motor ability, participation in physical activity, and generalized self-efficacy towards physical activity (10 items). Six questions address the physical ability of a child during physical education, intramural sports, interschool sports, lunch periods and recess. The other four questions address the performance of a child during four hypothetical situations in which physical activity is required (completing an obstacle course, learning a new motor skill, trying out for school teams, and participation in very active games during recess). Teachers have to rate physical ability and performance of the children on a five-point scale (1 = *well below average*, 5 = *well above average*). Although developed as a population-based tool to measure physical activity, it has been successfully used to screen for DCD (Faught et al., 2008).

The MOQ-T is a revision of the Dutch Groningen Motor Observation Scale; the MOQ-T is developed to identify children with DCD between 5 and 11 years of age. The questionnaire contains 18 items divided over two subscales: general motor functioning and handwriting (Schoemaker et al., 2008). Nine out of 18 items ask the teacher to rate the quality of motor performance in general (clumsiness, lack of fluency, inadequate timing); the other nine items require rating of the performance of specific movement skills (ball skills, balance, handwriting). Each item is rated on a four-point scale (1 = *not at all true for this child*; 4 = *really true for this child*). The MOQ-T has been used for over two decades in the Netherlands and has recently been translated into English and Japanese.

Parents can also provide important information about functional motor performance at home (Wilson, Kaplan, Crawford, Campbell, & Dewey, 2000). In general, parents are able to accurately rate the behaviour of their child, regardless of differences in socioeconomic status, geographic location, or parental well-being, if presented with well-constructed, clear questions (Glascoe, 2000). Study of the ability of parents to rate motor performance of their children obtained less favourable results in older studies (Gubbay, 1975), compared to more promising results in recent studies (Hoare, 1991; Pless, Persson, Sundelin, & Carlsson, 2001; Missiuna et al., 2006c). In this later group of studies, parents were generally able to accurately identify motor problems in children with DCD (Pless et al., 2001; Missiuna et al., 2006c). Moreover, Green et al. (2005) found a strong relationship between parent report on the Developmental Coordination Disorder Questionnaire (DCDQ) and therapists' identification of the child having DCD or being at risk of having DCD, which suggests that parent report may be useful in the identification of DCD.

To date, only two parent questionnaires have been developed specifically for the identification of DCD. The Developmental Coordination Disorder Questionnaire (DCDQ) is a parent questionnaire developed in Canada to identify problems with everyday motor functioning at home, at play, and at school for children from 8 to 14.6 years of age (Wilson et al., 2000). The original questionnaire contained 17 items rating motor coordination, divided over four distinct subscales: control during movement, fine motor/handwriting, gross motor control/planning, and general coordination. Recently, the DCDQ has been revised, and the number of items has been reduced to 15 out of 17 of the original items, divided over three subscales: control during movement, fine motor/handwriting, and general coordination (Wilson et al., 2009). For each item, parents have to compare the degree of coordination of their child with other children of the same age, and to rate this on a five-point, adjectival scale (1 = *not at all like your child*; 5 = *extremely like your child*). The DCDQ-07 was found to be valid for use in children between 5.0 and 15.0 years of age.

The ChAS-P (Rosenblum, 2006) is the parent version of the ChAS-T and measures four, distinct aspects of motor performance: fine and gross motor performance, organization of motor performance in space and time, and ADL performance (primarily related to eating and dressing). In contrast to the ChAS-T, which includes 21 items, the ChAS-P includes 27 items, among them items measuring ADL performance, which were difficult for teachers to observe (Rosenblum, 2006). The rating scales for each item are the same as in the teacher version.

Some instruments have been developed that take into account the appraisal of the children themselves. The Children's Self-Perceptions of Adequacy in and Predilection for Physical Activity (CSAPPA) considers physical activities and has potential as a screening instrument (Hay, 1992). The CSAPPA was developed to measure children's perceived adequacy in physical activities (good at sports, good at physical education, good at active games) and their tendency to select a physical activity as opposed to a sedentary activity (predilection in physical activities; Hay, 1992). The CSAPPA includes 19 items, each item consisting of two statements. Children are asked to choose the statement that best describes them from each pair of statements and have to indicate whether the selected statement is either *sort of true for him/her* or *really true for him/her*. The CSAPPA can be used for children between 8 and 16 years of age. Before the age of 7 or 8 years, children may have unrealistically high perceptions (Nicholls & Miller, 1984), so self-reports of children younger than 8 years of age may not be reliable.

The Perceived Efficacy and Goal Setting System (PEGS) has been designed to help clinicians learn about the child's perception of their own competence and to involve children in goal setting during intervention (Missiuna, Pollock, Law, Walter, & Cavey, 2006c). It is a modification of the original "All About Me" instrument, and its pictorial format of 24 tasks depicting daily tasks makes it appropriate for children from 6 to 9 years of age. The child's rating of his or her performance as "more competently" or "less competently" is scored and can be summed. In a study of 117 children with a variety of developmental disabilities (53 who had DCD), the children's perceptions were compared to those of their parents and teachers on questionnaires accompanying this measure. Regardless of DCD status, children tended to rate themselves as more competent, when compared to adult raters and to a measure of school functioning. This instrument is reported to function best as a way to assist children to set goals for their therapy and demonstrates good clinical utility for that purpose, but further research is needed to determine its value in the identification of DCD. It is interesting that the lack of agreement between parent- and child-report found in this study has also been reported in studies examining other measures (Dunford, Missiuna, Street, & Sibert, 2005; Green & Wilson, 2008).

Sensitivity and Specificity of Questionnaires Developed for Screening

The utility of questionnaires to accurately identify children with motor difficulties needs to be established before they can be recommended for use in clinical practice or for population-based screening. An important aspect of a questionnaire is its sensitivity, or the ability of a questionnaire to identify true cases of DCD. In order to minimize over-referral, a screening test should also have adequate specificity, or the ability to correctly identify children without DCD. For a screening test in which early diagnosis is beneficial, and when it is more desirable to identify all those at risk for having DCD, high sensitivity is preferable to higher specificity (Schoemaker, Smits-Engelsman, & Jongmans, 2003). This is especially true for a condition such as DCD where the psychological consequences of a false positive (screened positive in the absence of a condition) may be less than for a condition that carries a risk of mortality (e.g., cancer).

In order to determine the sensitivity and specificity of a screening tool, the scores, or diagnostic results, of a questionnaire need to be compared to a gold standard. A gold standard is an instrument with which the presence of a condition (i.e., DCD) can be determined with 100% certainty. Unfortunately, no empirically determined gold standard test for DCD exists with which we can compare the outcome of a screening questionnaire (Tan, Parker, & Larkin, 2001). In the absence of a gold standard, a standardized motor test is used to test for DCD, such as the MABC (Henderson & Sugden, 1992; Henderson et al., 2007), the Bruininks Test of Motor Proficiency (BOTMP; Bruininks, 1978; Bruininks & Bruininks, 2005), or the McCarron Assessment of Neuromuscular Development (MAND; 1982). The American Psychological Association (APA, 1985) requires a sensitivity of 80% and a specificity of 90% in order for a screening tool to be acceptable. There is usually a trade-off between sensitivity and specificity. If one does not want to miss any children with the disorder using a screening instrument, a more lenient cut-off criterion will be chosen, resulting in high sensitivity. However, with a more lenient cut-off criterion, the number of children without the disorder will become smaller, resulting in lower specificity.

The sensitivity and specificity of different questionnaires obtained in population-based studies are listed in Table 6.1; Table 6.2 shows the results obtained in studies in which at least 50% of the children who were included had been referred to clinical practice for motor difficulties, or where children with developmental problems were included.

In population-based studies, the results regarding teacher-based questionnaires are mixed. The sensitivity of the MABC Checklist was poor, whereas the sensitivity of the TEAF reached the required standard. Specificity of the TEAF was too low, which implies that the TEAF leads to over-referral. In contrast, specificity of the MABC Checklist was good. However, one should acknowledge that the values for sensitivity with the TEAF were computed differently than were the same values for the MABC Checklist. A receiver-operator characteristics (ROC) curve analysis was performed and cut-off scores for the TEAF were chosen in such a way that sensitivity reached the required standard of 80%; then, values for specificity belonging to this cut-off point were determined. If specificity had been set at the required standard of 90%, sensitivity would have been much lower (41%; Faught et al., 2008), which is too low to allow recommendation of the TEAF for population screening.

In our view, high sensitivity is considered to be more important for population screening than high specificity. A screening tool should

Table 6.1. Overview of Results Obtained in Population-Based Studies for the Sensitivity and Specificity of Different Screening Questionnaires

Author	Questionnaire	"GoldStandard"	N(age range)	Population-Based Studies		r
				Sensitivity	Specificity	
Teacher-Based Questionnaires						
Junaid et al. (2000)	MABC Checklist	MABC	103(7.2–8.11)	14.3%	97.8%	.51
Faught et al. (2008)	TEAF	BOTMP-SF	502(9.0–11.11)	85%	46%	–
Schoemaker et al. (2012)	MABC-2 Checklist	MABC-2	383(5.0–8.11)	41%	88%	–.38
Parent-Based Questionnaires				Sensitivity	Specificity	
Schoemaker et al. (2006)	DCDQ[1]	MABC	322(4.0–12.0)	28.9%	88.6%	–.26
Civetta & Hillier (2008)	DCDQ[1]	MABC	18DCD+39TD(7.0–8.11)	72%	62%	–.39
Tseng et al. (2010)	DCDQ-07[2]	MABC + BOTMP	114(6.0–9.0)	73%	54%	–
Pannekoek et al. (2012)	DCDQ-07[2]	MABC-2	87(12.0–14.11)	85.7%	77.5%	.34
Loh et al. (2009)	DCDQ[1]	MAND	129(9.0–12.0)	55%	74%	
Child-Based Questionnaires				Sensitivity	Specificity	
Hay et al. (2004)	CSAPPA	BOTMP-SF	206(11.5)[3]	90% (♂)88% (♀)	89% (♂)75% (♀)	–
Cairney et al. (2007)	CSAPPA	BOTMP-SF	546(11.5)[3]	91%	53%	–

[1] 17-item version.
[2] 15-item version.
[3] Mean age (no age range provided).

function as a "coarse sieve" to identify all children with DCD, even though some children without DCD may be falsely identified. The potential damage of false-positives is minimized by confirmatory testing, and high sensitivity is generally preferred (Hay, Hawes, & Faught, 2004). However, at a certain level of specificity, low rates are not acceptable for cost-effectiveness. An example illustrates our point: Suppose the prevalence of a disorder is 15% in a sample of 1,000 children. If the sensitivity of a screening tool is 80% and the specificity is 50%, 580 children will be positively screened (120 true positives and 460 false positives). This situation is not very efficient, as too many children will need further assessment to confirm the diagnosis.

Of all screening tools, the DCDQ is by far the one that has been translated most often and attracted research interest across different countries. Although sensitivity and specificity of the DCDQ vary largely across the five population-based studies reported, neither of the values for sensitivity nor specificity reached the required standard (80% and 90% respectively) in four of the five studies reported, regardless of the age range included or the kind of motor test used as reference standard. Only the most recent study with adolescents demonstrated acceptable sensitivity, but not specificity, of the DCDQ. Consequently, use of the DCDQ for population-based screening cannot be recommended.

The results regarding sensitivity of the only child-based questionnaire, the CSAPPA, are promising to date, as they reached the required standard in both studies reported. The results regarding specificity are contradictory, however, as they were found to be acceptable in one study (Hay et al., 2004), but too low in another (e.g., Cairney et al., 2007). Further research regarding sensitivity and specificity of the CSAPPA is needed before any conclusions can be drawn about its usefulness as a tool for population-based screening. The studies that have been done were limited to Canada, so implementation of the CSAPPA in research projects outside Canada is recommended to demonstrate the applicability of this tool for identification of children with DCD in other countries.

In a recent, large population-based study, both the CSAPPA and DCDQ were combined as a first step in the identification process of children with DCD. For both measures, the 5th percentile was used as cut-off criterion in order to minimize the number of false positives. However, even with such conservative cut-offs, 29% of the children identified by either the CSAPPA or the DCDQ did not have motor impairment scores (below 15th percentile) on the MABC (Missiuna et al., 2011).

Recently, a large literature search was undertaken in order to develop the European Guideline for assessment and intervention for children with DCD (Blank et al., 2012). Present studies of DCD questionnaires suggest that the sensitivity is very low when applied in the general population, such as regular schools. Therefore, one of the conclusions of the guideline is that "the use of questionnaires (e. g. DCDQ, MABC-Checklist) is not recommended for population-based screening for DCD" (Blank et al., 2012, p. 69). This recommendation is supported by the data presented above, although more research is needed regarding the usefulness of the CSAPPA for population-based screening. In addition, the TEAF was evaluated in only one study. Further studies regarding the TEAF in other countries, possibly with different tests used as the reference standard, are warranted.

A summary of the results of questionnaires used with clinical populations is shown in Table 6.2. For teacher-based questionnaires, the required standard of 80% sensitivity was reached only with the MOQ-T. However, the specificity of this questionnaire was too low and resulted in too many false positives. The Children Activity Scales (ChAS) were not sensitive enough to detect children at risk for DCD, irrespective of whether the scales were filled out by teachers or parents. Specificity of the ChAS is good, however. But as the ability of a screening test to detect children at risk for DCD is considered to be most important in clinical samples, use of the ChAS cannot be recommended at present. Given that these results are based on one study with a small sample of a limited age range, more research is needed before firm conclusions can be drawn about the usefulness of the ChAS as a screening tool.

The results regarding the ability of parents to detect children at risk for DCD with the DCDQ were promising when the MABC was used as the criterion standard, irrespective of whether the 15 or 17 item version was used (Schoemaker at al., 2006; Wilson et al., 2009). Less favourable sensitivity of the DCDQ was reported in one of the four studies (Crawford, Wilson, & Dewey, 2001); the inclusion of children with various developmental disabilities and learning disabilities might have been responsible for these results. Specificity of the DCDQ is still slightly too low, although generally higher than specificity when used in population based studies. The DCDQ and the MABC-2 Checklist are the two questionnaires that have been recommended in the European Guideline for DCD (Blank et al., 2012, p. 69), in particular to assist in the assessment of Criterion B (impact on ADL and academic achievement).

Table 6.2. Overview of Results Obtained in Clinical Populations for the Sensitivity and Specificity of Different Screening Questionnaires.

Author	Questionnaire	"Gold Standard"	N(age range)	Clinical Studies		R
Teacher-Based Questionnaires				Sensitivity	Specificity	
Schoemaker et al. (2003)	Checklist MABC	MABC	64 suspect of DCD(6.0–9.0)	62%	66%	–
Rosenblum(2006)	ChAS-T	MABC	30 TD[1] + 30 DCD(5.0–6.6)	67%	93%	.75
Schoemaker et al. (2008)	MOQ-T	MABC	91 TD[1] + 91 DCD(5.0–11.0)	80.5%	62%	.57
Parent-Based Questionnaires				Sensitivity	Specificity	
Wilson et al. (2000)	DCDQ[3]	MABC+BOTMP	224 LD+ADHD/155 TD(8.0–18.0)	86.4% DCD	70.9%	
Crawford et al. (2001)	DCDQ[3]	BOTMP	70 TD' + 64 DCD(8.0–17.0)	38%	90%	–
Schoemaker et al. (2006)	DCDQ[3]	MABC	55DCD + 55 TD	81.6%	84%	–.65
Wilson et al. (2009)	DCDQ-07[4]	MABC	55 TD[1]+ 87 DP[2]+ 90 DCD(5.1–15.6)	85%	71%	–.55
Rosenblum(2006)	ChAS-P	MABC	30 TD[1] + 30 DCD(5.0–6.6)	50%	90%	.51

[1] TD = Typically developing children.
[2] DP = Children with developmental problems (incl. DCD) or learning problems.
[3] 17-item version.
[4] 15-item version.

Measuring Issues in Screening

It is important to interpret the results regarding sensitivity and specificity of the various screening tools with caution, due to many factors: the lack of a gold standard, the different functions of tests and questionnaires, the way children are classified as DCD by the cut-off score chosen, the subjectivity of parent and teacher report, and the combination and order of tests administered. These issues are discussed below.

The major issue in measurement and screening is the lack of an accepted gold standard for identifying DCD (Henderson & Barnett, 1998; Larkin & Rose, 2005). In contrast to intellectual ability, no general factor called "motor ability' exists. Motor behaviour covers a multitude of specific, independent motor abilities, whereas standardized motor tests used for identification of DCD include only a limited selection of motor skills. To complicate matters further, the impairments of children with DCD are heterogeneous in both nature and severity. Consequently, it is possible that screening questionnaires and standardized motor tests detect different groups of children because each instrument may assess different motor behaviour and skills. A specific test or questionnaire might be good at detecting only a particular subtype of DCD (Tan, Parker, & Larkin, 2001). Children with motor problems identified by questionnaires may not necessarily have low scores on a motor test if the type of motor problem of a child is restricted to specific motor abilities not addressed by that test. Ideally, an instrument used as a gold standard for DCD should cover the whole range of motor problems that children with DCD might have. At present, however, no such instrument has been developed. Therefore, it is hardly surprising that the results regarding sensitivity and specificity of the screening questionnaires compared to standardized assessments are disappointing, at least when used for population-based screening.

An additional issue relates to how motor tests are administered in standardized situations, providing a "snap shot" of the child's performance, and usually consisting of tasks rarely part of children's everyday life (Netelenbos, 2005). This implies that the performance of motor tests does not need to reflect the child's home and school activities or ADL. A motor test measures capacity (the capacity to perform an activity in a standardized situation), whereas questionnaires represent capability (or what an individual can do in his or her natural environment; Civetta & Hillier, 2008; Holsbeeke, Ketelaar, Schoemaker, & Gorter, 2009). A child's capability may not necessarily be reflected by a child's capacity. According to Netelenbos (2005), it is likely that motor tests measuring functional activities in daily situations will result in higher correlations with teachers' or parents' ratings than the usual motor tests that measure underlying motor abilities with no obvious relation to daily activities. However, to date no tests measuring ADL have been developed for children with DCD.

In the majority of the questionnaires developed for screening purposes, parents and teachers are asked to rate the performance of a child on a specific motor skill. According to Faught et al. (2008), teachers and parents may find it easier to complete a screening instrument measuring the general aptitude for physical ability, than an instrument measuring specific motor skills. It would be interesting to design a concurrent validity study to investigate whether this theory is supported, by comparing an instrument measuring general aptitude for physical ability (such as the TEAF) with an instrument rating performance in specific motor skills (such as the MABC-2 Checklist). If the statement is supported, further development of screening instruments could take this finding into consideration.

Another factor affecting measurement in screening is that the classification of DCD in population-based studies investigating the accuracy of screening questionnaires is based upon the results of one standardized test only. However, performance on a motor test may be influenced by performance variables, such as anxiety, fatigue, or lack of motivation. Hence, a child who fails on a motor test does not necessarily have DCD. Likewise, a child may pass the test, but the child's movement quality is awkward and lacking in fluency (Civetta & Hillier, 2008). According to Henderson, Sugden, and Barnett (2007), performance on a single test should never be used in isolation to classify a child as DCD because the score reflects only the performance level attained at that given point in time. Application of all four DSM-IV diagnostic criteria is required to make a proper diagnosis of DCD. The accuracy of screening questionnaires to classify children as DCD or not DCD is enhanced if all the diagnostic criteria are applied. This was the case in the study by Schoemaker et al. (2006) regarding the DCDQ, in which sensitivity reached 81.6% and specificity approached 84%, the required standard (APA, 2000). However, the use of multiple tests for diagnosis can create other problems, as the error across different tests is compounded, placing limits on the ability to detect cases (see Chapter 7 for a discussion of this point).

The sometimes disappointing results regarding sensitivity and specificity of questionnaires are, of course, due to other factors. For example, the subjective nature of questionnaires also contributes to measurement error. In the case of teachers, they are not necessarily educated in observing and rating motor behaviour. In addition, they may not always have sufficient opportunities to observe the motor performance of their pupils. Piek and Edwards (1997), for instance, demonstrated that the ability of teachers to evaluate motor performance depends on whether they take the children for physical education. In their study, physical education teachers were able to identify 49% of the children with motor problems, whereas classroom teachers identified only 25%. Another factor affecting the ability of teachers to notice children with motor problems is the presence of comorbidity. Teachers appeared to report concern about motor difficulties more often when nondisruptive behaviours were present (Rivard, Missiuna, Hanna, & Wishart, 2007), but did not notice children with motor problems when disruptive classroom behaviour was present.

Similarly to teachers, parents may differ in their ability to rate the motor behaviour of their children. Some parents have very accurate perceptions of normal child development and their child's level of motor performance, whereas others have little understanding of their child's motor difficulties (Larkin & Rose, 2005). Another factor is whether they regularly observe their child in play or organized motor activities. Whether parents are reluctant to have "labels" applied to their child, compared to whether they are hoping to get a diagnosis and support for their child, will also influence how they report. The age of the child and whether the parents have been searching for help for a period of time might also influence their rating. Last, many clinicians believe that mothers and fathers will have different perspectives on how their child's performance compares to other children's and that, ideally, the report of both parents should be solicited. This has been observed in other assessments of child behaviour where fathers rate their children as having more problems than are identified by mothers (Davé, Nazareth, Senior, & Sherr, 2008).

The subjective nature of questionnaires is further illustrated by the finding that parents' and teachers' opinions regarding motor ability often differ from one another (Junaid, Harris, Fulmer, & Carswell, 2000). It is unclear whether the poor agreement is due to differences between parents and teachers in their ability to rate motor behaviour, or to differences in motor behaviour of the children as a function of different demands in either school or home settings, or to other sources of bias. But this lack of agreement is also seen in the low agreement between parents and teachers in reporting child behaviour (Grietens et al., 2004), especially between mothers and teachers.

Finally, the degree to which a questionnaire can discriminate children with DCD from those without the condition also depends on the cut-off score used for classification. Although much has been written (Geuze, Jongmans, Schoemaker, & Smits-Engelsman, 2001), there is still debate around which cut-off score of a measuring instrument is most appropriate for identification of DCD, the 5th or the 15th percentile. The DSM-IV criteria do not specify a cut-off point for motor impairment in DCD. In the absence of a demonstrable underlying medical condition, abnormality is mainly defined on statistical grounds: The diagnosis DCD is made if scores on a test exceed a certain criterion. If this criterion is too lenient, there is a risk for medical overconsumption, but if the criterion is too strict, cases with the disorder might be missed. In the medical tradition, often the 5th percentile is applied as a uniform cut-off criterion. In this situation, one implicitly assumes that prevalence is equal across various medical conditions. If motor ability is treated as a diagnostic characteristic, which follows a normal distribution, the decision as to which value will be considered abnormal is rather arbitrary.

So far, both cut-off criteria have been applied in clinical and experimental studies. Some authors encourage the use of the 15th percentile cut-off score based on clinical experience (Geuze et al., 2001; Larkin & Rose, 2005), whereas others argue against defining 15% of a population as abnormal because doing so may lead to medical overconsumption (Baxter, 2006). In 2006, a group of professionals from a wide range of disciplines reached consensus about the condition DCD, and the 5th percentile was recommended as the cut-off criterion for Criterion A in the Leeds Consensus Statement (Sugden et al., 2006). However, to complicate matters further, the 15th percentile has recently been recommended as the cut-off criterion in the European Guideline for DCD (Blank et al., 2012). One of the reasons to change to the 15th percentile as the cut-off criterion is the acknowledgment that any measuring instrument has some degree of measurement error, and it may be more appropriate to err on the side of a child possibly having DCD. It is clear that the issue of the cut-off criteria is an ongoing discussion and needs to be based upon current knowledge and research findings.

Multiple Assessment Procedure

It is clear that none of the questionnaires used for screening have sufficient sensitivity or specificity for population-based screening, and only the DCDQ'07 can be recommended for screening in populations at risk for DCD. In addition, there is not one standardized motor test that will suffice as a gold standard for the classification of DCD. For that reason, several authors have advocated a multiple assessment procedure for identification of children with DCD (Larkin & Rose, 2005; Schoemaker et al., 2008; Wright & Sugden, 1996). As recommended in the European Guideline for DCD, assessment that includes the administration of a standardized motor test should also take ADL into consideration (e.g. self-care and self-maintenance, academic and school productivity, prevocational and vocational activities, and leisure and play) and the views of the child, parents, teachers, and relevant others. As reported previously by Wright and Sugden (1996), and most recently by Missiuna et al. (2011a), if the functional impact of motor problems identified by parent or teacher report is taken into account using a multiple assessment procedure, the prevalence of DCD will significantly decrease. Use of a more lenient cut-off criteria (i.e., the 15th percentile) for all measuring instruments could reduce this effect, although there is a statistical explanation for this phenomenon that has to do with compounded errors rates across different tools (see Chapter 7 in this volume).

A multiple assessment process can also increase the validity of the assessment process while allowing us to assess the degree to which any one test increases our ability to predict DCD when that test is used in combination with other tests. Haynes and Lench (2003) define this as "incremental validity," or "the degree to which a measure explains or predicts a phenomenon of interest, relative to other measures" (p. 456). A measure is considered to have incremental validity when it increases the ability to predict the condition when used in combination with other tests. Therefore, incremental validity supplements, rather than replaces, traditional examinations of validity, including sensitivity, specificity, and predictive validity. This kind of validity may vary for several reasons. Using identification of DCD as an example, validity varies as a function of (1) the goals of assessment, whether for diagnosis of a condition, measurement of change over time, or evaluation of functional performance; (2) the order in which the different measures are given and whether meeting Criterion A or B is established first; (3) the criterion measures selected for comparison, especially when no gold standard exists; and (4) whether the target population being evaluated is population based or clinically referred (Haynes & Lench, 2003). This type of evaluation of each test, in relationship to each other, is essential for the cost-effective identification of DCD. The field of study of DCD may have reached a point in time when research can be designed to systematically vary the collection of assessment data for two or more randomly assigned groups of children in order to assess the accuracy of identification at each point of data collection (Hunsley & Meyer, 2003). Alternatively, a within-subject design could be used to examine clinicians' decisions when progressively more assessment data on a child are collected.

Conclusion

To date, several questionnaires have been developed that can assist in the identification of children with DCD. As reported here, they are not sensitive enough to be recommended for screening of DCD in the general population, although some hold promise in clinical diagnosis. However, present research findings regarding sensitivity and specificity of screening tools should be interpreted with caution due to the many methodological problems discussed above.

Notwithstanding some limitations with these measures, the questionnaires do provide important information about functional motor abilities of the children at home or at school. In addition to formal assessment with a standardized motor test, questionnaires can complement the identification process to ascertain that Criterion B of the diagnostic criteria has been met. Future research should be directed at investigating whether the accuracy of identification can be enhanced by combining several assessment tools, and in what manner this combination might be most effective.

REFERENCES

American Psychiatric Association. (2000). *DSM-IV-TR. Diagnostic and statistical manual of mental disorders* (4th ed., text rev.). Washington, DC: Author.
American Psychological Association. (1985). *Standards for educational and psychological tests*. Washington, DC: Author.
Baxter, P. (2006, Nov). Normality and abnormality. *Developmental Medicine and Child Neurology, 48*(11), 867. http://dx.doi.org/10.1017/S0012162206001885 Medline:17094217
Blank, R., Smits-Engelsman, B., Polatajko, H., & Wilson, P., & European Academy of Childhood Disability. (2012, Jan). European Academy of Childhood Disability (EACD): Recommendations on the definition,

diagnosis and intervention of developmental coordination disorder (long version). *Developmental Medicine and Child Neurology, 54*(1), 54–93. http://dx.doi.org/10.1111/j.1469-8749.2011.04171.x Medline:22171930

Bruininks, R.H. (1978). *Bruininks-Oseretsky Test of Motor Proficiency: Examiner's manual*. Circle Pines, MN: American Guidance Service.

Bruininks, R.H., & Bruininks, B.D. (2005). *Bruininks-Oseretsky Test of Motor Proficiency* (2nd ed.). Easel, TX: AGS Publishing.

Cairney, J., Veldhuizen, S., Kurdyak, P., Missiuna, C., Faught, B.E., & Hay, J. (2007, Nov). Evaluating the CSAPPA subscales as potential screening instruments for developmental coordination disorder. *Archives of Disease in Childhood, 92*(11), 987–991. http://dx.doi.org/10.1136/adc.2006.115097 Medline:17573409

Civetta, L.R., & Hillier, S.L. (2008, Spring). The developmental coordination disorder questionnaire and movement assessment battery for children as a diagnostic method in Australian children. *Pediatric Physical Therapy, 20*(1), 39–46. http://dx.doi.org/10.1097/PEP.0b013e31815ccaeb Medline:18300932

Crawford, S.G., Wilson, B.N., & Dewey, D. (2001). Identifying developmental coordination disorder: Consistency between tests. *Physical & Occupational Therapy in Pediatrics, 20*(2-3), 29–50. http://dx.doi.org/10.1080/J006v20n02_03 Medline:11345510

Davé, S., Nazareth, I., Senior, R., & Sherr, L. (2008, Dec). A comparison of father and mother report of child behaviour on the Strengths and Difficulties Questionnaire. *Child Psychiatry and Human Development, 39*(4), 399–413. http://dx.doi.org/10.1007/s10578-008-0097-6 Medline:18266104

Dunford, C., Missiuna, C., Street, E.C., & Sibert, J.R. (2005). Children's perceptions of the impact of developmental coordination disorder on activities of daily living. *British Journal of Occupational Therapy, 68*, 207–214.

Faught, B.E., Cairney, J., Hay, J., Veldhuizen, S., Missiuna, C., & Spironello, C.A. (2008, Apr). Screening for motor coordination challenges in children using teacher ratings of physical ability and activity. *Human Movement Science, 27*(2), 177–189. http://dx.doi.org/10.1016/j.humov.2008.02.001 Medline:18343517

Geuze, R.H., Jongmans, M.J., Schoemaker, M.M., & Smits-Engelsman, B.C.M. (2001, Mar). Clinical and research diagnostic criteria for developmental coordination disorder: A review and discussion. *Human Movement Science, 20*(1-2), 7–47. http://dx.doi.org/10.1016/S0167-9457(01)00027-6 Medline:11471398

Glascoe, F.P. (2000, Mar). Evidence-based approach to developmental and behavioural surveillance using parents' concerns. *Child: Care, Health and Development, 26*(2), 137–149. http://dx.doi.org/10.1046/j.1365-2214.2000.00173.x Medline:10759753

Green, D., Bishop, T., Wilson, B.N., Crawford, S., Hooper, R., Kaplan, B., & Baird, G. (2005). Is questionnaire-based screening part of the solution to waiting lists for children with developmental coordination disorder? *British Journal of Occupational Therapy, 68,* 2–10.

Green, D., & Wilson, B.N. (2008, Oct). The importance of parent and child opinion in detecting change in movement capabilities. *Canadian Journal of Occupational Therapy, 75*(4), 208–219. http://dx.doi.org/10.1177/000841740807500407 Medline:18975667

Grietens, H., Onghena, P., Prinzie, P., Gadeyne, E., Van Assche, V., Ghesquière, P., & Hellinckx, W. (2004). Comparison of mothers', fathers' and teachers' reports on problem behaviour in 5- to 6- year old children. *Journal of Psychopathology and Behavioral Assessment, 26*(2), 137–146. http://dx.doi.org/10.1023/B:JOBA.0000013661.14995.59

Gubbay, S.S. (1975). *The clumsy child.* London, England: Saunders & Co.

Hay, J. (1992). Adequacy in and predilection for physical activity in children. *Clinical Journal of Sport Medicine, 2*(3), 192–201. http://dx.doi.org/10.1097/00042752-199207000-00007

Hay, J.A., Hawes, R., & Faught, B.E. (2004, Apr). Evaluation of a screening instrument for developmental coordination disorder. *Journal of Adolescent Health, 34*(4), 308–313. http://dx.doi.org/10.1016/j.jadohealth.2003.07.004 Medline:15041000

Haynes, S.N., & Lench, H.C. (2003, Dec). Incremental validity of new clinical assessment measures. *Psychological Assessment, 15*(4), 456–466. http://dx.doi.org/10.1037/1040-3590.15.4.456 Medline:14692842

Henderson, S.E., & Barnett, A.L. (1998). The classification of specific motor coordination disorders in children: Some problems to be solved. *Human Movement Science, 17*(4-5), 449–469. http://dx.doi.org/10.1016/S0167-9457(98)00009-8

Henderson, S.E., & Hall, D. (1982, Aug). Concomitants of clumsiness in young schoolchildren. *Developmental Medicine and Child Neurology, 24*(4), 448–460. Medline:7117703

Henderson, S.E., & Sugden, D.A. (1992). *The Movement Assessment Battery for Children.* San Antonio, TX: Psychological Corporation.

Henderson, S.E., Sugden, D.A., & Barnett, A.L. (2007). *Movement Assessment Battery for Children-2 examiner's manual.* London, England: Harcourt Assessment.

Hoare, D. (1991). *Classification of movements dysfunctions in children: Descriptive and statistical approaches* (Unpublished doctoral thesis). University of Western Australia, Nedlands, W. Australia.

Holsbeeke, L., Ketelaar, M., Schoemaker, M.M., & Gorter, J.W. (2009, May). Capacity, capability, and performance: Different constructs or three of a kind? *Archives of Physical Medicine and Rehabilitation, 90*(5), 849–855. http://dx.doi. org/10.1016/j.apmr.2008.11.015 Medline:19406307

Hunsley, J., & Meyer, G.J. (2003, Dec). The incremental validity of psychological testing and assessment: Conceptual, methodological, and statistical issues. *Psychological Assessment, 15*(4), 446–455. http://dx.doi. org/10.1037/1040-3590.15.4.446 Medline:14692841

Junaid, K., Harris, S.R., Fulmer, K.A., & Carswell, A. (2000, Winter). Teachers' use of the MABC Checklist to identify children with motor coordination difficulties. *Pediatric Physical Therapy, 12*(4), 158–163. http://dx.doi. org/10.1097/00001577-200001240-00003 Medline:17091027

Kirby, A., Edwards, L., Sugden, D., & Rosenblum, S. (2010, Jan-Feb). The development and standardization of the Adult Developmental Co-ordination Disorders/Dyspraxia Checklist (ADC). *Research in Developmental Disabilities, 31*(1), 131–139. http://dx.doi.org/10.1016/j.ridd.2009.08.010 Medline:19819107

Larkin, D., & Rose, E. (2005). Assessment of developmental coordination disorder. In D.A. Sugden & M.E. Chambers (Eds.), *Children with developmental coordination disorder* (pp. 135–154). London, England: Whurr Publishers.

Loh, P.R., Piek, J.P., & Barrett, N.C. (2009, Jan). The use of the Developmental Coordination Disorder Questionnaire in Australian children. *Adapted Physical Activity Quarterly; APAQ, 26*(1), 38–53. Medline:19246772

Missiuna, C., Cairney, J., Pollock, N., Russell, D., Macdonald, K., Cousins, M., … Schmidt, L. (2011, Mar-Apr). A staged approach for identifying children with developmental coordination disorder from the population. *Research in Developmental Disabilities, 32*(2), 549–559. http://dx.doi.org/10.1016/j. ridd.2010.12.025 Medline:21216564

Missiuna, C., Gaines, R., & Soucie, H. (2006a, Aug 29). Why every office needs a tennis ball: A new approach to assessing the clumsy child. *Canadian Medical Association Journal, 175*(5), 471–473. http://dx.doi.org/10.1503/ cmaj.051202 Medline:16940261

Missiuna, C., Moll, S., Law, M., King, S., & King, G. (2006b, Feb). Mysteries and mazes: Parents' experiences of children with developmental coordination disorder. *Canadian Journal of Occupational Therapy, 73*(1), 7–17. Medline:16570837

Missiuna, C., Pollock, N., Law, M., Walter, S., & Cavey, N. (2006c, Mar-Apr). Examination of the Perceived Efficacy and Goal Setting System (PEGS) with children with disabilities, their parents, and teachers. *American Journal of Occupational Therapy., 60*(2), 204–214. http://dx.doi.org/10.5014/ajot.60.2.204 Medline:16596924

Morris, P.R., & Whiting, H.T.A. (1971). *Motor impairment and compensatory education*. London, England: G. Bell & Sons.

Netelenbos, J.B. (2005, Feb). Teachers' ratings of gross motor skills suffer from low concurrent validity. *Human Movement Science, 24*(1), 116–137. http://dx.doi.org/10.1016/j.humov.2005.02.001 Medline:15949584

Nicholls, J.G., & Miller, A.T. (1984). Development and its discontents: The differentiation of the concept of ability. In J.G. Nicholls (Ed.), *Advances in motivation and achievement: Vol. 3. The development of achievement motivation* (pp. 185–218). Greenwich, CT: JAI.

Pannekoek, L., Rigoli, D., Piek, J.P., Barrett, N.C., & Schoemaker, M. (2012, Jan). The revised DCDQ: Is it a suitable screening measure for motor difficulties in adolescents? *Adapted Physical Activity Quarterly; APAQ, 29*(1), 81–97. Medline:22190054

Piek, J.P., & Edwards, K. (1997, Mar). The identification of children with developmental coordination disorder by class and physical education teachers. *British Journal of Educational Psychology, 67*(1), 55–67. http://dx.doi.org/10.1111/j.2044-8279.1997.tb01227.x Medline:9114732

Pless, M., Persson, K., Sundelin, C., & Carlsson, M. (2001). Children with developmental co-ordination disorder: A qualitative study of parents' descriptions. *Advances in Physiotherapy, 3*(3), 128–135. http://dx.doi.org/10.1080/140381901750475375

Revie, G., & Larkin, D. (1993). Looking at movement: Problems with teacher identification of poorly coordinated children. *ACHPER National Journal, 40*, 4–9.

Rihtman, T., Wilson, B.N., & Parush, S. (2011). Development of the Little Developmental Coordination Disorder Questionnaire for preschoolers and preliminary evidence of its psychometric properties in Israel. Research in Developmental Disabilities, 32, 1378-1387.

Rivard, L.M., Missiuna, C., Hanna, S., & Wishart, L. (2007, Sep). Understanding teachers' perceptions of the motor difficulties of children with developmental coordination disorder (DCD). *British Journal of Educational Psychology, 77*(3), 633–648. http://dx.doi.org/10.1348/000709906X159879 Medline:17908379

Rosenblum, S. (2006, Nov). The development and standardization of the Children Activity Scales (ChAS-P/T) for the early identification of children with developmental coordination disorders. *Child: Care, Health and Development, 32*(6), 619–632. http://dx.doi.org/10.1111/j.1365-2214.2006.00687.x Medline:17018039

Saban, M.T., Ornoy, A., Grotto, I., & Parush, S. (2012, Jul-Aug). Adolescents and Adults Coordination Questionnaire: Development and psychometric properties. *American Journal of Occupational Therapy, 66*(4), 406–413. http://dx.doi.org/10.5014/ajot.2012.003251 Medline:22742688

Schoemaker, M.M., Flapper, B.C.T., Reinders-Messelink, H.A., & de Kloet, A. (2008, Apr). Validity of the Motor Observation Questionnaire for Teachers as a screening instrument for children at risk for developmental coordination disorder. *Human Movement Science, 27*(2), 190–199. http:// dx.doi.org/10.1016/j.humov.2008.02.003 Medline:18346804

Schoemaker, M.M., Flapper, B., Verheij, N.P., Wilson, B.N., Reinders-Messelink, H.A., & de Kloet, A. (2006, Aug). Evaluation of the Developmental Coordination Disorder Questionnaire as a screening instrument. *Developmental Medicine and Child Neurology, 48*(8), 668–673. http://dx.doi.org/10.1017/S001216220600140X Medline:16836779

Schoemaker, M.M., Niemeijer, A.S., Flapper, B.C.T., & Smits-Engelsman, B.C. (2012, Apr). Validity and reliability of the Movement Assessment Battery for Children-2 Checklist for children with and without motor impairments. *Developmental Medicine and Child Neurology, 54*(4), 368–375. http://dx.doi. org/10.1111/j.1469-8749.2012.04226.x Medline:22320829

Schoemaker, M.M., Smits-Engelsman, B.C.M., & Jongmans, M.J. (2003). Psychometric properties of the Movement ABC Checklist as a screening instrument for children with developmental coordination disorder. *British Journal of Educational Psychology, 73*(3), 425–441. http://dx.doi. org/10.1348/000709903322275911 Medline:14672152

Stephenson, E.A., & Chesson, R.A. (2008, May). "Always the guiding hand": Parents' accounts of the long-term implications of developmental co-ordination disorder for their children and families. *Child: Care, Health and Development, 34*(3), 335–343. http://dx.doi.org/10.1111/j.1365-2214.2007.00805.x Medline:18410640

Sugden, D.A., Chambers, M., & Utley, A. (2006). *Leeds Consensus Statement: Developmental coordination disorder as a specific learning difficulty.* Leeds, England: University of Leeds. Retrieved from www.dcd-uk.org/consensus.html

Tan, S.K., Parker, H.E., & Larkin, D. (2001). Concurrent validity of motor tests used to identify children with motor impairment. *Adapted Physical Activity Quarterly; APAQ, 18*, 168–182.

Tseng, M.-H., Fu, C.-P., Wilson, B.N., & Hu, F.-C. (2010, Jan-Feb). Psychometric properties of a Chinese version of the Developmental Coordination Disorder Questionnaire in community-based children. *Research in Developmental Disabilities, 31*(1), 33–45. http://dx.doi. org/10.1016/j.ridd.2009.07.018 Medline:19709853

Wilson, B.N., Crawford, S.G., Green, D., Roberts, G., Aylott, A., & Kaplan, B.J. (2009). Psychometric properties of the revised Developmental Coordination Disorder Questionnaire. *Physical & Occupational Therapy in Pediatrics, 29*(2), 182–202. http://dx.doi.org/10.1080/01942630902784761 Medline:19401931

Wilson, B.N., Kaplan, B.J., Crawford, S.G., Campbell, A., & Dewey, D. (2000, Sep-Oct). Reliability and validity of a parent questionnaire on childhood motor skills. *American Journal of Occupational Therapy, 54*(5), 484–493. http://dx.doi.org/10.5014/ajot.54.5.484 Medline:11006808

Wilson, B.N., Neil, K., Kamps, P.H., & Babcock, S. (2013, Mar). Awareness and knowledge of developmental co-ordination disorder among physicians, teachers and parents. *Child: Care, Health and Development, 39*(2), 296–300. http://dx.doi.org/10.1111/j.1365-2214.2012.01403.x Medline:22823542

Wright, H.C., & Sugden, D.A. (1996, Dec). A two-step procedure for the identification of children with developmental co-ordination disorder in Singapore. *Developmental Medicine and Child Neurology, 38*(12), 1099–1105. http://dx.doi.org/10.1111/j.1469-8749.1996.tb15073.x Medline:8973295

7 Methodological Issues in Field-Based DCD Research: Case Identification and Study Design

SCOTT VELDHUIZEN AND JOHN CAIRNEY

Several authors in this book have already noted the importance of conducting community- or school-based research to increase our understanding of the consequences of DCD and to test interventions to improve the quality of life of children with this disorder. Longitudinal studies, in particular, can do much to illuminate the long-term effects of DCD. Previous chapters have discussed their importance for research on participation in physical activity (Chapter 2), on participation and health-related fitness (chapter three), and on mental health (Chapter 4). In this chapter, we consider the challenges associated with conducting field research of this kind on children with DCD.

Problems in Field-Based Research

DCD is a difficult condition to study. It can be hard to identify accurately, especially in research settings. There are no unique symptoms or laboratory findings; instead, DCD represents one end of a continuum of functioning. DCD is also usually identified in childhood, which adds several complications: Apart from the practical and ethical difficulties of conducting research on children, childhood is a time of rapid change and development, which can create methodological challenges unusual in research on adult populations.

The first problem faced by any study on DCD is that of finding a group of affected children. There are essentially two ways to do this. One is to recruit a sample of children from treatment centres or specialized programs. This provides a group of children who have been diagnosed with DCD by a specialist, which seems to solve the problem of case ascertainment at a stroke. Clinic-based research, however, has two significant drawbacks. First, it is difficult to obtain large samples. Second, the children seen are, arguably, not representative of the larger population of children with DCD. They are generally more likely to be male, while general population samples have shown a sex ratio closer to 1:1 (e.g., Cairney, Hay, Faught, Mandigo, & Flouris, 2005). They are also likely to be relatively severe cases, and often have comorbid conditions, particularly ADHD, and it is often these other conditions that are the principal focus of clinical care (Dewey, Kaplan, Crawford, & Wilson, 2002).

The alternative to recruiting from clinics is to screen children from the general population. This avoids a host of selection biases and makes it possible to obtain a sample of almost any size (within the limits of the available funding). It brings with it, though, serious difficulties of case identification and study planning.

These problems are the subject of this chapter. We consider, first, the issue of case identification. Specific screening instruments, and some of the methodological issues surrounding the screening process, are discussed in Chapter 6; here, we consider the more general issue of operationalizing DCD criteria, with a view towards study design. Next, we discuss a few issues associated with the design of field-based studies of DCD and argue for a greater focus on longitudinal studies.

Case Identification

As discussed in Chapter 1 of this book, the definition, and indeed the name, of DCD was long in a state of flux. Relatively recently, a consensus has been reached (Blank, Smits-Engelsman, Polatajko, & Wilson, 2012; Sugden, Chambers, & Utley, 2006), and the mainstream of research has begun to use the criteria set out in the *Diagnostic and Statistical Manual of Mental Disorders* (DSM-IV and, more recently, DSM-V) by the American Psychiatric Association (2000). Although the resulting focus on DCD as an independent disorder of motor functioning may have its drawbacks (including, perhaps, the relative neglect of its associations with other problems or deficits; see Chapter 1), having a relatively stable definition of the disorder simplifies matters considerably. Among other things, it means that independent studies can be compared with less concern that they have identified completely different disorders.

The DSM criteria are discussed elsewhere (see Chapter 1), but, in brief, they are concerned with A) motor functioning, B) interference with activities of daily living, C) early onset of symptoms, and D) differential diagnosis. Most research studies concern themselves primarily with A, as this criterion represents the core deficit in DCD. Criterion

B attempts to confirm that the motor deficit is actually problematic, that is, that functional impairment is present; Criterion C, that it is present from childhood (and not acquired); and Criterion D, that other conditions, such as poor eyesight or neurological disorders, are not more responsible for the poor motor functioning.

Any field-based research project faces the problem of translating diagnostic criteria into screening and assessment procedures that can be applied on a large scale. If we assume an acceptance of DSM-V criteria, there remains the issue of how to translate them into a field-based screening program. We will discuss these criteria one at a time.

Criterion A

The acquisition and execution of coordinated motor skills is substantially below that expected given the individual's chronological age and opportunity for skill learning and use.

Many diseases and disorders are identifiable from signs or symptoms that do not occur in most people and which are accepted as pathological (e.g., cancer, psychosis). Motor functioning, though – insofar as it can be thought of as a single trait or ability at all (see, e.g., Albaret & de Castelnau, 2007) – occurs on a continuum. Clearly pathological motor impairments shade into normal functioning. This is true of many disease states and does not, of course, threaten the validity or the usefulness of this identification. It does, though, raise the question of where the line between normal functioning and potential disorder ought to be drawn.

There are several validated instruments (see Albaret & de Castelnau, 2007, and Blank et al., 2012, for reviews) that can measure general motor functioning, as well as tools that have been more specifically designed to assess motor impairment. Often, these tests compare the subject's performance to population norms and provide an estimate of the percentile in which the subject falls. Test developers and existing research generally use the 5th or the 15th percentiles as cut-points,[1] with children falling below these levels regarded as having motor difficulties that may be consistent with DCD. The 5th percentile was originally chosen, in part, because of existing estimates that significant motor

---

1 Those readers familiar with the latest version of the Movement ABC (2nd ed.) will know that there is actually no 15th percentile score; the manual recommends, therefore, use of the 16th.

coordination problems affected roughly 5% of the population. This approach makes measurement of prevalence a rather circular exercise, but is similar to definitions of other developmental conditions, in which some part of the tail of the population distribution is judged to represent people with meaningful deficits. The Leeds Consensus (Sugden et al., 2006), while recognizing the arbitrariness of this cut-point, recommends it "as being both reasonable and part of custom and practice in both clinical and research settings." The 15th percentile is also popular (see Geuze, Jongmans, Schoemaker, & Smits-Engelsman, 2001), however, because milder levels of impairment are often also of interest – and, of course, because identifying only one case of every 20 children screened can oblige researchers to recruit impractically large numbers of subjects.

SUGGESTIONS FOR CRITERION A

There are a number of important nuances in the assessment of motor skills and the identification of DCD. Many of these can be addressed only by using skilled assessors. Significant training and experience are necessary for the correct use of some instruments in any case, however. Many studies employ occupational therapists or other clinicians for this purpose (e.g., Missiuna et al., 2011). The judgment of such professionals is valuable, particularly if they are asked to note other conditions or circumstances that may be interfering with test performance.

It is also important, obviously, to have a research protocol that allows further investigation of issues raised, and a process for diagnosis that allows them to be taken into account. If the study protocol says that a child who fails certain motor tasks and shows signs of impairment has DCD, it will be difficult to know what to do with a note to the effect that some other problem seemed to be interfering with the assessment. The optimal approach should thus provide enough flexibility to take advantage of the skills of the assessors while remaining careful that different assessors are consistent in their approach. For larger studies, this may require monitoring of inter-rater reliability. It is important to note that reliability remains a concern when expert assessors are employed; time and effort in training and assessing are still required, just as they are with non-clinical assessors.

Beyond that, the important question in field-based research concerns the choice of instrument. To the discussions of this question elsewhere in this book, we would only add that the Movement-ABC has become a near-standard because of its apparently good accuracy, its flexibility, and its ability to incorporate professional judgment (Blank et al., 2012).

Criterion B

The motor skills deficit in Criterion A significantly and persistently
interferes with activities of daily living appropriate to chronological
age (e.g., self-care and self-maintenance) and impacts academic/school
productivity, prevocational and vocational activities, leisure, and play.

Criterion B addresses the problem of dividing disorder from mere poor
functioning. It requires interference with activities – some substantial
practical impact of poor motor functioning. This criterion is useful
clinically, and criteria like it occur throughout DSM (American Psychiatric Association, 2013), reminding clinicians to consider distress and
impairment when deciding whether a diagnosis is appropriate.

Unfortunately, this crucial criterion is quite difficult to translate into
field-based research because it requires a meaningful assessment of
each child's overall level of functioning. Unlike motor coordination
itself, this cannot be measured directly by a clinician or interviewer
who does not know the child well. Instead, it becomes necessary to
draw on the judgment and experience of teachers, parents, and the children themselves. Instruments such as the Developmental Coordination
Disorder Questionnaire (DCD-Q) (Wilson, Kaplan, Crawford, Campbell, & Dewey, 2000), the Teachers' Estimation of Activity Form (TEAF;
Faught et al., 2008), the Children's Self-Perceptions of Adequacy in and
Predilection for Physical Activity (CSAPPA) interview (Hay, Hawes, &
Faught, 2004), and the Movement-ABC checklist (Schoemaker, Smits-
Engelsman, & Jongmans, 2003) try to determine whether children have
experienced problems in active play or in activities of daily life. These
instruments, however, have typically been used for screening purposes,
rather than as part of an evaluation of impairment. The Leeds Consensus suggests an examination of handwriting skills, as this is important
for academic achievement, and some studies have also included assessments of problems with activities of daily living (ADL; Lingam, Hunt,
Golding, Jongmans, & Emond, 2009).

SUGGESTIONS FOR CRITERION B

Some studies have opted not to assess impairment (e.g., Cairney et al.,
2010a; Skinner & Piek, 2001); they have restricted themselves to a condition we might call *apparently poor motor functioning*. In some circumstances, this is acceptable. There is even a case to be made that including
functional impairment as a criterion confounds severity with diagnostic

classification. This can be problematic in circumstances where one may be interested in studying coping or resilience in children with poor motor coordination. For example, a child scoring below the 5th percentile on the Movement Assessment Battery for Children (MABC), and therefore meeting Criterion A, but who does not meet Criterion B, may have developed effective compensatory behavioural and/or motor adaptations that could provide important information for intervention and treatment. If this child were excluded for failing to meet all diagnostic criteria, this opportunity is lost. When functional outcomes are important, however, the incorporation of information on impairment seems essential. As the Leeds Consensus suggests, some studies have assessed handwriting, which is one important difficulty often experienced by children with DCD (Missiuna, Rivard, & Pollock, 2004).

The condition is thought, however, to affect both gross and fine motor coordination (Gibbs, Appleton, & Appleton, 2007), which suggests that some children with adequate handwriting could have limitations in other areas. Handwriting is also not, of course, a useful indicator among very young children, and difficulties that are present could also be associated with another condition, such as a learning disability, that is not itself an exclusion for DCD. Increasingly, children may also type more than they write, which may lead to poor penmanship among children without any genuine motor impairment.

Ideally, then, impairment should perhaps be broader than a test of handwriting. This moves the issue into the domain of the questionnaire. There are several of these, most reviewed in the chapter by Schoemaker and Wilson (see Chapter 6). In general, they are potential screening instruments that attempt to identify cases of DCD not by directly evaluating motor function, but by asking a key informer about apparent problems related to motor function. These instruments can provide an important adjunct to an evaluation such as the MABC, and they are capable of doing double duty: They not only address Criterion B but also can be used as preliminary screening instruments in their own right. This suggests an additional advantage to a two-stage screening approach, in which a low-cost questionnaire is used to identify potential cases who then receive a more expensive confirmatory evaluation with a test of motor functioning (e.g., Wright, Sugden, Ng, & Tan, 1994). Instead of regarding such a process simply as two-stage case identification, it may be thought of as one that addresses two different disorder criteria. This is perhaps an advantage for screens that address questions of practical impairment over those that focus more narrowly on functioning.

Criterion C

Onset of symptoms is in the early developmental period.

DSM-V notes that onset of DCD should, in keeping with the disorder's name, be early. For research on children, however, any disorder that is present can be said to have an early onset (even if this, in itself, does not make it certain that it is developmental rather than acquired).

For research on adolescents and adults, however, the issue deserves more consideration. It is not clear how common late-onset coordination problems are. Those that are clearly acquired (resulting from, e.g., brain injury or severe alcohol dependence) would, in any case, qualify for exclusion under Criterion D. So, the question is, perhaps, whether idiopathic late-onset coordination problems are common enough in various populations to worry researchers, and if so, what should be done about it.

A possibly more important reason to worry about age of onset among older individuals, however, is related to six weighty words added to DSM-V. Criterion A for DCD now states that motor skills must be below expected levels given an individual's age and *opportunity for skill learning and use*. DSM is mute on how this consideration might be operationalized. The older subjects get, however, the more interesting it becomes.

A final, and related, issue is that of things like body composition and inactivity. Unlike traumatic brain injury, these are extremely common; and with age, they may become increasingly important to measured coordination. The child with no movement difficulties at age 6, for example, might display poor gross motor coordination and balance as an obese teenager.

SUGGESTIONS FOR CRITERION C

Among very young children, all disorders are early onset, and opportunities for skill learning and use are probably not strongly differentiated.

For older populations, in particular those of adults, it may well be worthwhile incorporating age at onset into the process that considers differential diagnosis. Flawed recall is likely to prove troublesome, but the coordination disorder cannot otherwise be said to be developmental. Measuring an individual's past opportunities to develop motor skills, and then deciding exactly what to do with the results, however, seems ambitious for field-based research.

Criterion D

The motor skills deficits are not better explained by intellectual disability or visual impairment and are not attributable to a neurological condition affecting movement

A number of medical conditions can cause poor motor coordination, most of which are, as the DSM-V criterion implies, neurological. Screening for all such disorders is not possible in field-based studies. Instead, researchers have typically simply excluded children whose conditions are reported by teachers or parents, or which appear in administrative records. The conditions typically watched for are those with a clear effect on motor functioning that also have a high enough prevalence for there to be a fair probability of seeing them in the sample; these include muscular dystrophy and cerebral palsy. If the expertise of the assessors permits, it may also be desirable to allow exclusions based on clinical judgment. Although some movement abnormalities are consistent with DCD, more severe ones might legitimately prompt exclusion and referral for further assessment.

A further consideration concerns behavioural and emotional conditions. Hyperactivity or emotional distress are not exclusions for DCD, but they can make it difficult to accurately assess motor functioning. This is of particular concern because DCD often co-occurs with other common disorders of childhood – particularly attention deficit hyperactivity disorder (ADHD), but also mood and anxiety disorders (Cairney et al., 2010b; see also Chapter 4). Existing evidence suggests that almost half of all children diagnosed with ADHD also have significant coordination problems, and ADHD is likewise a common diagnosis among children with DCD (see Dewey et al., 2002; Kadesjo & Gillberg, 1998; and references above). (The closeness of this association underlies the long-standing debate about whether DCD should be regarded as an independent disorder at all, or whether it is better seen as one dimension of a broader disorder that includes attention, hyperactivity, perception, and perhaps internalizing disorders (Cairney et al., 2010b; Kaplan, Wilson, Dewey, & Crawford, 1998).)

The frequent co-occurrence of these disorders raises some interesting etiological questions. In field-based research, they also give rise to some important practical difficulties. Problems in attention can interfere with motor testing, as a child who is not focused may perform far below his or her capability. Similarly, depression might affect motivation, while anxiety can be associated with trembling, tics, or other psychomotor effects. Coordination testing that follows a strict protocol is problematic here; not only is it difficult to decide what is responsible for poor performance, some tests do not allow for judgments of this kind to be recorded. An important exception is the Movement-ABC, which allows more discretion on the part of testers. Obviously, however, this requires highly skilled testers and, as noted above, some effort is required to achieve and maintain consistency among multiple raters.

The final consideration with respect to competing diagnoses concerns intellectual disability. Treatments of this issue have undergone a minor shift in recent years. DSM-IV included a criterion specific to "mental retardation"; this was removed in DSM-V, but the concern it reflects surfaces in Criterion D, where intellectual disability is listed as a differential diagnosis.

This therefore remains a potential difficulty in field-based research. In the past, with DSM-IV's strictures in mind, a number of studies administered brief IQ tests with the purpose of entirely excluding those with full-scale IQs below 70 (e.g., Missiuna et al., 2011), and this threshold has recently been formally endorsed (Blank et al., 2012; Sugden et al., 2006). This is one point, however, on which many researchers deviate from DSM criteria, which state, even in version IV, only that motor difficulties should be incommensurate with the level of intellectual functioning. Neither DSM-IV nor DSM-V actually exclude children with an intellectual disability; they simply aim to avoid needlessly doubly diagnosing individuals in whom poor coordination is largely a symptom of another condition. In field-based research, the number of children with a serious intellectual disability is likely to be small, especially for studies recruiting from general school classes. It should, however, be considered alongside other conditions that may exclude DCD.

SUGGESTIONS FOR CRITERION D

In a general-population sample, we suggest, the most common physical health conditions that might be mistaken for DCD are likely to be known or observable. It is likely to be sufficient to ask parents, teachers, children, or other sources about *any condition* that affects motor functioning, and for the study design to allow for the exclusion of children with clear symptoms of other disorders. Some errors in this area may be unavoidable, but checking of administrative data, if available, and a few questions about other conditions is likely to be adequate. This is true, at least, of general medical conditions. Behavioural disorders, such as ADHD, present other difficulties. The challenge lies in determining whether there are independent motor coordination problems, or whether poor performance on tests of motor functioning is secondary to problems with attention, hyperactivity, or oppositional behaviour. In this situation, including information on impairment from a third party would be useful; in a research context, this suggests another advantage to the use of screening instruments that focus on functioning. Finally, as elsewhere, use of an instrument that can incorporate clinical judgment may ameliorate this problem – in the hands of an experienced clinician.

Excluding an evaluation of intellectual functioning is probably justifiable. Some studies drawn from school populations have argued that adequate performance in a regular class strongly suggests that a serious intellectual disability is not present – and, indeed, there is a case to be made that this is perhaps stronger evidence of normal-range IQ than performance on a single, short IQ test. Among very young children, this argument may become less compelling; but testing intelligence in this age range is also correspondingly more difficult, and it may be preferable to rely on the general reporting of competing diagnoses. Serious intellectual disability is, in any case, relatively uncommon (Larson et al., 2001), and it may therefore not represent a serious threat to the validity of a general population sample.

Difficulties with Assessing Multiple Criteria

Researchers have chosen to operationalize DSM criteria in various ways. Many studies have applied only Criterion A. Such studies can claim, however, only to have identified cases of poor motor coordination, and it has been persuasively argued that even field-based research really ought to take into account the other requirements laid out in DSM (Geuze et al., 2001; Lingam et al., 2009).

Deciding to include multiple measures, however, involves its own set of difficulties and compromises. One important study that has done so is the paper of Lingam, Hunt, Golding, Johgmans, and Emond (2009), which represents probably the most careful attempt to date to apply full DSM-IV criteria in a large, general-population sample of children. Its authors required a motor coordination score at or below the 5th percentile (DSM-IV Criterion A); academic problems related to handwriting and ADL impairments (DSM-IV Criterion B); the absence of any other recorded visual, developmental, or neurologic diagnosis

(DSM-IV Criterion C); and an IQ of 70 or higher (DSM-IV Criterion D). Only 1.8% of all children satisfied all these criteria, and the authors therefore reported this to be the prevalence of DCD in the population studied.

This is an appealingly thorough approach. When positive results on several imperfect assessments are required, however, the number of false negatives inevitably rises; the probability that a given case will come out negative on one or more of them can become startlingly large. The fact that a single negative result disqualifies a participant also means that the number of false positives is likely to be low. The final measured prevalence may therefore be substantially below the true value. As an example, we might imagine a situation in which four criteria have to be satisfied, with each measured by an instrument that has a sensitivity of 0.85 and a specificity of 0.85 in the study context. If the true prevalence of the condition is 5%, we can expect to accurately identify $0.05 * (1-(0.85^4)) = 2.39\%$ of participants as cases, and to have $0.95 * ((1-0.85)^4) = 0.05\%$ emerge as false positives. This study would thus be expected to yield a prevalence estimate of 2.43%, which is less than half the true value. This assumes, of course, that the probabilities in question are independent, which may not be the case. It remains true, however, that using multiple instruments in this way involves another, sometimes unappreciated, trade-off between sensitivity and specificity: It increases the latter at the cost of decreasing the former. The very low false positive rate means that the resulting sample will be comprised almost entirely of genuine cases, which is an important (and in some settings, perhaps crucial) advantage; but it also means that prevalence will probably be underestimated, that certain cases will be excluded (probably not at random, which creates doubts around representativeness), and that it will be necessary to screen a larger number of children in order to assemble a sample.

The ideal solution to problems of case identification is, of course, more accurate instruments. These, however, are not likely to be forthcoming. Accurately measuring something like motor functioning is difficult at the best of times, and field-based assessments of (often distracted) children are not the best of times. One thing that might reasonably be done, however, is to limit formal assessments of intellectual functioning and other competing diagnoses. Medical conditions can be reported or directly observed, while assessment of intellectual functioning can probably be omitted. Studies applying measures of functional limitations, meanwhile, should pay close attention to the sensitivity of their measures.

Other Considerations

In addition to co-occurring disorders, other characteristics of children may interfere with motor testing. There is now a sizeable body of evidence demonstrating that poor motor skills are associated with obesity, overweight, and poor cardiorespiratory fitness (e.g., Cairney, Hay, Veldhuizen, Missiuna, & Faught, 2009; Cairney et al., 2010a; Hands, 2008; Schott, Alof, Hultsch, & Meermann, 2007). It has been argued, however, that obesity may interfere with motor testing through its own effects on balance, agility, and fine motor coordination (Deforche et al., 2009; D'Hondt E, Deforche, De Bourdeaudhuji, & Lenoir, 2008; Goulding, Jones, Taylor, Piggot, & Taylor, 2003), and also that some children may be identified as cases of DCD when there is no real neurological impairment.

A related issue is the question of training. Most motor skill assessments include throwing and catching tasks, and performance on these items will reflect experience and skill, as well as the more intrinsic, deeper quality of motor coordination. These skills may be poorer in children with poor fitness or little experience in this type of play. Evaluations of some motor assessments have found, for example, that girls perform much more poorly than boys in throwing and catching tasks (Causgrove Dunn, 2000).

The Leeds Consensus (Sugden et al., 2006) notes the importance of using "culturally appropriate" motor testing, which will be an important consideration for some populations: If throwing and catching are not common in a child's play, it is not impossible that performance will be below norms because of unfamiliarity or lack of practice. Related issues include, for example, use of instruments that include shoelace-tying in cultures or climates where sandals are standard footwear. In these cases, it may be necessary either to revise existing tools or to develop adjusted scoring that removes problematic items. In either case, extensive psychometric work may unfortunately be necessary.

General Difficulties with Screening

When the diagnostic instruments are imperfect, which they always are, screening involves a basic trade-off between the correct identification of cases (sensitivity) and the exclusion of non-cases (specificity).

As noted elsewhere in this book (see Chapter 6), the accuracy of instruments used to identify cases of DCD in research tends to be modest. Sensitivities are rarely above 85%, and specificities rarely above 90%.

Moderate specificities, along with relatively low prevalences, mean that any research study must be prepared to deal with a high proportion of false positives from the initial screening. When the initial screening is the only form of case identification done, an instrument with high specificity seems essential, even if this comes at the cost of poor sensitivity and nonrandom loss of cases. Otherwise, the majority of children identified will be false positives; and it seems better to have a small, possibly unrepresentative sample of children with DCD than a sample of children who don't have DCD at all. When, as Schoemaker and Wilson (Chapter 6) suggest, two-stage case identification is done, the prospects for assembling a cohort that is both representative and has few false positives become considerably brighter.

Study Design: Advantages of Longitudinal Research

While a system for telling cases from non-cases is essential to field-based studies, a broader question in research design concerns the type of study to undertake. Much of the research on DCD has used cross-sectional designs. Children with DCD are identified, their functioning measured, and a comparison made either to population norms or to a group of children with typical motor functioning. The limitations of this approach are well known: It is not possible to study change over time, or to identify precedence of one thing over another. Several studies, for example, have examined the association between DCD and inactivity, obesity, and other health-related outcomes (e.g., Bouffard et al., 1996; Cairney et al., 2009, Cairney et al., 2010a). Generally, these take the view that DCD causes inactivity: Performance in play activities is poor because of poor motor coordination, and this discourages further participation, particularly as play activities become more complex and competitive as the child ages. It is also possible, however, that inactivity or obesity leads to a failure to develop some of the specific motor skills evaluated, which may include throwing, catching, and balancing. A cross-sectional design has little hope of providing convincing evidence one way or the other.

Longitudinal studies are, in general, more useful in a field like DCD research. When data are collected repeatedly on cases and matched controls, as in what epidemiologists call a *longitudinal case-control study*, it becomes possible to look not merely at a child's functioning at a single point in time, but at his or her trajectory over an entire period. This provides important information on course of illness and makes it possible to work out whether DCD precedes outcomes of interest.

One area of controversy in the field, for example, is whether poor motor functioning persists into adolescence and adulthood. Although a small number of studies have attempted to answer this question by following groups of children as they age, sample sizes have been small (e.g., Cantell, 1998). More important is the general assessment of outcomes. DCD is a concern not only because it is associated with functional problems at a given point in time but also because these problems may give rise, over the long term, to health problems, to low academic achievement, or to problems of psychosocial adjustment. Even in the absence of secure evidence on causality, which even longitudinal research cannot ordinarily provide, the knowledge that DCD functions as a precursor or warning of various outcomes can be invaluable. Longitudinal studies, and especially longer-term longitudinal studies, therefore have the potential to quantify the effects of the disorder in a way that other research cannot.

Another important, and less obvious, advantage of longitudinal designs concerns case ascertainment itself. As discussed elsewhere, screening for DCD is difficult. Agreement with reference measures tends to be relatively modest, and so are test–retest values, even when tests are conducted close together in time (Cools, Martelaer, Samaey, & Andries, 2009; Spironello, Hay, Missiuna, Faught, & Cairney, 2010). Part of the problem is that performance on a test of motor functioning will vary from day to day with the enthusiasm, mood, energy level, and focus of the child, not to mention possible chronobiological influences. Another is that performance will vary from month to month as a child's skills develop. And yet another is that *apparent* performance may vary as a child moves from one instrument-defined age category to another; a child age 13 years and 11 months may have good skills when compared to norms among children age 10 to 13 years, and poor ones when measured 2 months later against norms for those 14 to 18 years of age. Repeated testing of motor proficiency provides one way of addressing some of these difficulties. If the overall pattern of results from tests taken at different points in time, especially if spread over some significant developmental period, indicates that motor functioning is consistently poor, this is good evidence that the disorder is, in fact, present. Conversely, if repeated testing of children shows that wide variation between tests is common, it indicates serious problems with the testing protocol or suggests that motor functioning may not be as stable as generally assumed. Use of repeated testing may result in cases that change to non-cases, and vice versa, from measurement to measurement (and, unfortunately, from publication to publication), but also provides the opportunity to study cases of marginal or fluctuating functioning.

A review of longitudinal analytic methods is beyond the scope of this chapter, but hierarchical linear modelling (also known as mixed effects modelling and multilevel modelling) and latent trajectory analysis are two analytical approaches that are very useful with research designs of this type (for a detailed treatment of longitudinal modelling techniques, see, e.g., Singer & Willett, 2003). In brief, these methods allow for the measurement of change over time within and between subjects, and, in this case, between groups of children with and without DCD. Unlike techniques such as analysis of variance (ANOVA) and single-level regression, hierarchical linear modelling allows the researcher to take into account the non-independence of observations at the individual level (repeated measures on the same child over time), and at other levels of aggregation (e.g., children nested in classes, schools, or communities). At the same time, this family of statistical analyses produces estimates that are relatively easy to interpret.

Longitudinal Designs: When to Start?

DCD is generally regarded as a neurodevelopmental condition and, as such, is thought to be present from a very early age, perhaps from before birth (Flouris, Faught, Hay, & Cairney, 2005; Gubbay, 1975). Functional limitations are present beginning in early childhood and become markedly more important as academic and other demands increase: As the child with DCD grows, tasks such as tying shoelaces, printing, and playing sports present themselves, and these prove to be more difficult than for other children. More serious academic problems may present in later childhood, as schoolwork becomes more demanding, and it becomes necessary to take notes and produce written assignments. Other, secondary outcomes, such as obesity and inactivity, may also become apparent in middle childhood. Some secondary outcomes, such as certain psychosocial issues or health problems related to inactivity, may present much later in life, perhaps with a scatter of sequelae continuing to emerge into adulthood (Kirby, Edwards, & Sugden, 2011; Rasmussen & Gillberg, 2000).

It is, however, very difficult to follow a cohort from conception until middle age. Though there have been exceptions (e.g., Batty, Deary, Schoon, & Gale, 2007), studies must usually choose a beginning and an end that will cover only a small part of its subjects' lives. There are several considerations that apply in selecting the part of greatest interest. First, there is the question of practicality. It is probably not possible to accurately measure motor functioning before age 3 or 4, and it may not be possible to securely identify functional deficits until somewhat later. These difficulties notwithstanding, there is much to be said for attempting to study the condition in young children. At age 3, relatively few children are overweight or obese, comparatively few have exceptional emotional problems, and none are failing at school, which has not yet begun. Although the underlying motor deficit may be established at these ages, functional impairment, except in the most severe cases, is unlikely to be present. Identifying motor coordination problems in this period therefore provides a valuable opportunity to observe the *development* of functional problems – and thus of DCD itself – and, in some cases, to make inferences about the direction of causality. This is, moreover, an age of great neurological plasticity (Kolb & Gibb, 2011), and may be one at which experimental interventions might usefully be attempted.

Research on very young children is complex and difficult, however. Waiting until children are enrolled in school can dramatically simplify recruitment and is also likely to make it possible to identify cases more accurately. Research studies beginning at these ages, however, must be prepared for the fact that many functional deficits will already be present in affected children, and thus researchers may need to track smaller differences in outcomes with larger samples or over longer periods.

Study Design: One Possibility

Any field-based study will involve several compromises on the issues we have discussed. One design that seems reasonable, though, is as follows:

• Recruit children shortly after the beginning of formal schooling.
• Do initial screening with a short questionnaire focused on functional impairment.
• Follow this up with a direct assessment of motor functioning (e.g., the Movement-ABC).
• Exclude children not in regular classes or who have a documented relevant medical condition.
• Follow cases and controls regularly over a meaningful period.

This is by no means the only, or even the best, way to conduct field-base research in DCD. It does seem to us, though, to make one reasonable set of compromises. It includes measures of the two central criteria of DSM DCD, while addressing (albeit imperfectly) the two concerned with differential diagnosis. By including two measures, it ought to have an acceptably low proportion of false positives (though this will come at the cost of some loss of sensitivity). By recruiting children in the first years of schooling, it benefits from the advantages of using a school-based sample and assesses children old enough for testing to be practical and for some impairment to be observable – but young enough that important health, academic, social, and emotional outcomes will, in many cases, not yet have occurred.

Conclusion

Field-based DCD research projects must confront a number of methodological challenges. There are several decisions that must be made about study aims, design, and case ascertainment. In this chapter, we have offered opinions about these matters, suggesting, for example, that formal evaluation of exclusion criteria may be of doubtful benefit in some situations and that the field would benefit from a greater number of longitudinal studies. The last point is of particular relevance both to accurate identification of children with DCD and to the problem of secondary consequences. Repeated assessments of motor coordination, and its functional impact, can help separate false positives from true cases in a chronic, persistent disorder like DCD. Understanding the social, emotional, and physical outcomes associated with DCD is also only possible with longitudinal designs. As several chapters in this collection show, evidence for secondary consequences associated with DCD is compelling, but it is limited by a paucity of longitudinal data.

REFERENCES

Albaret, J.M., & de Castelnau, P. (2007). Diagnostic procedures for developmental coordination disorder. In R.H. Geuze (Ed.), *Developmental coordination disorder: A review of current approaches* (pp. 27–82). Marseille, France: Solal.
American Psychiatric Association. (2000). *Diagnostic and statistical manual of mental disorders* (4th ed., text rev.). Washington, DC: Author.
American Psychiatric Association. (2013). *Diagnostic and statistical manual of mental disorders* (5th ed.). Arlington, VA: American Psychiatric Publishing.

Batty, G.D., Deary, I.J., Schoon, I., & Gale, C.R. (2007, Nov). Mental ability across childhood in relation to risk factors for premature mortality in adult life: The 1970 British Cohort Study. *Journal of Epidemiology and Community Health, 61*(11), 997–1003. http://dx.doi.org/10.1136/jech.2006.054494 Medline:17933959

Blank, R., Smits-Engelsman, B., Polatajko, H., & Wilson, P., & European Academy of Childhood Disability. (2012, Jan). European Academy of Childhood Disability (EACD): Recommendations on the definition, diagnosis and intervention of developmental coordination disorder (long version). *Developmental Medicine and Child Neurology, 54*(1), 54–93. http://dx.doi.org/10.1111/j.1469-8749.2011.04171.x Medline:22171930

Bouffard, M., Watkinson, E.J., Thompson, L.P., Causgrove Dunn, J., & Romanow, S.K.E. (1996). A test of the activity deficit hypothesis with children with movement difficulties. *Adapted Physical Activity Quarterly; APAQ, 13*, 61–73.

Cairney, J., Hay, J.A., Faught, B.E., Mandigo, J., & Flouris, A. (2005). Developmental coordination disorder, self-efficacy toward physical activity and participation in free play and organized activities: Does gender matter? *Adapted Physical Activity Quarterly; APAQ, 22*(1), 67–82.

Cairney, J., Hay, J., Veldhuizen, S., Missiuna, C., & Faught, B.E. (2009, May). Comparing probable case identification of developmental coordination disorder using the short form of the Bruininks-Oseretsky Test of Motor Proficiency and the Movement ABC. *Child: Care, Health and Development, 35*(3), 402–408. http://dx.doi.org/10.1111/j.1365-2214.2009.00957.x Medline:19397603

Cairney, J., Hay, J., Veldhuizen, S., Missiuna, C., Mahlberg, N., & Faught, B.E. (2010a, Aug 10). Trajectories of relative weight and waist circumference among children with and without developmental coordination disorder. *Canadian Medical Association Journal, 182*(11), 1167–1172. http://dx.doi.org/10.1503/cmaj.091454 Medline:20584932

Cairney, J., Veldhuizen, S., & Szatmari, P. (2010b, Jul). Motor coordination and emotional-behavioral problems in children. *Current Opinion in Psychiatry, 23*(4), 324–329. http://dx.doi.org/10.1097/YCO.0b013e32833aa0aa Medline:20520549

Cantell, M.H. (1998). *Developmental coordination disorder in adolescence: Perceptuo-motor, academic and social outcomes of early motor delay* (Research Report No. 112). Research Reports on Sports and Health. Jyväskylä, Finland: LIKES Research Center, University of Jyväskylä.

Causgrove Dunn, J. (2000). Goal orientations, perceptions of the motivational climate, and perceived competence of children with movement difficulties. *Adapted Physical Activity Quarterly; APAQ, 17*, 1–19.

Cools, W., Martelaer, K.D., Samaey, C., & Andries, C. (2009). Movement skill assessment of typically developing preschool children: A review of seven movement skill assessment tools. *Journal of Sports Science and Medicine, 8*(2), 154–168. Medline:24149522

Deforche, B.I., Hills, A.P., Worringham, C.J., Davies, P.S., Murphy, A.J., Bouckaert, J.J., & De Bourdeaudhuij, I.M. (2009). Balance and postural skills in normal-weight and overweight prepubertal boys. *International Journal of Pediatric Obesity: IJPO, 4*(3), 175–182. http://dx.doi.org/10.1080/17477160802468470 Medline:18972242

Dewey, D., Kaplan, B.J., Crawford, S.G., & Wilson, B.N. (2002, Dec). Developmental coordination disorder: Associated problems in attention, learning, and psychosocial adjustment. *Human Movement Science, 21*(5-6), 905–918. http://dx.doi.org/10.1016/S0167-9457(02)00163-X Medline:12620725

D'Hondt, E., Deforche, B., De Bourdeaudhuij, I., & Lenoir, M. (2008, Jul 25). Childhood obesity affects fine motor skill performance under different postural constraints. *Neuroscience Letters, 440*(1), 72–75. http://dx.doi.org/10.1016/j.neulet.2008.05.056 Medline:18541379

Faught, B.E., Cairney, J., Hay, J., Veldhuizen, S., Missiuna, C., & Spironello, C.A. (2008, Apr). Screening for motor coordination challenges in children using teacher ratings of physical ability and activity. *Human Movement Science, 27*(2), 177–189. http://dx.doi.org/10.1016/j.humov.2008.02.001 Medline:18343517

Flouris, A.D., Faught, B.E., Hay, J., & Cairney, J. (2005, Jul). Exploring the origins of developmental disorders. *Developmental Medicine and Child Neurology, 47*(7), 436. http://dx.doi.org/10.1017/S0012162205000848 Medline:15991861

Geuze, R.H., Jongmans, M.J., Schoemaker, M.M., & Smits-Engelsman, B.C. (2001, Mar). Clinical and research diagnostic criteria for developmental coordination disorder: A review and discussion. *Human Movement Science, 20*(1-2), 7–47. http://dx.doi.org/10.1016/S0167-9457(01)00027-6 Medline:11471398

Gibbs, J., Appleton, J., & Appleton, R. (2007, Jun). Dyspraxia or developmental coordination disorder? Unravelling the enigma. *Archives of Disease in Childhood, 92*(6), 534–539. http://dx.doi.org/10.1136/adc.2005.088054 Medline:17515623

Goulding, A., Jones, I.E., Taylor, R.W., Piggot, J.M., & Taylor, D. (2003, Apr). Dynamic and static tests of balance and postural sway in boys: Effects of previous wrist bone fractures and high adiposity. *Gait & Posture, 17*(2), 136–141. http://dx.doi.org/10.1016/S0966-6362(02)00161-3 Medline:12633774

Gubbay, S.S. (1975). *The clumsy child: A study of developmental apraxic and agnosic ataxia.* London, England: W.B. Saunders.

Hands, B. (2008, Apr). Changes in motor skill and fitness measures among children with high and low motor competence: A five-year longitudinal study. *Journal of Sports Science & Medicine, 11*(2), 155–162. http://dx.doi. org/10.1016/j.jsams.2007.02.012 Medline:17567536.

Hay, J.A., Hawes, R., & Faught, B.E. (2004, Apr). Evaluation of a screening instrument for developmental coordination disorder. *Journal of Adolescent Health, 34*(4), 308–313. http://dx.doi.org/10.1016/j.jadohealth.2003.07.004 Medline:15041000

Kadesjö, B., Gillberg, C. (1998). Attention deficits and clumsiness in Swedish 7-year-old children. *Developmental Medicine & Child Neurology, 40*(12): 796–804.

Kaplan, B.J., Wilson, B.N., Dewey, D., & Crawford, S.G. (1998). DCD may not be a discrete disorder. *Human Movement Science, 17*(4–5), 471–490. http:// dx.doi.org/10.1016/S0167-9457(98)00010-4

Kirby, A., Edwards, L., & Sugden, D. (2011, Jul-Aug). Emerging adulthood in developmental co-ordination disorder: Parent and young adult perspectives. *Research in Developmental Disabilities, 32*(4), 1351–1360. Medline:21334175

Kolb, B., & Gibb, R. (2011, Nov). Brain plasticity and behaviour in the developing brain. *Journal of the Canadian Academy of Child and Adolescent Psychiatry, 20*(4), 265–276. Medline:22114608

Larson, S.A., Lakin, C., Anderson, L., Lee, N.K., Lee, J.H., & Anderson, D. (2001). Prevalence of mental retardation and developmental disabilities: Estimates from the 1994/1995 National Health Interview Survey disability supplements. *American Journal of Mental Retardation, 106*(3), 231–252. http:// dx.doi.org/10.1352/0895-8017(2001)106<0231:POMRAD>2.0.CO;2

Lingam, R., Hunt, L., Golding, J., Jongmans, M., & Emond, A. (2009, Apr). Prevalence of developmental coordination disorder using the DSM-IV at 7 years of age: A UK population-based study. *Pediatrics, 123*(4), e693–e700. http://dx.doi.org/10.1542/peds.2008-1770 Medline:19336359

Missiuna, C., Cairney, J., Pollock, N., Russell, D., Macdonald, K., Cousins, M., … Schmidt, L. (2011, Mar-Apr). A staged approach for identifying children with developmental coordination disorder from the population. *Research in Developmental Disabilities, 32*(2), 549–559. http://dx.doi.org/10.1016/j. ridd.2010.12.025 Medline:21216564

Missiuna, C., Rivard, L., & Pollock, N. (2004). They're bright but can't write: Developmental coordination disorder in school aged children. *TEACHING Exceptional Children Plus, 1*(1), 3.

Rasmussen, P., & Gillberg, C. (2000, Nov). Natural outcome of ADHD with developmental coordination disorder at age 22 years: A controlled, longitudinal, community-based study. *Journal of the American Academy of Child and Adolescent Psychiatry, 39*(11), 1424–1431. http://dx.doi. org/10.1097/00004583-200011000-00017 Medline:11068898

Schoemaker, M.M., Smits-Engelsman, B.C.M., & Jongmans, M.J. (2003). Psychometric properties of the Movement Assessment Battery for Children-Checklist as a screening instrument for children with developmental coordination disorder. *British Journal of Educational Psychology, 73*(3), 425–441. http://dx.doi.org/10.1348/000709903322275911 Medline:14672152

Schott, N., Alof, V., Hultsch, D., & Meermann, D. (2007, Dec). Physical fitness in children with developmental coordination disorder. *Research Quarterly for Exercise and Sport, 78*(5), 438–450. http://dx.doi.org/10.1080/02701367.2007.10599444 Medline:18274216

Singer, J.D., & Willett, J.B. (2003). *Applied longitudinal data analysis: Modeling change and event occurrence.* New York, NY: Oxford University Press. http://dx.doi.org/10.1093/acprof:oso/9780195152968.001.0001

Skinner, R.A., & Piek, J.P. (2001, Mar). Psychosocial implications of poor motor coordination in children and adolescents. *Human Movement Science, 20*(1-2), 73–94. http://dx.doi.org/10.1016/S0167-9457(01)00029-X Medline:11471399

Spironello, C., Hay, J., Missiuna, C., Faught, B.E., & Cairney, J. (2010). Concurrent and construct validation of the short form of the Bruininks-Oseretsky Test of Motor Proficiency and the Movement-ABC administered under field conditions. *Child: Health, Care and Development, 36*(4), 499–507. http://dx.doi.org/10.1111/j.1365-2214.2009.01066.x

Sugden, D.A., Chambers, M., & Utley, A. (2006). Leeds Consensus Statement. Available online at http://dcd.canchild.ca/en/dcdresources/consensusstatements.asp (downloaded 14 May 2011).

Wilson, B.N., Kaplan, B.J., Crawford, S.G., Campbell, A., & Dewey, D. (2000, Sep-Oct). Reliability and validity of a parent questionnaire on childhood motor skills. *American Journal of Occupational Therapy., 54*(5), 484–493. http://dx.doi.org/10.5014/ajot.54.5.484 Medline:11006808

Wright, H.C., Sugden, D.A., Ng, R., & Tan, J. (1994). Identification of movement problems in Singapore: Usefulness of the M-ABC Checklist. *Adapted Physical Activity Quarterly; APAQ, 11*, 150–157.

SECTION FOUR

Intervention and Reflections on the Future

8 Strategic Management of Children with Developmental Coordination Disorder

CHERYL MISSIUNA, HELENE J. POLATAJKO,
AND NANCY POLLOCK

"Only when you make the right changes to your thinking do other things begin to turn out right."

John Maxwell

The Challenge

Developmental coordination disorder (DCD) is a chronic health condition that affects a child's ability to perform everyday tasks at home, at school and at play (American Psychiatric Association, 2000; Barnett, 2008; Missiuna, Moll, King, King, & Law, 2007; Summers, Larkin, & Dewey, 2008; Wang, Tseng, Wilson, & Hu, 2009). It is likely that there is a child with DCD in nearly every primary school classroom in the world, and yet, we know that few educational or health care systems acknowledge or understand it (Barnett, 2008; Gaines, Missiuna, Egan, & McLean, 2008b; Rodger & Mandich, 2005). Twenty-five years of research has produced compelling evidence that the motor problems of children with DCD are lifelong (Cousins & Smyth, 2003; Fitzpatrick & Watkinson, 2003; Kirby, Sugden, Beveridge, & Edwards, 2008; Losse et al., 1991; Missiuna, Moll, King, Stewart, & Macdonald, 2008a) and that these motor difficulties are strongly associated with the subsequent development of physical and mental health difficulties, including decreased physical fitness (Schott, Alof, Hultsch, & Meermann, 2007; Tsiotra, Nevill, Lane, & Koutedakis, 2009), obesity (Cairney, Hay, Faught, & Hawes, 2005a; Cairney et al., 2010b; Wagner et al., 2011; Zhu, Wu, & Cairney, 2011), anxiety (Cairney, Veldhuizen, & Szatmari, 2010c; Piek, Barrett, Smith, Rigoli, & Gasson, 2010; Piek, Bradbury, Elsley, & Tate, 2008), depression (Cairney et al., 2010c; Missiuna et al., 2014;

Piek et al., 2010; Piek, Bradbury, Elsley, & Tate, 2008; Piek et al., 2007), low self-esteem (Cocks, Barton, & Donelly, 2009; Engel-Yeger & Hanna Kasis, 2010), and also academic failure (Lingam, Golding, Jongmans, Hunt, Ellis, & Emond, 2010; Roberts et al., 2011; Stephenson & Chesson, 2008). The secondary consequences and lifelong impact of DCD have been clearly outlined in previous chapters (Chapters 1 through 4) and lead to our compelling conclusion: Future management of children with DCD must be much more strategic than it has previously been and must take into consideration what is already known.

In this chapter, we will provide an overview of the approaches that have been taken over the years to intervene with children with DCD. Using evidence from the emergent literature, we will then argue for a new, population-based approach. In our discussion, which we have organized in a "what we now know, what we should do" format, we argue for a more strategic management of the needs of children with DCD based on a staged or "levelled" approach. The approach supports children who are experiencing motor challenges differently depending upon a variety of factors, including their age, severity, need, intensity of service provision, location, and target of the intervention. We then provide a Canadian example of this type of population-based approach that involves management within the school system. We will finish the chapter by outlining future considerations for the management of children with DCD and proposing directions for research.

Approaches to Date

Over the years, we have seen the development and evaluation of many different approaches to intervention for children with DCD. Some of the early models, including sensory integration (Ayres, 1972; Ayres, 1979), kinaesthetic training (Laszlo & Bairstow, 1985; Laszlo, Bairstow, Bartrip, & Rolfe, 1988), and perceptual motor intervention (Lord & Hulme, 1987a, 1987b) have been referred to as process-oriented or "bottom-up" interventions because they address movement problems by emphasizing the building of foundational skills (Mandich, Polatajko, Macnab, & Miller, 2001). These interventions reflect traditional theories of motor development and are based on the theoretical belief that changing underlying deficits will improve motor performance (Mandich et al., 2001). Several comprehensive systematic reviews on the effectiveness of these approaches have found them to produce minimal change, at best, in functional outcomes and have shown no clear advantage of one type of intervention over another (Forsyth et al., 2007; Hillier, 2007; Polatajko & Cantin, 2005).

In more recent years, dynamic systems theories have guided the development of newer approaches to intervention. Theorists such as Thelen (1995) proposed that changes in motor performance rely on many variables that are task- and environment-specific. This task-oriented way of thinking emphasizes that intervention must be contextually based, must occur in everyday situations, and must be of significance to the child. More recent interventions for children with DCD reflect these beliefs and now tend to emphasize the development of specific motor skills rather than underlying skill components (Rivard, Missiuna, Pollock, & David, 2011). Also described in the literature as top-down because of their emphasis on learning specific tasks (Mandich et al., 2001), these intervention approaches utilize motor learning principles, such as Neuromotor Task Training (NTT), and may also emphasize the role of cognitive processes in the learning of new movement skills, such as Cognitive Orientation to daily Occupational Performance (CO-OP; Levac, Wishart, Missiuna, & Wright, 2009).

In NTT and other task-specific interventions, learning is directed by a physical or occupational therapist who provides verbal instructions, visual prompts, or physical assistance to help the child get the feeling of and learn efficient movement (Schoemaker & Smits-Engelsman, 2005). In CO-OP, the child is actively involved in choosing the tasks and goals and is guided to solve the performance problem. The target is motor skill acquisition through cognitive strategy use. Focus and attention are directed towards the difficult aspects of the task performance experienced by the individual child. In using cognitive strategies, researchers anticipate that there will be generalization and transfer to other tasks that encompass similar difficulties (Polatajko & Mandich, 2004). Promising support for task-focused interventions such as NTT and CO-OP are reported in the literature and will be reviewed in more detail later in this chapter. Sugden (2007) summarized current approaches to intervention for children with DCD and highlighted the movement in the field towards recognizing "the importance of more functional approaches that address the tasks a child wants to achieve (e.g., scoring goals, riding a bike), in the contexts they wish to achieve them" (p. 470).

The intervention approaches described to this point – whether emphasizing a change in impairment or a change in performance of motor activities – focus on the individual child who has DCD as the target of the intervention. There are many situations in which the most appropriate target of intervention is the individual child and, as will be demonstrated, the top-down approaches used in recent years to assist children with DCD to learn motor skills are well justified and appropriate for this purpose. There are several reasons, however, to consider the need for "management" of children with DCD that extends beyond the individual child to encompass the family, the school, and the community.

Strategic Management

The premise that serves as the foundation for this section and our proposed strategic approach is that *DCD is a learning-based motor problem.* This statement is not an attempt to imply causation, but reflects our belief that DCD involves a disruption in the child's ability to learn new motor skills, to transfer learned skills to subsequent tasks, and to generalize that learning to new settings. In order to understand the importance of this statement, one needs to differentiate motor *learning,* the permanent acquisition of a skilled movement, from motor *performance,* which is the performance of a motor skill at one particular moment in time. Children with DCD show inconsistent motor performance because they have difficulty with motor learning, with transfer (the influence that the acquisition of one motor skill has on the learning of the next motor skill), and with generalization (the performance of a specific motor skill that has been learned in another context; Polatajko & Mandich, 2004). The management of children with DCD that we are proposing in this chapter is based upon this core assumption. We will now outline the evidence that provides a rationale for a strategic, levelled approach to management of children with DCD.

Level 1: Management at a School/Population Level

What We Now Know: The prevalence of DCD is very high

Research performed in countries around the world has looked at prevalence, gender distribution, and populations within which there is a high likelihood of children having DCD. Studies have confirmed that large numbers of children are affected by DCD (Forsyth et al., 2007; Gillberg, 1998; Iloeje, 1987; Kadesjö & Gillberg, 1999; Lingam, Hunt, Golding, Jongmans, & Emond, 2009; Wright & Sugden, 1996). In fact, many researchers would suggest that there is a child in every classroom who has DCD. While Lingam and colleagues (2009) proposed that only 1.7% of children had DCD, the American Psychiatric Association (APA) suggests 5% to 6% of school-age children had DCD, and studies in some countries have found even higher numbers (Cheng, Chen, Tsai, Chen, & Cherng, 2009; Faught et al., 2008; Gubbay, 1975; Iloeje, 1987; Kadesjö & Gillberg, 1999; Sugden & Sugden, 1991; Tsiotra et al., 2006; van Dellen, Vaessen, & Schoemaker, 1990). It has commonly been accepted that boys with DCD outnumber girls in a 2:1 ratio (APA, 2000); however, population-based studies of children with DCD suggest that more equal numbers of boys and girls may be affected (Cairney et al., 2007; Edwards et al., 2011; Missiuna et al., 2011a; Roberts et al., 2011). The numbers of children who present with motor coordination difficulties is even higher among children who are of low birthweight or born prematurely (Dewey et al., 2011; Edwards et al., 2011; Goyen & Lui, 2009; Holsti, Grunau, & Whitfield, 2002; Roberts et al., 2011). While it would be easy to dispute any findings regarding the prevalence, gender distribution, or methods through which these figures were ascertained, it is impossible to argue with the statement that very large numbers of children, both boys and girls, are affected by DCD in every country in which there have been studies.

What We Now Know: When children with DCD are recognized and referred, waitlists are unwieldy

We know that in countries where children with DCD have been recognized and referred for provision of service, the high prevalence of DCD means that waiting lists are ridiculously long. Recent studies have illustrated for example that in any given health care region, hundreds of children with probable DCD may await assessment from 1 to 4 years (Deloitte, 2010; Dunford, Street, O'Connell, Kelly, & Sibert, 2004; Peters, Henderson, & Dookun, 2004). We also know that many children with DCD are never identified at all (Missiuna et al., 2008a) and that these unidentified or under-identified children may experience very stressful periods at school (Engel-Yeger & Hanna Kasis, 2010; Missiuna et al., 2007; Missiuna, Moll, Law, King, & King, 2006b) and have difficulty with social participation, bullying, and secondary mental health issues (Campbell, Missiuna, Rivard, & Pollock, 2012a; Campbell, Missiuna, & Vaillancourt, 2012b; Piek, Barrett, Allen, Jones, & Louise, 2005), as outlined in earlier chapters. Clearly, we will never be able to identify and intervene with all children with DCD at the appropriate time if they are managed individually, one child at a time.

———————

Level 1: Given the large numbers of children with DCD and long waiting lists, we need to be intervening at a population level, particularly in schools, to create environments that facilitate the learning of motor skills. These environments will be helpful to all children but are absolutely essential for children with DCD.

———————

What We Should Do: Strategic Management Level 1

In order to address the needs of this large population of children and to reduce waitlists and poor access to service, we need to move from focusing on the one child in the classroom who likely has DCD towards a more general focus on enhancing the knowledge of educators who work with all school-age children, building their capacity regarding children who have similar motor challenges. If educators are to be supported in recognizing and working with children with DCD, they first need to have more knowledge about typical motor development, of the motor skills that are expected of children at different ages, and of how to promote these motor skills through general, curriculum-based activities. As a first step, educators would learn to implement "universal design for learning" motor skills in the same way that classrooms have been developed to have a universal design that encourages literacy. Universal Design for Learning (UDL) focuses on enabling performance development in the classroom through promotion of changes within the physical and social environment (Campbell & Skarakis-Doyle, 2007). This approach emphasizes designing educational materials and methods that enable goals to be met by children who may differ widely in their abilities and in the extent to which they are able to fully participate in the curriculum (Campbell, Missiuna, Pollock, & Gaines, 2011; Orkwis, 2003). Children who are participating in a classroom that is designed to facilitate motor skill development may or may not have DCD; they may be children who simply have not had prior opportunity to develop specific motor skills. It makes sense, though, that these types of classrooms will be very supportive to children who do have DCD.

In order to set up an environment that facilitates motor skill development, educators will need to enhance their capacity to understand developmental differences in motor development and to actually teach motor-based skills to all children. There are methods to optimize classroom layout, to design activity centres, or to teach large-group lessons for the class as a whole about motor skills such as printing, tying shoes, or putting on a jacket. In a school that has universal design for motor learning, educators will learn to recognize when the curricular tasks that they are using require motor skills (e.g., cutting out shapes during a math activity) and will actually teach those skills, in the same way as they teach numeracy and literacy. Collaborative dialogue may occur between educators and health professionals to facilitate thinking about the varied ways in which children might receive instruction about skills that are motor based (Campbell & von Stauffenberg, 2009).

Studies asking parents of children with DCD about their concerns frequently identify decreased social and physical participation in school settings (Rodger & Mandich, 2005; Segal, Mandich, Polatajko, & Cook, 2002). Children with DCD have reduced interest in physical activities and may begin to withdraw from, and avoid, motor and physical education activities at an early age (Bouffard, Watkinson, Thompson, Dunn, & Romanow, 1996; Watkinson et al., 2001). Due to difficulties with self-care, children are often slow to get to the playground for recess, restricting their physical participation and further diminishing their opportunities for social interactions. Using creative UDL principles, educators would create a noncompetitive environment that encourages children with a variety of motor abilities to participate during physical education classes and on the playground. Motor skills that need to be acquired in order for all children to be successful (e.g., throwing and catching balls, using swings) would be taught without any assumption that children arrive at school knowing how to perform these skills.

While we believe that management of large numbers of children with DCD must encompass UDL in schools to support motor skill development, we recognize that this is only the first level of a strategic approach.

Level 2: Management at a Group Level

What We Now Know: Children with DCD do not learn motor skills spontaneously, by trial and error, or vicariously by observing others

If children with DCD were able to learn purely by being placed in an environment that facilitated motor skill development, then Level 1 management would be sufficient. We have more than two decades of evidence, however, that suggests that children with DCD have a learning-based motor problem that leads them to be unable to benefit solely from exposure within this environment. As early as 1987, Marchiori, Wall, and Bedingfield illustrated that when provided with 1,200 trials in a closed environment, children with DCD achieved only minimal improvement in their ability to shoot hockey pucks. Missiuna (1994) showed that performance of an extremely simple movement could be improved through much repetition but that the level of performance never reached that of age-matched controls. Using functional magnetic resonance imaging (fMRI), Zwicker and colleagues demonstrated how much more energy children with DCD need to use in both the initial learning and performance of a new motor skill, relative to their peers (Zwicker, Missiuna, Harris, & Boyd, 2010b). Their brain activation is clearly different, as are the neural networks that are recruited during the learning process. Data suggest that there is a neurobiological correlate for the impaired learning of motor skills in children with DCD (Zwicker, Missiuna, & Boyd, 2009; Zwicker, Missiuna, Harris, & Boyd, 2011a). While this work is groundbreaking, it needs to be confirmed with a larger sample of children with DCD.

Work is progressing to determine why children with DCD have so much difficulty learning motor skills by imitation, or by trial and error. It has been hypothesized that children with DCD may have inadequate forward modelling of movements so they are unable to form, access, or update their internal models of what a movement should involve; this results in poor error correction and ultimately affects their motor learning (Smits-Engelsman, Wilson, Westenberg, & Duysens, 2003; see also Chapter 5 in this volume for an in-depth discussion of forward modelling deficits). Other work examining motor adaptation – the ability of children with DCD to adapt their performance to changing environmental contexts – has reached a similar conclusion. In these studies, children with motor difficulties have shown poor adaptation to gradual changes in environmental stimuli (Brookes, Nicolson, & Fawcett, 2007; Cantin, Polatajko, Thach, & Jaglal, 2007). While we still do not have a definitive answer as to the nature of the difficulties, this work affirms the premise of this chapter that children with DCD have a learning-based motor problem.

What We Now Know: Children with DCD need to be identified early, before secondary conditions begin to emerge

The increased risk for children with DCD of secondary health issues and academic failure highlights the need to identify children who actually do have DCD as early as possible (Missiuna, Rivard, & Bartlett, 2003). Early identification may facilitate sharing of knowledge with teachers and parents about how to make tasks easier and how to ensure that activities are matched to children's capabilities. In this way, children with DCD can be provided with optimally challenging situations that emphasize mastery and avoid multiple failed attempts (Missiuna, Rivard, & Pollock, 2004). Parents have described a trajectory of deterioration for their untreated children, from difficulty with self-care and academic activities when a child is young, to lowered self-esteem and social problems and, by adolescence, the onset of mental health issues (Missiuna et al., 2007). Longitudinal studies following children with DCD through middle childhood and adolescence (see Chapter 1 in this volume) have also demonstrated that children with DCD are less physically active (Cairney, Hay, Veldhuizen, Missiuna, & Faught, 2010a), differ in their activity preferences (Cairney et al., 2005b), are overrepresented among children who are overweight and obese (Cairney et al., 2010b), and appear to be at greater risk for cardiovascular difficulties (Faught, Hay, Cairney, & Flouris, 2005). Clearly, it is necessary to identify children with DCD before such problems begin (see Chapter 3 in this volume for an in-depth review of these studies).

Early identification of children with DCD is possible by several groups of professionals, including occupational therapists, physiotherapists, physicians, pediatricians, and psychologists. Teachers or parents could be informed and educated by these health professionals, or they themselves could be the source of the identification of DCD (Sugden & Chambers, 2003). Kirby, Davies, and Bryant (2005) argue that teachers are among the professionals who will most consistently come into contact with children with DCD; however, their study confirmed that teachers often know little about the disorder, even though it is likely that at least one child in every elementary school classroom will have DCD (Carslaw, 2011). Classroom teachers are in an excellent position both to identify and to support children with DCD. Teachers spend hours every day with the children and have a built-in normative group for comparison. They meet with parents and so have an opportunity to discuss their observations of the child in the classroom and to problem-solve difficulties seen in the school and home environments. Physical education teachers, when present in a school, may also be very knowledgeable about motor development, skill acquisition, and motor learning. Studies in the past that involved teacher identification using screening tools and checklists have not shown these methods to be very promising (e.g., Piek & Edwards, 1997). Kourtessis et al. (2008) found, however, that after 8 hours of lectures about DCD, both physical education teachers and early childhood educators had an enhanced ability to identify children with DCD. It is probable that teachers can learn to identify children with DCD if provided with the right type of educational sessions or job-embedded learning (Missiuna et al., 2012a), but this will need further investigation.

Level 2: Given that children with DCD do not learn motor skills spontaneously, by observation, trial and error or practice, we need to be teaching specific, functional motor skills that are needed to encourage participation. Teachers are capable, with the right training, of identifying children whose motor skill development is delayed, and of teaching specific motor skills to groups of these children.

What We Should Do: Strategic Management Level 2

There is evidence that children with DCD may benefit from specific skill training. A great deal of work has been conducted by Smits-Engelsman and colleagues, who have developed and investigated Neurorehabilitation Training Toolkit or NTT, a therapeutic program that utilizes motor learning teaching principles (Niemeijer, Schoemaker, & Smits-Engelsman, 2006; Niemeijer, Smits-Engelsman, & Schoemaker, 2007; Schoemaker & Smits-Engelsman, 2005; Wilson, 2005). In NTT, the emphasis is on directly teaching the fundamental motor skills of childhood by creating an environment that promotes and supports learning. Skill performance is considered from the perspective of limiting factors and breakdown points of the movement. Task difficulty is then reduced so that the child can manage the performance and experience success. For example, a child would be taught to catch a ball by using progressively smaller balls at progressively larger distances.

A study by Tsai (2009) used a context-based intervention to investigate the efficacy of table-tennis training on treating the known difficulties of children with DCD with motor coordination and also with volitional shifts of attention. Forty-three children 9–10 years of age were screened and divided into DCD ($n = 27$) and typically developing (TD, $n = 16$) groups. Children with DCD were then quasi-randomly assigned to either a DCD-training group who underwent a 10-week table-tennis training program 3 times a week or a DCD non-training group. Table-tennis training was reported to result in significant improvement of both attentional and motor functions for the children with DCD. The study demonstrated that exercise intervention employed within the school setting may benefit attention and motor performance in children with DCD. Future research efforts need to replicate these results and should continue to clarify whether the performance gains could be maintained over time (Tsai, 2009).

Other research studies have been conducted with groups of children with DCD in school settings. A meta-analysis by Pless and Carlsson (2000) looked at the results of 13 intervention studies conducted from 1970 to 1996. These authors concluded that motor skill interventions were most effective when applied with children over 5 years of age, using a focus on specific skill training, conducted in a group setting or home program, with an intervention frequency of at least 3 times per week. It seems that this approach lends itself to a school environment either as a method of teaching specific motor skills in physical education classes or in after-school groups that target children with motor learning difficulties. Mannisto, Cantell, Huovinen, Kooistra, and Larkin (2006) demonstrated that 5–7-year-old children with both borderline and more severe motor coordination difficulties benefited from an intervention that targeted specific motor skills and that was delivered weekly during group sessions in a school setting. A similar approach was used by Tsai, Wang, and Tseng (2012), who trained groups of children in the motor skills used in soccer; improvement was noted in task performance in the group of children with DCD who received the training but, not surprisingly, did not occur in the group who were not trained. Similar to Tsai's (2009) work, this study also reported improvements in children's ability to inhibit impulsive responses in a laboratory task.

Children who have DCD will need to be taught the specific motor skills that they require for active participation in school and in the community. There may be children with motor coordination challenges for whom this level of management will be sufficiently facilitatory that no other intervention will be needed. Many other children who have poorly developed motor skills will also benefit from targeted physical activity groups in which motor learning principles are used to guide the teaching. We presume, however, that most children with DCD will also require adaptation of tasks and accommodation of their academic program.

Level 3: Management of Individual Children in the Context of the Classroom

What We Now Know: The underlying motor impairment is not going to go away

As indicated above, the rationale for intervening at the level of the individual child with DCD is fairly obvious. Longitudinal research clearly demonstrates that without intervention, children with DCD do not "grow out of" the disorder. There is strong evidence that the motor problems of childhood persist into adolescence and adulthood (Cantell & Kooistra, 2002; Cousins & Smyth, 2003; Fitzpatrick & Watkinson, 2003; Hellgren, Gillberg, Gillberg, & Enerskog, 1993; Losse et al., 1991; Rasmussen & Gillberg, 2000). There needs to be some adjustments and accommodation made for individual children with DCD if they are to be successful. Given that children spend the majority of their time in school, the classroom is a logical place for this management to occur.

What We Now Know: When children with DCD learn a motor skill, it does not transfer

While there is strong evidence that if taught using motor learning principles, children with DCD are able to learn a motor skill, present but less compelling is the evidence of this skill generalizing and transferring so that it and like tasks can be performed in other environments. Missiuna (1994) demonstrated that a simple movement was able to be transferred and applied in a different task but that children with DCD had more difficulty doing so than did age-matched control children. Generalization to a completely new environment was not examined. Zwicker, Missiuna, Harris, and Boyd (2011) had children practise a motor skill outside the fMRI machine and found that even after 4 days of practice, children with DCD were recruiting brain regions as if this was a new motor skill and did not transfer the learning that had occurred; in contrast, typically developing children transferred the learning that had occurred outside the machine and were able to perform the learned task easily once inside the fMRI machine. Alloway and Warn (2008) showed that with a program of task-specific motor exercises, significant improvement in motor skills and in visuospatial working memory were achieved by the intervention group; however, this effect did not transfer to other skill areas. All of these studies have highlighted the difficulty that children with DCD seem to have with transfer and generalization of motor skills.

The approach that we are proposing aligns well with the summary provided by Mahoney and Perales (2006):

> Early motor intervention procedures are not adequately meeting the goals envisioned for this endeavour. We argue that there are two interrelated reasons why this may be occurring. The first is that parents, who are the people with the greatest opportunities to promote children's motor learning are not being asked to become active participants in their children's motor intervention. The second is that contemporary models of motor intervention have been focusing on motor learning activities that are incompatible with contemporary theories and research on early motor learning. (p. 67)

Findings such as these are not surprising. Well-known theorists in human movement science have noted that transfer occurs very rarely, in and of itself, following acquisition of a specific motor skill (Schmidt & Lee, 2005) and that concerted efforts have to be made in the teaching process to support generalization and transfer (Geusgens, Winkens, van Heugten, Jolles, & van den Heuvel, 2007). A rigorous systematic review and meta-analysis of the DCD literature conducted by Wilson, Ruddock, Smits-Engelsman, Polatajko, and Blank (2013) pointed out that while training effects are commonly shown at a task-specific level, transfer is seldom shown. The notorious difficulty in demonstrating generalization and transfer may explain why these are seldom addressed in research. A striking exception is research on the CO-OP approach, which has included an exploration of generalization and transfer and has provided important evidence of its ability to affect both generalization and transfer (Hyland & Polatajko, 2012; Polatajko & Cantin, 2005). However, this is a specialized approach that goes beyond what can be provided in the classroom.

Support for our propositions can be seen in the expert consensus provided by the European Academy for Childhood Disability International Consensus Guidelines (Blank, Smits-Engelsman, Polatajko, & Wilson, 2012). These guidelines emphasize the importance of working on actually doing motor tasks in the environments in which the tasks are required.

Level 3: Given that the motor impairment is lifelong, we need to be accommodating for motor learning difficulties in order to encourage children's participation in classrooms and in physical activity environments in the community. The fact that children do not transfer or generalize learning well suggests that accommodations and individual skill teaching need to occur in the environment in which the motor skill will be used.

What We Should Do: Strategic Management Level 3

Teachers are in an ideal position to support students who learn differently but who often require support in order to do so effectively. While many different professionals have consulted to teachers over the years, typically through assessing the child individually and then making recommendations, the evidence shows that it is often difficult for teachers to implement the recommendations within the classroom (Friend, 2000; Sayers, 2008; Villeneuve, 2009). Recent evidence supports a move to more collaborative consultation and coaching models where the teacher and consultant work together in the classroom, determine shared goals and understandings of the student's challenges, and through the use of a response to intervention (RtI) model determine the most effective strategies to help the student succeed (Hanft & Shepherd, 2008). The RtI approach is becoming widely accepted within the educational literature as a more contextually relevant and effective practice in contrast to a focus on identifying individual children and referring them for special education services (Ardoin, Witt, Connell, & Koenig, 2005; Shores & Bender, 2007). The use of RtI within the classroom in combination with a collaborative relationship between the teacher and the consultant also serves to develop the capacity of the teacher to support not only an individual student but also other students with similar difficulties. The specialized knowledge does not remain with the consultant, but is translated, trialed, and implemented together with the teacher (Rush, Shelden, & Hanft, 2003).

Children with DCD can often perform effectively despite their motor difficulties if some accommodations are in place. Teachers are usually familiar with formulating individualized plans for children with other neurodevelopmental disorders and can learn to accommodate for the difficulties experienced by children with DCD as well. With greater understanding, educators will be able to design alternative methods that are not motor based to address curriculum goals (e.g., using stamps and stickers instead of paper and pencil to complete a worksheet).

To promote a general strategy to adapt tasks and accommodate for motor difficulties, teachers can be encouraged to access resources that will encourage them to adjust, or "M.A.T.C.H.," tasks to fit the needs of individual children with DCD. Teachers can Modify the task, Alter their expectations, Teach strategies, Change the environment, and Help by understanding (Missiuna et al., 2004). Modifying the task involves changing the aspects of the activity that are too difficult for the child. This often involves changing the types of tools and materials used (e.g., catching a larger ball, using a pencil grip, writing math questions on graph paper). Altering expectations puts the emphasis on the ultimate goal of the activity, rather than the process. For example, if the curriculum goal is the development of narrative writing, the child might use a computer rather than write by hand. As noted earlier, children with DCD need to be taught explicitly using specific strategies rather than be expected to learn through observation or experience only. For example, the use of scissors may need to be broken down into steps, and the role of each hand, the finger placement, and directional cues may need to be taught to a young child. Changing the environment can make a child very quickly more successful, for example, by providing a properly fitted desk and chair, ensuring that the child has the end locker to reduce crowding while dressing, or allowing the youngster to lean against a bookcase during circle times on the floor. The most powerful strategy is for the adults around the child to help through their understanding of why the child is struggling so that they can implement strategies, support the child's participation, and prevent the child from becoming discouraged.

Although teachers can often modify or adapt academic activities in the classroom where motor performance is not the primary focus, it may not be as easy to decrease the motor requirements in physical education classes. Strategies can be used, however, to encourage children with DCD to progress within their own range of abilities, to foster self-esteem, and to promote the value of physical activity for long-term fitness and health (Missiuna & Rivard, 2010; Rivard & Missiuna, 2004).

Level 4: Management of Individual Children Who Are Complex

What We Now Know: Many children with DCD have comorbidities

It has long been recognized that the presence of co-occurring conditions in children with DCD increases the probability of negative outcomes (Bouffard et al., 1996; Rasmussen & Gillberg, 2000; Schoemaker & Kalverboer, 1994). Strong associations have been demonstrated between DCD and attention deficit hyperactivity disorder (ADHD); speech and articulation difficulties (specific language impairment); and language-based learning disabilities (LD), in particular, reading disability (Dewey, Kaplan, Crawford, & Wilson, 2002; Gaines & Missiuna, 2007; Hill, 2001; Jongmans, Smits-Engelsman, & Schoemaker, 2003; Kadesjö & Gillberg, 1998; Piek & Dyck, 2004; Pitcher, Piek, & Hay, 2003; Rasmussen & Gillberg, 2000; Tervo, Azuma, Fogas, & Fiechtner, 2002; Webster, Majnemer, Platt, & Shevell, 2005). The presence of these comorbidities can make the type of environmentally focused management that has been proposed in the lower levels much more challenging.

What We Now Know: Children with DCD often experience secondary consequences

In addition to the complexity that may be added due to the high rates of comorbidities, earlier chapters in this book have documented the very strong evidence suggesting a trajectory from early motor impairment to secondary difficulties with academics (Missiuna et al., 2007), social participation (Chen & Cohn, 2003), bullying (Piek et al., 2005), physical fitness (Schott et al., 2007; Tsiotra et al., 2009), and mental health (Cairney et al., 2010c; Cocks et al., 2009; Engel-Yeger & Hanna Kasis, 2010; Missiuna et al., 2014; Piek et al., 2010; Piek et al., 2008; Piek et al., 2007). This picture of the numerous secondary consequences associated with DCD seems dire, but we know that the potential also exists for positive trajectories and pathways of resilience (Missiuna et al., 2008a). Intervention that takes into consideration all of these comorbidities and sequelae likely needs to be individualized. Given the environmental and task supports that we are recommending be put into place at earlier levels of management, however, very few children with DCD should need to become involved with specialists.

Level 4: Some children with DCD who are complex and/or have comorbidities will need specialized intervention. Recognizing that DCD is a motor-based learning problem, the optimal approach will be to use motor learning principles and to have a caregiver involved who will support transfer and generalization in home and community environments.

What We Should Do: Strategic Management Level 4

Long-term outcomes in children with DCD are influenced not only by the severity of impairment and co-occurring conditions but also by early identification, the presence of supportive environments, and the strengths of individuals with DCD, including their coping mechanisms. It is self-esteem and these coping mechanisms that may need to be addressed through a more individualized approach, particularly with children who are 8 years of age and above. All of the evidence-based principles that have been outlined with regard to DCD as a learning-based motor problem, however, also need to be reflected as core facets of any individual intervention that is provided. Evidence has been shown for the effectiveness of the cognitive CO-OP approach (Polatajko et al., 2001a). This approach guides the child in discovering verbally-based strategies that help them problem-solve in new movement situations (Mandich et al., 2001; Martini & Polatajko, 1998; Miller, Polatajko, Missiuna, Mandich, & Macnab, 2001; Polatajko, Mandich, Miller, & Macnab, 2001a; Sangster, Beninger, Polatajko, & Mandich, 2005). CO-OP emphasizes a child-centred approach with goals that are child chosen, ecologically valid, and performed in a realistic context. It is a 10-session treatment approach that teaches the child to solve his or her own performance problems through a metacognitive process of identifying a goal, setting a plan, carrying out that plan, checking to see how the plan has worked, and if necessary, adapting the plan in an iterative fashion. Practice focuses on the child's ability to learn, apply, generate, evaluate, and monitor task-specific cognitive strategies with emphasis on facilitating transfer and generalization of the newly learned skills.

The CO-OP approach has repeatedly been demonstrated to be an effective intervention for school-age children with DCD (Banks, Rodger, & Polatajko, 2008; Bernie & Rodger, 2004; Chan, 2007; Mandich & Miller, 2005; Miller et al., 2001; Polatajko & Mandich, 2004; Rodger & Brandenburg, 2009; Rodger & Liu, 2008; Sangster et al., 2005; Sugden, 2007; Wilson, 2005), and even very young children (Taylor, Fayed, & Mandich, 2007). Hyland and Polatajko (2012) have recently presented clear evidence that over the course of intervention, children become better at self-monitoring their performance and correcting it. It is significant that the children most often use strategies that increase their awareness and understanding of task requirements, supporting the theory that DCD is a learning problem that affects the motor domain (Banks et al., 2008) and requires specialized attention. Emerging evidence suggests that this specialized attention may be delivered in a group format (Green, Chambers, & Sugden, 2008), but further research is required to determine whether the learning generalizes to other environments. If a child's needs are sufficiently complex to warrant this specialized intervention, then the intervention should be delivered outside the classroom, but always with the involvement of the appropriate significant other to support generalization and transfer. In the case of CO-OP, having parents watching and taking part has been an integral part of the approach since its inception (Polatajko et al., 2001a).

In summary, we are proposing that strategic management of children with DCD should stage intervention along four levels, progressing from general facilitation of motor skill development and learning through to more intense and specialized intervention that occurs outside the classroom but involves appropriate significant others who have the best opportunities to encourage transfer and generalization of skills (see Figure 8.1). Decisions about the level, or intensity, of intervention required for any individual child may depend on factors such as the child's age, severity of the motor difficulties, and evidence of secondary consequences. A strategic approach, however, should provide supportive and effective management for many children with DCD who might otherwise go unnoticed until secondary mental or physical health difficulties have emerged; see Table 8.1.

A Canadian Example of "Levelled" Management

Over the past 3 years, an innovative service delivery model for children with DCD has been tested in Ontario, Canada. It is a conceptually- and empirically-based model of service that aligns well with the premise of DCD as a learning-based motor problem and with the recommendations outlined thus far for a levelled approach to be used to manage large numbers of children. The service that has been tested is delivered by occupational therapists in school settings and is called Partnering for Change (P4C). The name emphasizes the partnership of the therapist with educators and parents to change the life and daily environment of a child. Children with DCD are the population of concern, but therapists do not work one-to-one with individual children. Instead, service delivery occurs indirectly, in the environment, through a partnership between the therapist, educator, and parent. P4C focuses on Capacity building through Collaboration and Coaching in Context (the four Cs). Instead of direct service, the core activities of the occupational therapist are relationship building and knowledge translation, with the school as the target of the intervention. The therapist collaborates with educators and coaches them in the strategies that are needed to facilitate learning of new motor skills for all children. Therapists encourage explicit teaching

Figure 8.1

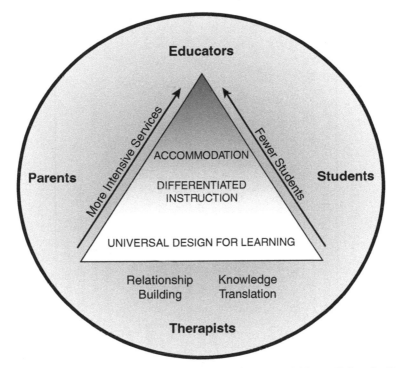

PARTNERING FOR CHANGE: P4C

Building Capacity though Collaboration and Coaching in Context

Educators

Parents

Students

More Intensive Services

Fewer Students

ACCOMMODATION

DIFFERENTIATED
INSTRUCTION

UNIVERSAL DESIGN FOR LEARNING

Relationship   Knowledge
Building   Translation

Therapists

©Missiuna, Pollock, Campbell, Levac and Whalen, CanChild, McMaster University, 2011.

of motor skills and demonstrate techniques that can be used with classes or groups of children. When children are having difficulty with particular tasks, therapists work collaboratively in the context of the classroom to problem-solve ways to accommodate for motor skill challenges. Educators use the term "differentiated instruction" to describe the accommodations they make to activities to improve the ability of the child with DCD to participate fully in the classroom. Knowledge translation focuses on helping educators understand motor skill development and the motor learning issues of children with DCD. The model was developed based on

Table 8.1 A Strategic, Levelled Approach to Management of Children with DCD

Level/Stage of Intervention	What We Now Know	What We Should Do: Strategic Management	Target for Capacity Building	Knowledge Required to Support Child
School/ Population of Children	High prevalence of children with DCDLong waitlists for individual intervention	Universal design of classrooms and schools to encourage motor learning	General Public/ Educators	Increased awareness of DCD as a common, chronic health condition
Class/Group of Children with Motor Learning Difficulties	Children do not learn motor skills spontaneously, by imitation, or by trial and errorChildren with DCD need to be identified at an early age	Direct teaching of motor skills needed by all children through group interventionTeachers identify children who are not learning through exposure	Educators/ Community Leaders	Understanding of specific issues of children with DCD, how to identify DCD, and strategies to encourage learning and participation
Children with DCD	DCD is a lifelong impairment that does not go away. Children do not transfer or generalize learned motor skills	Accommodation to increase participation is requiredDirect, individual teaching of motor skills and provision of strategies, in context	Educators/ Primary Care Physicians	Strategies to accommodate tasks and classroom environments to support children with DCDKnowledge about diagnosing DCD, awareness of secondary consequences and comorbid conditions
Complex Childwith DCD	Many children with DCD have co-occurring conditions and experience secondary consequences	Specialized/individualized interventionStrategies address learning-based motor problem, in context	Family/ Caregivers	Indepth understanding of DCD, issues and management of their childAdvocacy and sharing of information with others

both theory and research about the needs of children with DCD, and about the type of strategies that are useful to enhance children's participation in school settings (Missiuna et al., 2012b).

The overall goals of P4C are to facilitate earlier identification of children with DCD, build the capacity of teachers and parents to manage DCD, and improve children's participation in school and at home. A feasibility study recently examined the receptivity of teachers and schools to this intervention and measured the uptake of knowledge about DCD by both teachers and parents. All participants reported the project to be successful (Missiuna et al., 2012a), and the occupational therapists who delivered this model unequivocally recommended it as a preferred method of providing service to this population of children in school settings (Campbell et al., 2012a). Further research is required to determine the extent to which this model can build capacity over the long term.

A Comprehensive Approach to Management of Children with DCD

While Partnering for Change is one example of a promising approach for strategic management of many children with DCD in school settings, the school is only one environment of concern. In addition to the individualized intervention (e.g., CO-OP) that may need to be provided to a few children, we argue that there is a need for change through building capacity to support children within family environments, by health professionals such as their family physician, and through education of other members of the community.

Building Capacity to Support Children with DCD

Supportive Families

Similar to the strategic, levelled approach that we are proposing for management of children with DCD, sharing of information and promoting greater understanding of children with DCD can also be envisioned as a staged or levelled approach. The most intense or direct focus for sharing of information about DCD needs to be on the families and caregivers who require "deep" knowledge about DCD. Families need to have in-depth understanding of the characteristics of children with DCD and of why they experience difficulty learning new motor tasks.

Helping parents to understand their child's strengths and limitations is an important component of secondary prevention and chronic disease management. Family and cultural expectations can be inconsistent with a child's motor abilities. Parents who expect their child to demonstrate proficiency in competitive sports or dance, for example, or who value perfect penmanship, can induce frustration in the child and increase stress for everyone. Education about DCD can help families and children match interests and skills with expectations that lead to success. If parents are able to look at a play situation in their neighbourhood or community recreation program and understand which motor skills are interfering with their child's ability to participate, the situation can be adapted to maximize their child's participation (Mahoney & Perales, 2006; Rivard et al., 2011).

Families may also benefit from knowledge about resources that they can access and share with others in order to advocate on behalf of their child. The CanChild website (www.canchild.ca) now provides an online workshop to familiarize families with information about DCD and also provides resources in many languages that families can download at no cost in order to share information about their child with educators, physicians, and other members of the community (e.g., Missiuna et al., 2011b).

Supportive Physicians

Another important individual to engage in the strategic management of children with DCD is the primary care physician, pediatrician, or general practitioner, who is apt to be a stable presence in the child's life over many years. These physicians are conceivably the first line of health professional contact for children with DCD and could facilitate early recognition of this chronic health condition (Gaines, Missiuna, Egan, & McLean, 2008a). Many primary care physicians are unfamiliar with DCD; however, Gaines, Missiuna, Egan, and McLean (2008a) succeeded in effectively educating a group of physicians through an educational outreach and collaborative care project on DCD. Physicians who participated reported that they were likely to use newly learned DCD screening measures (Missiuna, Gaines, & Soucie, 2006a) and to provide educational material to families in the future (Gaines et al., 2008a). Carslaw (2011) stressed the importance of physicians being aware of the implications of DCD and of practical strategies that can be used by a family to create a supportive environment for their child with DCD. Family physicians and pediatricians must also have knowledge that demonstrates an understanding of DCD as a chronic health condition that will need to be monitored to recognize the onset of – and possibly prevent – secondary physical and mental health consequences.

Supportive Communities

In order to encourage the physical and social participation of children with DCD, adults in the community who interact regularly with children to encourage their participation (e.g., sports instructors, camp counselors) also need to have some awareness about DCD. Information that is specific to any particular child can be shared by families; however, general knowledge about how to teach motor skills and how children with DCD learn most effectively needs to be imparted to instructors of martial arts, swimming, skating, arts and crafts, and to a variety of other after-school activity leaders.

Supportive Societies

Finally, at the most basic level, the general public needs increased awareness about DCD as a health condition that affects large numbers of individuals in our society, both children and adults. Providing this level of knowledge to the public will require the advocacy of families, educators, health professionals, policy makers, and individuals with DCD themselves.

Conclusions

The strategic levelled approach to management that we are proposing is grounded in the premise that children with DCD have a learning-based motor problem and that the negative characteristics that we observe when children are older are secondary consequences. We are recommending this approach on the proposition that diagnosing children with DCD early and supporting them within an integrated system will be protective; however, at this point there is not sufficient evidence to support this proposition. What is still needed is longitudinal research, which involves following children who are identified before age 5 and who are well supported in school, home, and community settings. We are aware of the many environments in which children with DCD struggle and believe strongly that there is a need for a multi-layered approach that extends beyond the individual child and family and encompasses the school, the family, primary care physicians, and all of the individuals in the community who interact with children as they grow and develop.

REFERENCES

Alloway, T.P., & Warn, C. (2008, Oct). Task-specific training, learning, and memory for children with developmental coordination disorder: A pilot study. *Perceptual and Motor Skills, 107*(2), 473–480. http://dx.doi.org/10.2466/pms.107.2.473-480 Medline:19093608

American Psychiatric Association. (2000). *Diagnostic and statistical manual of mental disorders*(4th ed., text rev.). Arlington, VA: American Psychiatric Publishing.

Ardoin, S.P., Witt, J.C., Connell, J.E., & Koenig, J.L. (2005). Application of a three-tiered response to intervention model for instructional planning, decision making, and the identification of children in need of services. *Journal of Psychoeducational Assessment, 23*(4), 362–380. http://dx.doi.org/10.1177/073428290502300405

Ayres, A.J. (1972). *Sensory integration and learning disorders.* Los Angeles, CA: Western Psychological Services.

Ayres, A.J. (1979). *Sensory integration and the child.* Los Angeles, CA: Western Psychological Services.

Banks, R., Rodger, S., & Polatajko, H.J. (2008). Mastering handwriting: How children with developmental coordination disorder succeed with CO-OP. *OTJR: Occupation, Participation, & Health, 28,* 100–109.

Barnett, A.L. (2008). Motor assessment in developmental coordination disorder: From identification to intervention. *International Journal of Disability Development and Education, 55*(2), 113–129. http://dx.doi.org/10.1080/10349120802033436

Bernie, C., & Rodger, S. (2004). Cognitive strategy use in school-aged children with developmental coordination disorder. *Physical & Occupational Therapy in Pediatrics, 24*(4), 23–45. http://dx.doi.org/10.1300/J006v24n04_03 Medline:15669668

Blank, R., Smits-Engelsman, B., Polatajko, H., Wilson, P., & European Academy of Childhood Disability. (2012, Jan). European Academy of Childhood Disability (EACD): Recommendations on the definition, diagnosis and intervention of developmental coordination disorder (long version).

Developmental Medicine and Child Neurology, 54(1), 54–93. http://dx.doi. org/10.1111/j.1469-8749.2011.04171.x Medline:22171930

Bouffard, M., Watkinson, E.J., Thompson, L.P., Dunn, J.L.C., & Romanow, S.K.E. (1996). A test of the activity deficit hypothesis with children with movement difficulties. *Adapted Physical Activity Quarterly; APAQ*, 13, 61–73.

Brookes, R.L., Nicolson, R.I., & Fawcett, A.J. (2007, Apr 9). Prisms throw light on developmental disorders. *Neuropsychologia*, 45(8), 1921–1930. http:// dx.doi.org/10.1016/j.neuropsychologia.2006.11.019 Medline:17266997

Cairney, J., Hay, J.A., Faught, B.E., & Hawes, R. (2005a, Apr). Developmental coordination disorder and overweight and obesity in children aged 9–14 y. *International Journal of Obesity*, 29(4), 369–372. http://dx.doi.org/10.1038/ sj.ijo.0802893 Medline:15768042

Cairney, J., Hay, J.A., Faught, B.E., Wade, T.J., Corna, L., & Flouris, A. (2005b, Oct). Developmental coordination disorder, generalized self-efficacy toward physical activity, and participation in organized and free play activities. *Journal of Pediatrics*, 147(4), 515–520. http://dx.doi.org/10.1016/j. jpeds.2005.05.013 Medline:16227039

Cairney, J., Hay, J.A., Veldhuizen, S., Missiuna, C., & Faught, B.E. (2010a, Mar). Developmental coordination disorder, sex, and activity deficit over time: A longitudinal analysis of participation trajectories in children with and without coordination difficulties. *Developmental Medicine and Child Neurology*, 52(3), e67–e72. http://dx.doi.org/10.1111/j.1469-8749.2009.03520.x Medline:20015253

Cairney, J., Hay, J., Veldhuizen, S., Missiuna, C., Mahlberg, N., & Faught, B.E. (2010b, Aug 10). Trajectories of relative weight and waist circumference among children with and without developmental coordination disorder. *Canadian Medical Association Journal*, 182(11), 1167–1172. http://dx.doi. org/10.1503/cmaj.091454 Medline:20584932

Cairney, J., Veldhuizen, S., Kurdyak, P., Missiuna, C., Faught, B.E., & Hay, J. (2007, Nov). Evaluating the CSAPPA subscales as potential screening instruments for developmental coordination disorder. *Archives of Disease in Childhood*, 92(11), 987–991. http://dx.doi.org/10.1136/adc.2006.115097 Medline:17573409

Cairney, J., Veldhuizen, S., & Szatmari, P. (2010c, Jul). Motor coordination and emotional-behavioral problems in children. *Current Opinion in Psychiatry*, 23(4), 324–329. http://dx.doi.org/10.1097/YCO.0b013e32833aa0aa Medline:20520549

Campbell, W., Missiuna, C., Pollock, N., & Gaines, R. (2011, April). *Partnering for Change: An innovative service delivery model for implementing response to intervention.* Poster presented at the annual conference of the Canadian

Association of Speech-Language Pathologists and Audiologists, Montreal, Quebec.

Campbell, W.N., Missiuna, C.A., Rivard, L.M., & Pollock, N.A. (2012a, Feb). "Support for Everyone": Experiences of occupational therapists delivering a new model of school-based service. *Canadian Journal of Occupational Therapy*, 79(1), 51–59. http://dx.doi.org/10.2182/cjot.2012.79.1.7 Medline:22439292

Campbell, W., Missiuna, C., & Vaillancourt, T. (2012b). Peer victimization and depression in children with and without motor coordination difficulties. *Psychology in the Schools*, 49(4), 328–341. http://dx.doi.org/10.1002/pits.21600

Campbell, W.N., & Skarakis-Doyle, E. (2007, Nov-Dec). School-aged children with SLI: The ICF as a framework for collaborative service delivery. *Journal of Communication Disorders*, 40(6), 513–535. http://dx.doi.org/10.1016/j.jcomdis.2007.01.001 Medline:17343872

Campbell, S.B., & von Stauffenberg, C. (2009, Jan). Delay and inhibition as early predictors of ADHD symptoms in third grade. *Journal of Abnormal Child Psychology*, 37(1), 1–15. http://dx.doi.org/10.1007/s10802-008-9270-4 Medline:18787941

Cantell, M., & Kooistra, L. (2002). Long-term outcomes of developmental coordination disorder. In S. Cermak & D. Larkin (Eds.), *Developmental coordination disorder* (pp. 23–38). Albany, NY: Delmar.

Cantin, N., Polatajko, H.J., Thach, W.T., & Jaglal, S. (2007, Jun). Developmental coordination disorder: Exploration of a cerebellar hypothesis. *Human Movement Science*, 26(3), 491–509. http://dx.doi.org/10.1016/j.humov.2007.03.004 Medline:17509709

Carslaw, Helen. (2011). Developmental coordination disorder. InnovAiT, 4(2) 87–90. http://dx.doi.org/10.1093/innovait/inq184.

Chan, D.Y.K. (2007). The application of Cognitive Orientation to daily Occupational Performance (CO-OP) in children with developmental coordination disorder (DCD) in Hong Kong: A pilot study. *Hong Kong Journal of Occupational Therapy*, 17(2), 39–44. http://dx.doi.org/10.1016/S1569-1861(08)70002-0

Chen, H.F., & Cohn, E.S. (2003). Social participation for children with developmental coordination disorder: Conceptual, evaluation and intervention considerations. *Physical & Occupational Therapy in Pediatrics*, 23(4), 61–78. Medline:14750309

Cheng, H.C., Chen, H.Y., Tsai, C.L., Chen, Y.J., & Cherng, R.J. (2009, Sep-Oct). Comorbidity of motor and language impairments in preschool children of Taiwan. *Research in Developmental Disabilities*, 30(5), 1054–1061. http://dx.doi.org/10.1016/j.ridd.2009.02.008 Medline:19297128

Cocks, N., Barton, B., & Donelly, M. (2009). Self-concept of boys with developmental coordination disorder. *Physical & Occupational Therapy in Pediatrics, 29*(1), 6–22. http://dx.doi.org/10.1080/01942630802574932 Medline:19197755

Cousins, M., & Smyth, M.M. (2003, Nov). Developmental coordination impairments in adulthood. *Human Movement Science, 22*(4-5), 433–459. http://dx.doi.org/10.1016/j.humov.2003.09.003 Medline:14624827

Deloitte. (2010). *Review of school health support services: Final report.* Toronto, ON: Ministry of Health and Long-Term Care.

Dewey, D., Creighton, D.E., Heath, J.A., Wilson, B.N., Anseeuw-Deeks, D., Crawford, S.G., & Sauve, R. (2011). Assessment of developmental coordination disorder in children born with extremely low birth weights. *Developmental Neuropsychology, 36*(1), 42–56. http://dx.doi.org/10.1080/875 65641.2011.540535 Medline:21253990

Dewey, D., Kaplan, B.J., Crawford, S.G., & Wilson, B.N. (2002). Developmental coordination disorder: Associated problems in attention, learning, and psychosocial adjustment. *Human Movement Science. Special Current Issues in Motor Control and Coordination, 21,* 905–918.

Dunford, C., Street, E., O'Connell, H., Kelly, J., & Sibert, J.R. (2004, Feb). Are referrals to occupational therapy for developmental coordination disorder appropriate? *Archives of Disease in Childhood, 89*(2), 143–147. http://dx.doi.org/10.1136/adc.2002.016303 Medline:14736629

Edwards, J., Berube, M., Erlandson, K., Haug, S., Johnstone, H., Meagher, M., … Zwicker, J.G. (2011, Nov). Developmental coordination disorder in school-aged children born very preterm and/or at very low birth weight: A systematic review. *Journal of Developmental and Behavioral Pediatrics, 32*(9), 678–687. http://dx.doi.org/10.1097/DBP.0b013e31822a396a Medline:21900828

Engel-Yeger, B., & Hanna Kasis, A. (2010, Sep). The relationship between developmental co-ordination disorders, child's perceived self-efficacy and preference to participate in daily activities. *Child: Care, Health and Development, 36*(5), 670–677. http://dx.doi.org/10.1111/j.1365-2214.2010.01073.x Medline:20412146

Faught, B.E., Cairney, J., Hay, J., Veldhuizen, S., Missiuna, C., & Spironello, C.A. (2008, Apr). Screening for motor coordination challenges in children using teacher ratings of physical ability and activity. *Human Movement Science, 27*(2), 177–189. http://dx.doi.org/10.1016/j.humov.2008.02.001 Medline:18343517

Faught, B.E., Hay, J.A., Cairney, J., & Flouris, A. (2005, Nov). Increased risk for coronary vascular disease in children with developmental coordination disorder. *Journal of Adolescent Health, 37*(5), 376–380. http://dx.doi.org/10.1016/j.jadohealth.2004.09.021 Medline:16227122

Fitzpatrick, D.A., & Watkinson, E.J. (2003). The lived experience of physical awkwardness: Adults' retrospective views. *Adapted Physical Activity Quarterly; APAQ, 20,* 279–297.

Forsyth, K., Howden, S., Maciver, D., Owen, C., Shepherd, C., & Rush, R. (2007). *Developmental co-ordination disorder: A review of evidence and models of practice employed by allied health professionals in Scotland – Summary of key findings.* Edinburg, Scotland: NHS Quality Improvement, Scotland.

Friend, M. (2000). Perspective: Myths and misunderstandings about professional collaboration. *Remedial and Special Education, 21*(3), 130–132. http://dx.doi.org/10.1177/074193250002100301

Gaines, R., & Missiuna, C. (2007, May). Early identification: Are speech/language-impaired toddlers at increased risk for developmental coordination disorder? *Child: Care, Health and Development, 33*(3), 325–332. http://dx.doi.org/10.1111/j.1365-2214.2006.00677.x Medline:17439447

Gaines, R., Missiuna, C., Egan, M., & McLean, J. (2008a). Educational outreach and collaborative care enhances physician's perceived knowledge about developmental coordination disorder. *BMC Health Services Research, 8*(1), 21. http://dx.doi.org/10.1186/1472-6963-8-21 Medline:18218082

Gaines, R., Missiuna, C., Egan, M., & McLean, J. (2008b, Oct). Interprofessional care in the management of a chronic childhood condition: Developmental coordination disorder. *Journal of Interprofessional Care, 22*(5), 552–555. http://dx.doi.org/10.1080/13561820802039037 Medline:24567970

Geusgens, C.A., Winkens, I., van Heugten, C.M., Jolles, J., & van den Heuvel, W.J. (2007, Jul). Occurrence and measurement of transfer in cognitive rehabilitation: A critical review. *Journal of Rehabilitation Medicine, 39*(6), 425–439. http://dx.doi.org/10.2340/16501977-0092 Medline:17624476

Gillberg, C. (1998). Hyperactivity, inattention and motor control problems: Prevalence, comorbidity and background factors. *Folia Phoniatrica et Logopaedica, 50*(3), 107–117. http://dx.doi.org/10.1159/000021456 Medline:9691527

Goyen, T.A., & Lui, K. (2009, Apr). Developmental coordination disorder in "apparently normal" schoolchildren born extremely preterm. *Archives of Disease in Childhood, 94*(4), 298–302. http://dx.doi.org/10.1136/adc.2007.134692 Medline:18838419

Green, D., Chambers, M.E., & Sugden, D.A. (2008, Apr). Does subtype of developmental coordination disorder count: Is there a differential effect on outcome following intervention? *Human Movement Science, 27*(2), 363–382. http://dx.doi.org/10.1016/j.humov.2008.02.009 Medline:18400322

Gubbay, S.S. (1975). *The clumsy child: A study of developmental apraxic and agnosic ataxia.* Philadelphia, PA: W.B. Saunders .

Hanft, B., & Shepherd, J. (2008). *Collaborating for student success: A guide for school-based occupational therapy*. Bethesda, MD: AOTA Press.

Hellgren, L., Gillberg, C., Gillberg, I.C., & Enerskog, I. (1993, Oct). Children with deficits in attention, motor control and perception (DAMP) almost grown up: General health at 16 years. *Developmental Medicine and Child Neurology, 35*(10), 881–892. http://dx.doi.org/10.1111/j.1469-8749.1993. tb11565.x Medline:8405717

Hill, E.L. (2001, Apr–Jun). Non-specific nature of specific language impairment: A review of the literature with regard to concomitant motor impairments. *International Journal of Language & Communication Disorders, 36*(2), 149–171. http://dx.doi.org/10.1080/13682820010019874 Medline:11344592

Hillier, S. (2007). Intervention for children with developmental coordination disorder: A systematic review. *Internet Journal of Allied Health Sciences and Practice, 5*(3), 1–11.

Holsti, L., Grunau, R.V.E., & Whitfield, M.F. (2002, Feb). Developmental coordination disorder in extremely low birth weight children at nine years. *Journal of Developmental and Behavioral Pediatrics, 23*(1), 9–15. http://dx.doi. org/10.1097/00004703-200202000-00002 Medline:11889346

Hyland, M., & Polatajko, H.J. (2012). Enabling children with Developmental Coordination Disorder to self-regulate through the use of Dynamic Performance Analysis: Evidence from the CO-OP approach. *Human Movement Science, 31*(4), 987–998. http://dx.doi.org/10.1016/j. humov.2011.09.003 Medline:22153327

Iloeje, S.O. (1987, Aug). Developmental apraxia among Nigerian children in Enugu, Nigeria. *Developmental Medicine and Child Neurology, 29*(4), 502–507. http://dx.doi.org/10.1111/j.1469-8749.1987.tb02510.x Medline:3678629

Jongmans, M.J., Smits-Engelsman, B.C.M., & Schoemaker, M.M. (2003, Nov–Dec). Consequences of comorbidity of developmental coordination disorders and learning disabilities for severity and pattern of perceptual-motor dysfunction. *Journal of Learning Disabilities, 36*(6), 528–537. http:// dx.doi.org/10.1177/00222194030360060401 Medline:15493435

Kadesjö, B., & Gillberg, C. (1998, Dec). Attention deficits and clumsiness in Swedish 7-year-old children. *Developmental Medicine and Child Neurology, 40*(12), 796–804. http://dx.doi.org/10.1111/j.1469-8749.1998.tb12356.x Medline:9881675

Kadesjö, B., & Gillberg, C. (1999, Jul). Developmental coordination disorder in Swedish 7-year-old children. *Journal of the American Academy of Child and Adolescent Psychiatry, 38*(7), 820–828. http://dx.doi.org/10.1097/00004583-199907000-00011 Medline:10405499

Kirby, A., Davies, R., & Bryant, A. (2005). Do teachers know more about specific learning difficulties than general practitioners? *British Journal of Special Education, 32*(3), 122–126. http://dx.doi.org/10.1111/j.0952-3383.2005.00384.x

Kirby, A., Sugden, D., Beveridge, S., & Edwards, L. (2008). Developmental coordination disorder (DCD) in adolescents and adults in further and higher education. *Journal of Research in Special Educational Needs, 8*(3), 120–131. http://dx.doi.org/10.1111/j.1471-3802.2008.00111.x

Kourtessis, T., Tsigilis, N., Maheridou, M., Ellinoudis, T., Kiparissis, M., & Kioumourtzoglou, E. (2008). The influence of a short intervention program on early childhood and physical education teachers' ability to identify children with developmental coordination disorders. *Journal of Early Childhood Teacher Education, 29*(4), 276–286. http://dx.doi.org/10.1080/10901020802470002

Laszlo, J.I., & Bairstow, P.J. (1985). *Perceptual motor behaviour: Developmental assessment and therapy.* London: Holt, Rinehart and Winston.

Laszlo, J.I., Bairstow, P.J., Bartrip, J., & Rolfe, V.T. (1988). Clumsiness or perceptuo-motor dysfunction? In A.M. Colley & J.R. Beech (Eds.), *Cognition and action in skilled behaviour* (pp. 293–310). Amsterdam, the Netherlands: North Holland. http://dx.doi.org/10.1016/S0166-4115(08)60629-9

Levac, D., Wishart, L., Missiuna, C., & Wright, V. (2009, Winter). The application of motor learning strategies within functionally based interventions for children with neuromotor conditions. *Pediatric Physical Therapy, 21*(4), 345–355. http://dx.doi.org/10.1097/PEP.0b013e3181beb09d Medline:19923975

Lingam, R., Golding, J., Jongmans, M.J., Hunt, L.P., Ellis, sM., & Emond, A. (2010, Nov). The association between developmental coordination disorder and other developmental traits. *Pediatrics, 126*(5), e1109–e1118. http://dx.doi.org/10.1542/peds.2009-2789 Medline:20956425

Lingam, R., Hunt, L., Golding, J., Jongmans, M., & Emond, A. (2009, Apr). Prevalence of developmental coordination disorder using the DSM-IV at 7 years of age: A UK population-based study. *Pediatrics, 123*(4), e693–e700. http://dx.doi.org/10.1542/peds.2008-1770 Medline:19336359

Lord, R., & Hulme, C. (1987a, Apr). Perceptual judgments of normal and clumsy children. *Developmental Medicine and Child Neurology, 29*(2), 250–257. http://dx.doi.org/10.1111/j.1469-8749.1987.tb02143.x Medline:3582795

Lord, R., & Hulme, C. (1987b, Dec). Kinaesthetic sensitivity of normal and clumsy children. *Developmental Medicine and Child Neurology, 29*(6), 720–725. http://dx.doi.org/10.1111/j.1469-8749.1987.tb08816.x Medline:3691972

Losse, A., Henderson, S.E., Elliman, D., Hall, D., Knight, E., & Jongmans, M. (1991, Jan). Clumsiness in children – Do they grow out of it? A 10-year follow-up study. *Developmental Medicine and Child Neurology, 33*(1), 55–68. http://dx.doi.org/10.1111/j.1469-8749.1991.tb14785.x Medline:1704864

Mahoney, G., & Perales, F. (2006, Jul). The role of parents in early motor intervention. *Down's Syndrome: Research and Practice, 10*(2), 67–73. http://dx.doi.org/10.3104/reviews.307 Medline:16869364

Mandich, A., & Miller, L. (2005). *Enabling the participation of children with motor problems: The CO-OP approach.* London, ON: Research Alliance for Children with Special Needs.

Mandich, A.D., Polatajko, H.J., Macnab, J.J., & Miller, L.T. (2001). Treatment of children with developmental coordination disorder: What is the evidence? *Physical & Occupational Therapy in Pediatrics, 20*(2-3), 51–68. http://dx.doi.org/10.1080/J006v20n02_04 Medline:11345512

Mannisto, J., Cantell, M., Huovinen, T., Kooistra, L., & Larkin, D. (2006). A school-based movement programme for children with motor learning difficulty. *European Physical Education Review, 12*(3), 273–287. http://dx.doi.org/10.1177/1356336X06069274

Marchiori, G.E., Wall, A.E., & Bedingfield, E.W. (1987). Kinematic analysis of skill acquisition in physically awkward boys. *Adapted Physical Activity Quarterly; APAQ, 4*, 305–315.

Martini, R., & Polatajko, H.J. (1998). Verbal self-guidance as a treatment approach for children with developmental coordination disorder: A systematic replication study. *OTJR: Occupation, Participation and Health, 18*(4), 157–181.

Miller, L.T., Polatajko, H.J., Missiuna, C., Mandich, A.D., & Macnab, J.J. (2001, Mar). A pilot trial of a cognitive treatment for children with developmental coordination disorder. *Human Movement Science, 20*(1-2), 183–210. http://dx.doi.org/10.1016/S0167-9457(01)00034-3 Medline:11471396

Missiuna, C. (1994). Motor skill acquisition in children with developmental coordination disorder. *Adapted Physical Activity Quarterly; APAQ, 11*, 214–235.

Missiuna, C., Cairney, J., Pollock, N., Campbell, W., Russell, D.J., Macdonald, K., Schmidt, L., Heath, N., Veldhuizen, S., & Cousins, M. (2014, May). Psychological distress in children with developmental coordination disorder and attention-deficit hyperactivity disorder. *Research in Developmental Disabilities. 35*(5), 198–207. Medline: 24559609

Missiuna, C., Cairney, J., Pollock, N., Russell, D., Macdonald, K., Cousins, M., ... Schmidt, L. (2011a, Mar-Apr). A staged approach for identifying children with developmental coordination disorder from the population. *Research in Developmental Disabilities, 32*(2), 549–559. http://dx.doi.org/10.1016/j.ridd.2010.12.025 Medline:21216564

Missiuna, C., Gaines, R., & Soucie, H. (2006a, Aug 29). Why every office needs a tennis ball: A new approach to assessing the clumsy child. *Canadian Medical Association Journal, 175*(5), 471–473. http://dx.doi.org/10.1503/cmaj.051202 Medline:16940261

Missiuna, C., Moll, S., King, S., King, G., & Law, M. (2007). A trajectory of troubles: Parents' impressions of the impact of developmental coordination disorder. *Physical & Occupational Therapy in Pediatrics, 27*(1), 81–101. Medline:17298942

Missiuna, C., Moll, S., King, G., Stewart, D., & Macdonald, K. (2008a, Jun). Life experiences of young adults who have coordination difficulties. *Canadian Journal of Occupational Therapy, 75*(3), 157–166. http://dx.doi. org/10.1177/000841740807500307 Medline:18615927

Missiuna, C., Moll, S., Law, M., King, S., & King, G. (2006b, Feb). Mysteries and mazes: Parents' experiences of children with developmental coordination disorder. *Canadian Journal of Occupational Therapy, 73*(1), 7–17. Medline:16570837

Missiuna, C., Pollock, N., Campbell, W.N., Bennett, S., Hecimovich, C., Gaines, R., . . ., & Molinaro, E. (2012a, Sep-Oct). Use of the Medical Research Council Framework to develop a complex intervention in pediatric occupational therapy: Assessing feasibility. *Research in Developmental Disabilities, 33*(5), 1443–1452. http://dx.doi.org/10.1016/j.ridd.2012.03.018 Medline:22522203

Missiuna, C., Pollock, N., Egan, M., DeLaat, D., Gaines, R., & Soucie, H. (2008b, Feb). Enabling occupation through facilitating the diagnosis of developmental coordination disorder. *Canadian Journal of Occupational Therapy, 75*(1), 26–34. http://dx.doi.org/10.2182/cjot.07.012 Medline:18323365

Missiuna, C.A., Pollock, N.A., Levac, D.E., Campbell, W.N., Whalen, S.D., Bennett, S.M., ... Russell, D.J. (2012b, Feb). Partnering for change: An innovative school-based occupational therapy service delivery model for children with developmental coordination disorder. *Canadian Journal of Occupational Therapy, 79*(1), 41–50. http://dx.doi.org/10.2182/cjot.2012.79.1.6 Medline:22439291

Missiuna, C., & Rivard, L. (2010). *Children with coordination difficulties: A flyer for physical educators.* Hamilton, ON: CanChild Centre for Childhood Disability Research.

Missiuna, C., Rivard, L., & Bartlett, D. (2003, Spring). Early identification and risk management of children with developmental coordination disorder. *Pediatric Physical Therapy, 15*(1), 32–38. http://dx.doi.org/10.1097/01. PEP.0000051695.47004.BF Medline:17057429

Missiuna, C., Rivard, L., & Pollock, N. (2004). They're bright but can't write: Developmental coordination disorder in school aged children. *TEACHING Exceptional Children Plus, 1*(1), Article 3. Retrieved July 10, 2014, from http://escholarship.bc.edu/education/tecplus/vol1/iss1/3.

Missiuna, C., Rivard, L., & Pollock, N. (2011b). *Children with developmental coordination disorder: At home, at school, and in the community* [booklet] (5th ed.). Hamilton, ON: CanChild Centre for Childhood Disability Research.

Niemeijer, A.S., Schoemaker, M.M., & Smits-Engelsman, B.C. (2006, Sep). Are teaching principles associated with improved motor performance in children with developmental coordination disorder? A pilot study. *Physical Therapy, 86*(9), 1221–1230. http://dx.doi.org/10.2522/ptj.20050158 Medline:16959670

Niemeijer, A.S., Smits-Engelsman, B.C., & Schoemaker, M.M. (2007, Jun). Neuromotor task training for children with developmental coordination disorder: A controlled trial. *Developmental Medicine and Child Neurology, 49*(6), 406–411. http://dx.doi.org/10.1111/j.1469-8749.2007.00406.x Medline:17518923

Orkwis, R. (2003). *Universally designed instruction.* Arlington, VA: ERIC Clearinghouse on Disabilities and Gifted Education.

Peters, J.M., Henderson, S.E., & Dookun, D. (2004, Sep). Provision for children with developmental co-ordination disorder (DCD): Audit of the service provider. *Child: Care, Health and Development, 30*(5), 463–479. http://dx.doi.org/10.1111/j.1365-2214.2004.00442.x Medline:15320923

Piek, J.P., Barrett, N.C., Allen, L.S., Jones, A., & Louise, M. (2005, Sep). The relationship between bullying and self-worth in children with movement coordination problems. *British Journal of Educational Psychology, 75*(3), 453–463. http://dx.doi.org/10.1348/000709904X24573 Medline:16238876

Piek, J.P., Barrett, N.C., Smith, L.M., Rigoli, D., & Gasson, N. (2010, Oct). Do motor skills in infancy and early childhood predict anxious and depressive symptomatology at school age? *Human Movement Science, 29*(5), 777–786. http://dx.doi.org/10.1016/j.humov.2010.03.006 Medline:20650535

Piek, J.P., Bradbury, G.S., Elsley, S.C., & Tate, L. (2008). Motor coordination and social–emotional behaviour in preschool-aged children. *International Journal of Disability Development and Education, 55*(2), 143–151. http://dx.doi.org/10.1080/10349120802033592

Piek, J.P., & Dyck, M.J. (2004, Oct). Sensory-motor deficits in children with developmental coordination disorder, attention deficit hyperactivity disorder and autistic disorder. *Human Movement Science, 23*(3-4), 475–488. http://dx.doi.org/10.1016/j.humov.2004.08.019 Medline:15541530

Piek, J.P., & Edwards, K. (1997, Mar). The identification of children with developmental coordination disorder by class and physical education teachers. *British Journal of Educational Psychology, 67*(1), 55–67. http://dx.doi.org/10.1111/j.2044-8279.1997.tb01227.x Medline:9114732

Piek, J.P., Rigoli, D., Pearsall-Jones, J.G., Martin, N.C., Hay, D.A., Bennett, K.S., & Levy, F. (2007, Aug). Depressive symptomatology in child and adolescent twins with attention-deficit hyperactivity disorder and/or developmental coordination disorder. *Twin Research and Human Genetics, 10*(4), 587–596. http://dx.doi.org/10.1375/twin.10.4.587 Medline:17708700

Pitcher, T.M., Piek, J.P., & Hay, D.A. (2003, Aug). Fine and gross motor ability in males with ADHD. *Developmental Medicine and Child Neurology, 45*(8), 525–535. http://dx.doi.org/10.1111/j.1469-8749.2003.tb00952.x Medline:12882531

Pless, M., & Carlsson, M. (2000). Effects of motor skill intervention on developmental coordination disorder: A meta-analysis. *Adapted Physical Activity Quarterly; APAQ, 17,* 381–401.

Polatajko, H.J., & Cantin, N. (2005, Dec). Developmental coordination disorder (dyspraxia): An overview of the state of the art. *Seminars in Pediatric Neurology, 12*(4), 250–258. http://dx.doi.org/10.1016/j.spen.2005.12.007 Medline:16780296

Polatajko, H.J., & Mandich, A. (2004). *Enabling occupation in children: The Cognitive Orientation to daily Occupational Performance (CO-OP) approach.* Ottawa, ON: Canadian Association of Occupational Therapists Publications ACE.

Polatajko, H.J., Mandich, A.D., Miller, L.T., & Macnab, J.J. (2001a). Cognitive Orientation to daily Occupational Performance (CO-OP): Part II, The evidence. *Physical & Occupational Therapy in Pediatrics, 20*(2-3), 83–106. http://dx.doi.org/10.1080/J006v20n02_06 Medline:11345514

Polatajko, H.J., Mandich, A.D., Missiuna, C., Miller, L.T., Macnab, J.J., Malloy-Miller, T., & Kinsella, E.A. (2001b). Cognitive Orientation to daily Occupational Performance (CO-OP): Part III, The protocol in brief. *Physical & Occupational Therapy in Pediatrics, 20*(2–3), 107–123. http://dx.doi.org/10.1080/J006v20n02_07 Medline:11345506

Rasmussen, P., & Gillberg, C. (2000, Nov). Natural outcome of ADHD with developmental coordination disorder at age 22 years: A controlled, longitudinal, community-based study. *Journal of the American Academy of Child and Adolescent Psychiatry, 39*(11), 1424–1431. http://dx.doi.org/10.1097/00004583-200011000-00017 Medline:11068898

Rivard, L., & Missiuna, C. (2004). *Encouraging participation in physical activities for children with developmental coordination disorder.* Hamilton, ON: CanChild Centre for Childhood Disability Research.

Rivard, L., Missiuna, C., Pollock, N., & David, K.S. (2011). Developmental coordination disorder (DCD). In S. Campbell, M. Orlin, & R. Palisano (Eds.), *Physical therapy for children* (4th ed., pp. 498–538). St. Louis, MO: Elsevier.

Roberts, G., Anderson, P.J., Davis, N., De Luca, C., Cheong, J., & Doyle, L.W.; Victorian Infant Collaborative Study Group. (2011, Jan). Developmental coordination disorder in geographic cohorts of 8-year-old children born extremely preterm or extremely low birthweight in the 1990s. *Developmental Medicine and Child Neurology, 53*(1), 55–60. http://dx.doi.org/10.1111/j.1469-8749.2010.03779.x Medline:21039437

Rodger, S., & Brandenburg, J. (2009, Feb). Cognitive Orientation to (daily) Occupational Performance (CO-OP) with children with Asperger's syndrome who have motor-based occupational performance goals. *Australian Occupational Therapy Journal, 56*(1), 41–50. http://dx.doi.org/10.1111/j.1440-1630.2008.00739.x Medline:20854488

Rodger, S., & Liu, S. (2008). Cognitive Orientation to (daily) Occupational Performance: Changes in strategy and session time use over the course of intervention. *OTJR: Occupation, Participation and Health, 28*(4), 168–179. http://dx.doi.org/10.3928/15394492-20080901-03

Rodger, S., & Mandich, A. (2005, Jul). Getting the run around: Accessing services for children with developmental co-ordination disorder. *Child: Care, Health and Development, 31*(4), 449–457. http://dx.doi.org/10.1111/j.1365-2214.2005.00524.x Medline:15948882

Rush, D.D., Shelden, M.L., & Hanft, B. (2003). Coaching families and colleagues: A process for collaboration in natural settings. *Infants and Young Children, 16*(1), 33–47. http://dx.doi.org/10.1097/00001163-200301000-00005

Sangster, C.A., Beninger, C., Polatajko, H.J., & Mandich, A. (2005, Apr). Cognitive strategy generation in children with developmental coordination disorder. *Canadian Journal of Occupational Therapy, 72*(2), 67–77. http://dx.doi.org/10.1177/000841740507200201 Medline:15881046

Sayers, B.R. (2008). Collaboration in school settings: A critical appraisal of the topic. *Journal of Occupational Therapy, Schools, & Early Intervention, 1*(2), 170–179. http://dx.doi.org/10.1080/19411240802384318

Schmidt, R.A., & Lee, T.D. (2005). *Motor control and learning: A behavioural emphasis* (4th ed.). Champaign, IL: Human Kinetics.

Schoemaker, M.M., & Kalverboer, A. (1994). Social and affective problems of children who are clumsy: How early do they begin. *Adapted Physical Activity Quarterly; APAQ, 11*, 130–140.

Schoemaker, M.M., & Smits-Engelsman, B.C.M. (2005). Neuromotor task training: A new approach to treat children with DCD. In D.A. Sugden & M. Chambers (Eds.), *Children with developmental coordination disorder* (pp. 212–227). London, England: Whurr Publishers.

Schott, N., Alof, V., Hultsch, D., & Meermann, D. (2007, Dec). Physical fitness in children with developmental coordination disorder. *Research Quarterly for Exercise and Sport, 78*(5), 438–450. http://dx.doi.org/10.1080/02701367.2007.10599444 Medline:18274216

Segal, R., Mandich, A., Polatajko, H., & Cook, J.V. (2002, Jul-Aug). Stigma and its management: A pilot study of parental perceptions of the experiences of children with developmental coordination disorder. *American Journal*

of Occupational Therapy., *56*(4), 422–428. http://dx.doi.org/10.5014/
ajot.56.4.422 Medline:12125831

Shores, C., & Bender, W. (2007). Response to intervention. In W.N. Bender &
C. Shores (Eds.), *Response to intervention: A practical guide for every teacher*
(pp. 1–19). Thousand Oaks, CA: Corwin Press.

Smits-Engelsman, B.C.M., Wilson, P.H., Westenberg, Y., & Duysens, J. (2003,
Nov). Fine motor deficiencies in children with developmental coordination
disorder and learning disabilities: An underlying open-loop control deficit.
Human Movement Science, 22(4-5), 495–513. http://dx.doi.org/10.1016/j.
humov.2003.09.006 Medline:14624830

Stephenson, E.A., & Chesson, R.A. (2008, May). "Always the guiding hand":
Parents' accounts of the long-term implications of developmental coordination disorder for their children and families. *Child: Care, Health
and Development, 34*(3), 335–343. http://dx.doi.org/10.1111/j.1365-
2214.2007.00805.x Medline:18410640

Sugden, D. (2007, Jun). Current approaches to intervention in children
with developmental coordination disorder. *Developmental Medicine
and Child Neurology, 49*(6), 467–471. http://dx.doi.org/10.1111/j.1469-
8749.2007.00467.x Medline:17518935

Sugden, D.A., & Chambers, M.E. (2003, Dec). Intervention in children with
developmental coordination disorder: The role of parents and teachers.
British Journal of Educational Psychology, 73(4), 545–561. http://dx.doi.
org/10.1348/000709903322591235 Medline:14713377

Sugden, D., & Sugden, L. (1991, Nov). The assessment of movement skill
problems in 7- and 9-year-old children. *British Journal of Educational
Psychology, 61*(3), 329–345. http://dx.doi.org/10.1111/j.2044-8279.1991.
tb00990.x Medline:1786212

Summers, J., Larkin, D., & Dewey, D. (2008, Apr). Activities of daily living
in children with developmental coordination disorder: Dressing, personal
hygiene, and eating skills. *Human Movement Science, 27*(2), 215–229. http://
dx.doi.org/10.1016/j.humov.2008.02.002 Medline:18348898

Taylor, S., Fayed, N., & Mandich, A. (2007). CO-OP intervention for young
children with developmental coordination disorder. *OTJR: Occupation,
Participation, & Health, 27*(4), 124–130.

Tervo, R.C., Azuma, S., Fogas, B., & Fiechtner, H. (2002, Jun). Children with
ADHD and motor dysfunction compared with children with ADHD only.
Developmental Medicine and Child Neurology, 44(6), 383–390. http://dx.doi.
org/10.1111/j.1469-8749.2002.tb00832.x Medline:12088306

Thelen, E. (1995, Feb). Motor development: A new synthesis. *American
Psychologist, 50*(2), 79–95. http://dx.doi.org/10.1037/0003-066X.50.2.79
Medline:7879990

Tsai, C.L. (2009, Nov-Dec). The effectiveness of exercise intervention on inhibitory control in children with developmental coordination disorder: Using a visuospatial attention paradigm as a model. *Research in Developmental Disabilities, 30*(6), 1268–1280. http://dx.doi.org/10.1016/j.ridd.2009.05.001 Medline:19497707

Tsai, C.L., Wang, C.H., & Tseng, Y.T. (2012, Jun). Effects of exercise intervention on event-related potential and task performance indices of attention networks in children with developmental coordination disorder. *Brain and Cognition, 79*(1), 12–22. http://dx.doi.org/10.1016/j.bandc.2012.02.004 Medline:22387276

Tsiotra, G.D., Flouris, A.D., Koutedakis, Y., Faught, B.E., Nevill, A.M., Lane, A.M., & Skenteris, N. (2006, Jul). A comparison of developmental coordination disorder prevalence rates in Canadian and Greek children. *Journal of Adolescent Health, 39*(1), 125–127. http://dx.doi.org/10.1016/j.jadohealth.2005.07.011 Medline:16781974

Tsiotra, G.D., Nevill, A.M., Lane, A.M., & Koutedakis, Y. (2009, May). Physical fitness and developmental coordination disorder in Greek children. *Pediatric Exercise Science, 21*(2), 186–195. Medline:19556624

van Dellen, T., Vaessen, W., & Schoemaker, M. (1990). Clumsiness: Definition and selection of subjects. In A.F. Kalverboer (Ed.), *Developmental biopsychology: Experimental and observational studies in children at risk* (pp. 135–152). Ann Arbour, MI: University of Michigan Press.

Villeneuve, M. (2009, Jul). A critical examination of school-based occupational therapy collaborative consultation. *Canadian Journal of Occupational Therapy, 76*(Spec. No.), 206–218. Medline:19757726

Wagner, M.O., Kastner, J., Petermann, F., Jekauc, D., Worth, A., & Bös, K. (2011, Sep-Oct). The impact of obesity on developmental coordination disorder in adolescence. *Research in Developmental Disabilities, 32*(5), 1970–1976. http://dx.doi.org/10.1016/j.ridd.2011.04.004 Medline:21596520

Wang, T.N., Tseng, M.H., Wilson, B.N., & Hu, F.C. (2009, Oct). Functional performance of children with developmental coordination disorder at home and at school. *Developmental Medicine and Child Neurology, 51*(10), 817–825. http://dx.doi.org/10.1111/j.1469-8749.2009.03271.x Medline:19416344

Watkinson, E.J., Dunn, J.C., Cavaliere, N., Calzonetti, K., Wilhelm, L., & Dwyer, S. (2001). Engagement in playground activities as a criterion for diagnosing developmental coordination disorder. *Adapted Physical Activity Quarterly; APAQ, 18*(1), 18–34.

Webster, R.I., Majnemer, A., Platt, R.W., & Shevell, M.I. (2005, Jan). Motor function at school age in children with a preschool diagnosis of developmental language impairment. *Journal of Pediatrics, 146*(1), 80–85. http://dx.doi.org/10.1016/j.jpeds.2004.09.005 Medline:15644827

Wilson, P.H. (2005, Aug). Practitioner review: Approaches to assessment and treatment of children with DCD: an evaluative review. *Journal of Child Psychology and Psychiatry, and Allied Disciplines, 46*(8), 806–823. http://dx.doi.org/10.1111/j.1469-7610.2005.01409.x Medline:16033630

Wilson, P.H., Ruddock, S., Smits-Engelsman, B., Polatajko, H., & Blank, R. (2013, Mar). Understanding performance deficits in developmental coordination disorder: A meta-analysis of recent research. *Developmental Medicine and Child Neurology, 55*(3), 217–228. http://dx.doi.org/10.1111/j.1469-8749.2012.04436.x Medline:23106668

Wright, H.C., & Sugden, D.A. (1996, Dec). A two-step procedure for the identification of children with developmental co-ordination disorder in Singapore. *Developmental Medicine and Child Neurology, 38*(12), 1099–1105. http://dx.doi.org/10.1111/j.1469-8749.1996.tb15073.x Medline:8973295

Zhu, Y.C., Wu, S.K., & Cairney, J. (2011, Mar-Apr). Obesity and motor coordination ability in Taiwanese children with and without developmental coordination disorder. *Research in Developmental Disabilities, 32*(2), 801–807. http://dx.doi.org/10.1016/j.ridd.2010.10.020 Medline:21109392

Zwicker, J.G., Missiuna, C., & Boyd, L.A. (2009, Oct). Neural correlates of developmental coordination disorder: A review of hypotheses. *Journal of Child Neurology, 24*(10), 1273–1281. http://dx.doi.org/10.1177/0883073809333537 Medline:19687388

Zwicker, J.G., Missiuna, C., Harris, S.R., & Boyd, L.A. (2011a, Apr). Brain activation associated with motor skill practice in children with developmental coordination disorder: an fMRI study. *International Journal of Developmental Neuroscience, 29*(2), 145–152. http://dx.doi.org/10.1016/j.ijdevneu.2010.12.002 Medline:21145385

Zwicker, J.G., Missiuna, C., Harris, S.R., & Boyd, L.A. (2010b, Sep). Brain activation of children with developmental coordination disorder is different than peers. *Pediatrics, 126*(3), e678–e686. http://dx.doi.org/10.1542/peds.2010-0059 Medline:20713484

Zwicker, J.G., Missiuna, C., Harris, S.R., & Boyd, L.A. (2011, Apr). Brain activation associated with motor skill practice in children with developmental coordination disorder: An fMRI study. *International Journal of Developmental Neuroscience, 29*(2), 145–152. http://dx.doi.org/10.1016/j.ijdevneu.2010.12.002 Medline:21145385

9 Final Reflections

JOHN CAIRNEY

As the chapters in this collection show, developmental coordination disorder (DCD) is associated with a variety of physical and mental health outcomes and has a significant impact on social functioning, especially in relation to participation in social activities and active play. We have reviewed the neurocognitive deficits in children with DCD, and how these may affect participation and provide clues to how we might intervene on an individual level. In addition, the authors have discussed the challenges associated with screening and with conducting research on children with DCD, describing some new approaches to intervention that fall outside conventional paradigms of service delivery.

The research reviewed leaves little doubt that DCD is a serious condition that has a profound impact on the lives of children who have it. Yet, as the authors of these chapters acknowledge, our work on consequences is not done yet. Derived in part from the chapters that compose this work, I offer here some general reflections.

Research on Participation and Physical and Mental Health in DCD Has Increased Dramatically over the Past Decade

While concern about the consequences of DCD is not new, the reviews in each of the chapters highlights the significant amount of work that has been produced in the areas of physical, mental, and social participation in just the last 10 years or so: Since the mid-2000s, a substantial body of work has been published, documenting a variety of negative health and social outcomes in children with motor coordination problems.

In addition to quantity, the quality of these studies has also shown steady improvement. For example, the number of longitudinal studies tracking change in children with DCD has increased dramatically. Longitudinal data have increased our understanding of the persistence of DCD over time (e.g., Cantell, Smyth, & Ahonen, 2003), the disorder's impact on health-related fitness (e.g., Cairney, Hay, Veldhuizen, & Faught, 2011; Hands, 2008), and the emotional and behavioural problems that may result (e.g., Lingam, Jongmans, Ellis, Hunt, Golding, & Emond, 2012).

While some of these studies, such as the Avon Longitudinal Study of Parents and Children (ALSPAC; Lingam et al., 2012) and the PHAST (Cairney et al., 2011) sample large numbers of children, others do not (Cantell et al., 2003; Hands, 2008). Small sample sizes in prospective studies present several challenges. Small samples are particularly vulnerable to the negative effects of attrition. As children are lost to follow-up, both the representativeness of the original cohort and the statistical power to detect group differences are compromised. Large studies, however, are expensive, especially in the case of disorders like DCD where identification of cases generally relies on large-scale screening efforts. It is little wonder that studies like PHAST and ALSPAC are so rare.

The co-occurrence of DCD with other conditions such as attention deficit hyperactivity disorder (ADHD) and even with conditions such as autism means that partnering with other researchers interested in neurodevelopmental disorders may be the best way to address the challenges of doing this kind of work. Large-scale collaborations across researchers in our field could also prove extremely useful. For example, there has yet to be a collaborative, international, multisite study of DCD. Such initiatives have proven useful in the study of other disorders where the prevalence is relatively low, and/or where it is difficult to identify cases. Now that we have both the Leeds Consensus (Sugden, Chambers, & Utley, 2006) and European Academy of Childhood Disability (Blank, Smits-Engelsman, Polatajko, & Wilson, 2012) consensus statements for case identification, it is not difficult to imagine an international study where researchers from different countries assemble cohorts of children with DCD based on these common criteria and where samples can be pooled for analysis. Such an endeavour would overcome the small sample size problem and, in doing so, provide a unique opportunity to study small subgroups of interest (e.g., girls with DCD and ADHD), as well as to engage in comparative, cross-national investigations. This may also provide a practical solution to a common funding problem experienced by many researchers in the field of DCD: Relative to the funding for other disorders, the share of funding resources for DCD research is small. Pooling funding resources across several countries may be one solution.

Beyond the practicality of such partnerships, the co-occurrence of DCD with other neurodevelopmental, emotional, and behavioural problems and physical health conditions necessitates a focus on comorbidity, especially if we are to better understand secondary consequences. Examining the interrelatedness of disorders in childhood, including DCD, is essential to understand short- and long-term developmental trajectories in children.

Increasing utilization of longitudinal designs is not the only evidence of increased quality. The incorporation of new disciplinary perspectives and the use of state-of-the-art technologies, especially in the area of neuroscience, represent two new developments that offer exciting possibilities. One example of this is the work of Jan Piek and her colleagues and the use of the Australian twin registry (see Chapter 4). While DCD research has been multidisciplinary for some time, the scope of disciplinarity has been limited largely to psychologists, movement (kinesiology) and rehabilitation scientists. The incorporation of new disciplines such as genomics can only increase our understanding of this complex disorder. To that end, it would be interesting to consider how other disciplines, for example, anthropology, sociology, and economics, might also enrich our understanding. Social context, for example, is likely to play an even more important role in how DCD is experienced than we currently know. I use "context" here to refer, broadly, to environmental factors such as family, school, and community or neighbourhood. It strikes me that we know very little about how these different aspects of social context influence the association between DCD and outcomes such as participation or physical activity, or mental and social functioning. In addition, what influence does culture have on the lived experience of DCD? Cross-cultural comparisons could offer greater insight into the influence of social factors on its consequences. Similarly, I am not aware of any study of the economic impact of DCD. Even in intervention studies, there is at best only a passing reference to the cost of therapy, and no discussion of the money that can be saved through prevention of secondary consequences. In the current economic climate, it is unlikely that there will be any new money to help children with DCD unless a compelling economic case for intervention can be made. This would by necessity include an estimate of the cost of DCD to individual, families, and society as a whole and an estimate of the benefits of a cost-effective intervention for dealing with the problem.

At a different level of analysis, fMRI offers a unique opportunity to understand the neurological mechanisms associated with DCD.

Only recently have we begun to use this technology for this purpose (Zwicker, Missiuna, Harris, & Boyd, 2010a; Zwicker, Missiuna, Harris, & Boyd, 2010b). However, I am intrigued by Peter Wilson's argument for longitudinal research in the area of neurocognitive processing. The dominant paradigm for this work – experimental research – provides important snapshots that highlight deficits in children with DCD. They tell us little, however, about how these processes may change over time. Such knowledge is critical to understanding neurological adaptations to DCD-related deficits. While we are tracking the impact of DCD at a functional (behavioural) level, we could also be exploring developmental change in neurocognitive processing.

Towards a Focus on Mechanisms

I believe we have yet to fully understand the mechanisms that connect DCD to secondary consequences. While there are notable exceptions in the areas of physical activity (e.g, Cairney et al., 2005; Poulsen, Ziviani, & Cuskelly, 2008; Poulsen, Ziviani, Cuskelly, & Smith, 2007) and mental health (e.g., Rigoli, Piek, & Kane, 2012), most of the work in the field has focused on establishing differences in outcomes (e.g., prevalence of depression) between children with and without the condition. This is understandable: If there is no evidence that children are at greater risk for obesity or depression, there is little point investigating possible mechanisms that may link coordination difficulties to these secondary concerns. To be clear, when I refer to mechanisms, I am talking about factors that connect DCD to outcomes. For example, if we believe inactivity to be the reason children with DCD are at greater risk for obesity and poor physical health in general, then we are specifying a mechanism – inactivity. A graphical depiction of this simple pathway is shown in Figure 9.1.

Another way of describing this is by using the term *model*. Specifically, here we have specified a model, where inactivity is hypothesized to mediate the association between DCD and physical health status. Of course, we can imagine a model much more complex than that depicted here. Additional circles representing the impact of gender, parental attitudes towards physical activity, self-efficacy towards physical ability, are a few examples of factors that could be added. Although the insertion of these new factors would certainly increase the complexity of the model, it also provides a closer approximation to reality, as there are likely many factors (at multiple levels) that influence physical activity behaviours in children with DCD.

Figure 9.1. Pathway connecting DCD to physical inactivity and poor health.

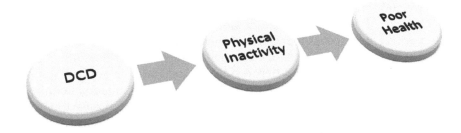

Statistically, one way to test whether this is so is to use a technique known as structural equation modelling (SEM), which in addition to estimating the effect of individual pathways in a model allows the researchers to evaluate the "fit" of the whole model to the data. In other words, does the hypothesized model fit with what is actually observed in the data? SEM offers other advantages as well, and these have been described in numerous publications since the technique found its way into the health sciences (e.g., Bollen, 1989; Streiner, 2006). Building and testing a model is quite a bit more complex than simply describing associations using bivariate statistical analyses (e.g., children with DCD are less active than their peers, children with DCD are more likely to be obese), or even estimating adjusted effects using procedures such as multivariable regression analysis. This kind of model building has been done before in DCD research (e.g., Cairney et al., 2005; Causgrove Dunn, 2000; Rigoli et al., 2012), but I argue that when characterized in this way, our understanding of the mechanisms that link DCD outcomes remain largely theoretical, and that we need more empirical testing of the pathways that connect DCD to important secondary outcomes. I will elaborate further on possible directions using two examples in subsequent sections.

Practically speaking, while the testing of pathways is important for science, in that it allows us to test our assumptions about DCD and its consequences, it is also important for the development of interventions. Understanding the process allows us to proceed systematically in the creation of interventions that target specific parts of the causal chain.

Interconnections between Secondary Outcomes

Part of furthering our understanding of pathways that connect DCD to secondary outcomes must include analyses of the interconnections that exist between the outcomes themselves. Throughout this collection, entire chapters have been devoted to participation, emotional-behavioural problems, inactivity, and cardiovascular health, but often with little or very general discussion of how these "outcomes" are themselves interconnected. The link between depression and obesity can illustrate the usefulness of such an approach. It has been known for some time that obesity and depression are correlated in adults (Atlantis & Baker, 2008; Luppino, de Wit, Bouvy, Stijnen, Cuijpers, Penninx & Zitman, 2010), as are depression and cardiovascular disease (Suls & Bunde, 2005). There is growing evidence of these associations in children and adolescents (Goodman & Whitaker, 2002). It is reasonable therefore to ask, whether the obese child with DCD is at even greater risk for depression, owing to the "double jeopardy" of facing two conditions, both motor coordination problems and obesity, than either an obese child without DCD or a child with DCD who is in the normal weight range. To my knowledge, there has yet to be a study exploring the connections between mental health problems and physical health problems in children with DCD. Similarly, low levels of participation, be it in recreational physical activity or in social activities such as being part of a choir or going to summer camp, are associated with physical (obesity), social (isolation), and emotional (depression) outcomes. Again, very little has been done to trace these pathways in the extant literature.

A focus on interconnections has practical value not only for understanding secondary consequences but also for designing interventions. For example, if the sedentary, obese child with DCD is indeed more likely to be depressed and socially withdrawn, then we need to consider all these factors when intervening. While physical inactivity can be a risk factor for depression (Dunn, Trivedi, & O'Neal, 2001; Paffenbarger, Lee, & Leung, 1994), depression also is a formidable barrier to engaging in physical activity (Sallis & Owen, 1999). Interventions, then, must consider a broad range of psychological factors that influence motivation, beyond the salient ones for typically developing children (e.g., self-efficacy, perceived behavioural control).

A Case for Coping and Resiliency

One of the pitfalls of studying secondary consequences related to DCD is that we tend to focus on negative outcomes. While this is both understandable and necessary, we cannot forget that many children with DCD are not inactive, overweight, depressed, or anxious. Many children with DCD learn to compensate for the challenges they face and lead happy, engaged lives. As much as we need to understand the factors that place children with DCD at risk for negative social, psychological, and physical outcomes, we should also devote attention to understanding the factors that keep children healthy in the face of the challenges that DCD offers. We refer to such factors often in terms of resiliency and coping. While not exactly the same, both orientate us to thinking about personal characteristics and environmental (social, ecological) resources that protect children from risks and work to maintain or even increase well-being. There is surprisingly little focus on this in the extant research literature on DCD. However, models do exist in other areas that can help to inform our efforts. In the mental health literature, for example, one popular theoretical framework is the stress process model (Pearlin, 1989). This model includes both risks (e.g., stress exposures) and protective factors at the individual (e.g, self-esteem, mastery) and social/environmental (e.g., social support) levels. A core feature of the model is the emphasis on stress-buffering effects of these protective factors. In the case of DCD, we might ask, does the presence of supportive parents and/or other positive role models in the child's social network offset negative interactions with peers (e.g., being teased or bullied)? What are the factors that lead to a well-developed sense of self-worth in children with DCD? The challenge will be to avoid thinking in terms of opposites: The absence of depression does not necessarily equate to happiness. To understand resiliency, we need to take seriously the proposition that the factors that keep a child well may be different than the risks that can lead to illness. In the next few years, I suspect, we will see more work in this important, otherwise neglected area.

Screening and the Identification of Cases of DCD

The chapter by Marina Schoemaker and Brenda Wilson provides a comprehensive review on issues related to screening for DCD in children. While the number of screening measures has certainly increased over the past few decades, the problem remains that very few, if any, of the tools we have at our disposal meet the usual standards for use as screens in general population samples. While these tools (e.g., DCDQ) often show good to very good specificity, they have poor to moderate (at best) levels of sensitivity. This means that they are efficient at screening out negative cases (children who do not have DCD), but less so at identifying children with the disorder. At present, it would be difficult to endorse any of the current tools at our disposal as effective screeners for DCD in the general population. Yet, early identification and intervention to prevent secondary problems is widely agreed upon as a necessary course of action in our field.

It seems that, at this point in time, we have several options open. The first is to abandon the hope of general population–based screening for DCD. I suspect that to many in the field, this is not a desirable option. Second is to continue to develop or refine existing tools to increase screening accuracy. There are several major problems here, many of which have already been outlined in previous chapters (Chapters 6 and 7). Among other things, development and/or refinement of tools is time intensive and costly; it almost never happens at a pace that is acceptable to those who work with children and want something now. Moreover, there is reason to question whether the approaches to test development we have used so far will yield the kind of results we would hope for (more on that below). A third option, noted by Schoemaker and Wilson (Chapter 6), is that we begin to investigate whether using multiple tools together (e.g., DCDQ and the MABC Checklist, or the DCDQ and the TEAF), increases sensitivity and specificity. There is merit to this proposal, but caution is warranted. With something as complex as DCD, why not use multiple assessments, possibly from different informants (e.g., parents, teachers, children themselves), to identify cases? The challenge is that when we combine different tests together, we may also be combining their errors (see Chapter 7). Practically, this means we may in fact have even worse results using this approach because of compounded errors across tests. On the other hand, it may be useful to use more contemporary psychometric approaches, such as item-response theory, to test to see if using different items, derived from a number of different measures, produces a set of items that is optimal for case identification. While this could minimize the problem of compounded errors, it still may not produce a measure that would be sufficient for population-based screening.

Up to this point, the focus on developing screening tools has been exclusively based on the use of survey-based measures: parents, teachers, or, more rarely, children themselves answer questions about the subject's motor ability. This approach is likely preferred because of the perceived (and real) benefits of surveys over other methods (e.g., direct assessment using a test such as the MABC). At the same time, much has been written about the challenges of using proxy reporting, especially parents and teachers, who may find it difficult to assess the child's motor ability relative to typically developing children. Another concern, which is less often identified, is compliance. In the case of teachers, can we really expect a teacher, given competing interests and limited time and resources, to complete a questionnaire on every child in his or her class each and every year? Now imagine that we ask teachers to complete several surveys on the same child. I seriously doubt this is a viable option for school-based screening interventions. I believe we need to rethink our approach in this regard. Pen-and-paper tests have been the mainstay of psychometric test development for decades; however, computer and media technology allows us to progressively think about the format we use for testing. Take, for example, the use of pictures or videos. A challenge in surveys is finding the appropriate wording or terminology to describe a scenario (e.g., problems with throwing a ball accurately, balancing on a beam). Instead of trying to capture this idea with words, we could use a web-based or tablet app that shows video images of children with and without DCD performing a number of motor tasks. A brief video presentation on the features of DCD could orientate the test taker (e.g., teacher or parent) to the problem. Use of multimedia can also enhance the experience and overcome the problem of relying solely on the interpretation of word-based descriptions. Another model altogether is the Partnering for Change (P4C) framework described by Missiuna and her colleagues in Chapter 8. Here, the focus is on educating teachers and getting support from professional groups when questions concerning a child's motor development arise. Screening is part of the intervention, though the focus is not so much on case identification as it is on learning to differentiate typical from atypical motor development; the format is very different from how we typically think about it. In either case, we need to begin to think more creatively about this problem.

Paradigm Shift in Treatment: From the Individual to the Population, from the Cause to the Consequence

Missiuna and her colleagues (see Chapter 8) leave little doubt that while there will also be an important place for one-on-one intervention with children with DCD, the problem of need–resource imbalance (i.e., there are many more children with DCD than there are professionals to provide clinical services) necessitates other kinds of interventions. The P4C model is one example, and the initial evidence in support of its utility is compelling. Other kinds of interventions, such as motor skill development interventions in preschool and the early grades (possibly for prevention) or group-based, after-school programs for kids struggling with motor coordination problems (secondary interventions), are other models that need to be tested. Indeed, the crux of the matter in all these proposals is the need for systematic, rigorous evaluation of the interventions. Many of these designs will be complex, multilevel interventions targeting populations and not individual children. Evaluation of complex interventions is a tricky business, and we need to be mindful that evaluations using designs such as randomized control trials are often not possible.

There also seems to be a shift, again well captured in the Partnering for Change model, away from the causes of DCD and towards mitigation of its consequences. Accommodation and modification of physical environments are among the ways we can enhance well-being and participation in children with DCD, rather than targeting, for example, neurological mechanisms that may underlie the problem. This does not mean we should abandon the search for causes and/ or for interventions at the individual level. However, the imperative to intervene now is strong, and if we cannot address the underlying causes of DCD, perhaps we can reduce or eliminate its negative consequences. As I have already noted, until we understand the pathways connecting DCD to outcomes, we may not be targeting the right mechanisms. Linking the study of secondary consequences to intervention research holds the most promise for improving the lives of children with DCD.

Conclusion

A stated purpose of this book was to raise awareness of the secondary outcomes associated with DCD. The pages contained within leave little doubt that DCD is a troubling disorder associated with many negative outcomes at multiple levels. At the same time, while we have learned much, there is much work still left to do. The contributors hope that the content of this book will stimulate further research into the consequences of DCD and lead to the development and testing of new interventions for dealing with the worrying cascade of impairments to which it gives rise.

REFERENCES

Atlantis, E., & Baker, M. (2008, Jun). Obesity effects on depression: Systematic review of epidemiological studies. *International Journal of Obesity, 32*(6), 881–891. http://dx.doi.org/10.1038/ijo.2008.54 Medline:18414420

Blank, R., Smits-Engelsman, B., Polatajko, H., Wilson, P., & European Academy of Childhood Disability. (2012, Jan). European Academy of Childhood Disability (EACD): Recommendations on the definition, diagnosis and intervention of developmental coordination disorder (long version). *Developmental Medicine and Child Neurology, 54*(1), 54–93. http://dx.doi. org/10.1111/j.1469-8749.2011.04171.x Medline:22171930

Bollen, K.A. (1989). *Structural equations with latent variables.* New York, NY: Wiley.

Cairney, J., Hay, J.A., Faught, B.E., Wade, T.J., Corna, L., & Flouris, A. (2005, Oct). Developmental coordination disorder, generalized self-efficacy toward physical activity, and participation in organized and free play activities. *Journal of Pediatrics, 147*(4), 515–520. http://dx.doi.org/10.1016/j.jpeds.2005.05.013 Medline:16227039

Cairney, J., Hay, J., Veldhuizen, S., & Faught, B.E. (2011, Dec). Trajectories of cardiorespiratory fitness in children with and without developmental coordination disorder: A longitudinal analysis. *British Journal of Sports Medicine, 45*(15), 1196–1201. http://dx.doi.org/10.1136/bjsm.2009.069880 Medline:20542967

Cantell, M.H., Smyth, M.M., & Ahonen, T.P. (2003, Nov). Two distinct pathways for developmental coordination disorder: Persistence and resolution. *Human Movement Science, 22*(4-5), 413–431. http://dx.doi. org/10.1016/j.humov.2003.09.002 Medline:14624826

Causgrove Dunn, J. (2000). Goal Orientations, perceptions of the motivational climate, and perceived competence of children with movement difficulties. *Adapted Physical Activity Quarterly; APAQ, 17*(1), 1–19.

Dunn, A.L., Trivedi, M.H., & O'Neal, H.A. (2001, Jun). Physical activity dose-response effects on outcomes of depression and anxiety. *Medicine and Science in Sports and Exercise, 33*(6 Suppl), S587–S597, discussion 609–610. http://dx.doi.org/10.1097/00005768-200106001-00027 Medline:11427783

Goodman, E., & Whitaker, R.C. (2002, Sep). A prospective study of the role of depression in the development and persistence of adolescent obesity. *Pediatrics, 110*(3), 497–504. http://dx.doi.org/10.1542/peds.110.3.497 Medline:12205250

Hands, B. (2008, Apr). Changes in motor skill and fitness measures among children with high and low motor competence: A five-year longitudinal study. *Journal of Science and Medicine in Sport, 11*(2), 155–162. http://dx.doi. org/10.1016/j.jsams.2007.02.012 Medline:17567536

Lingam, R., Jongmans, M.J., Ellis, M., Hunt, L.P., Golding, J., & Emond, A. (2012, Apr). Mental health difficulties in children with developmental coordination disorder. *Pediatrics, 129*(4), e882–e891. http://dx.doi.org/10.1542/peds.2011-1556 Medline:22451706

Luppino, F.S., de Wit, L.M., Bouvy, P.F., Stijnen, T., Cuijpers, P., Penninx, B.W., & Zitman, F.G. (2010, Mar). Overweight, obesity, and depression: A systematic review and meta-analysis of longitudinal studies. *Archives of General Psychiatry, 67*(3), 220–229. http://dx.doi.org/10.1001/archgenpsychiatry.2010.2 Medline:20194822

Paffenbarger, R.S., Jr., Lee, I.M., & Leung, R. (1994). Physical activity and personal characteristics associated with depression and suicide in American college men. *Acta Psychiatrica Scandinavica*, (377), 16–22. http://dx.doi.org/10.1111/j.1600-0447.1994.tb05796.x Medline:8053361

Pearlin, L.I. (1989, Sep). The sociological study of stress. *Journal of Health and Social Behavior, 30*(3), 241–256. http://dx.doi.org/10.2307/2136956 Medline:2674272

Poulsen, A.A., Ziviani, J.M., & Cuskelly, M. (2008). Leisure time physical activity energy expenditure in boys with developmental coordination disorder: The role of peer relations self-concept perceptions. *OTJR: Occupation, Participation and Health, 28*(1), 30–39. http://dx.doi.org/10.3928/15394492-20080101-05

Poulsen, A.A., Ziviani, J.M., Cuskelly, M., & Smith, R. (2007, Jul-Aug). Boys with developmental coordination disorder: Loneliness and team sports participation. *American Journal of Occupational Therapy, 61*(4), 451–462. http://dx.doi.org/10.5014/ajot.61.4.451 Medline:17685178

Rigoli, D., Piek, J.P., & Kane, R. (2012, Apr). Motor coordination and psychosocial correlates in a normative adolescent sample. *Pediatrics, 129*(4), e892–e900. http://dx.doi.org/10.1542/peds.2011-1237 Medline:22451714

Sallis, J.F., & Owen, N. (1999). *Physical activity and behavioral medicine.* Thousand Oaks, CA: Sage.

Streiner, D.L. (2006, Apr). Building a better model: An introduction to structural equation modelling. *Canadian Journal of Psychiatry, 51*(5), 317–324. Medline:16986821

Sugden, D.A., Chambers, M., & Utley, A. (2006). Leeds Consensus Statement. Available online at http://dcd.canchild.ca/en/dcdresources/consensusstatements.asp (downloaded 14 May 2011).

Suls, J., & Bunde, J. (2005, Mar). Anger, anxiety, and depression as risk factors for cardiovascular disease: The problems and implications of overlapping affective dispositions. *Psychological Bulletin, 131*(2), 260–300. http://dx.doi.org/10.1037/0033-2909.131.2.260 Medline:15740422

Zwicker, J.G., Missiuna, C., Harris, S.R., & Boyd, L.A. (2010a), Apr). Brain activation associated with motor skill practice in children with developmental coordination disorder: An fMRI study. *International Journal of Developmental Neuroscience, 29*(2), 145–152

Zwicker, J.G., Missiuna, C., Harris, S.R., & Boyd, L.A. (2010b), Apr). Brain activation associated with motor skill practice in children with developmental coordination disorder: An fMRI study. *International Journal of Developmental Neuroscience, 29*(2), 145–152. http://dx.doi.org/10.1016/j.ijdevneu.2010.12.002 Medline:21145385

Zwicker, J.G., Missiuna, C., Harris, S.R., & Boyd, L.A. (2010b, Sep). Brain activation of children with developmental coordination disorder is different than peers. *Pediatrics, 126*(3), e678–e686. http://dx.doi.org/10.1542/peds.2010-0059 Medline:20713484

Contributors

John Cairney, PhD (Editor & Contributor). John is the McMaster Family Medicine Professor of Child Health Research and Director of the Infant and Child Health (INCH) Research Lab, in the Department of Family Medicine at McMaster University, Hamilton, Ontario, Canada. He is also Professor in the Departments of Psychiatry and Behavioural Neurosciences, Kinesiology, and Clinical Epidemiology and Biostatistics at McMaster. John is also a scientist at the CanChild Centre for Childhood Disability Research and core member of the Offord Centre for Child Studies.

Batya Engel-Yeger, PhD. Batya is Chair of the Occupational Therapy Department in the Faculty of Social Welfare and Health Sciences at the University of Haifa, Israel.

Cheryl Missiuna, PhD, OT(Reg). Cheryl is Professor in the School of Rehabilitation Sciences at McMaster University, Hamilton, Ontario, Canada. At the time of writing of this book, she was the Director of the CanChild Centre for Childhood Disability Research.

Jan P. Piek, PhD. Jan is currently Professor Emeritus of Developmental Psychology in the School of Psychology and Speech Pathology at Curtin University in Perth, Australia.

Helene J. Polatajko, PhD. Helene is Professor in the Department of Occupational Science and Occupational Therapy at the University of Toronto, Toronto, Ontario, Canada.

Nancy Pollock, MSc. Nancy is an Associate Clinical Professor in the School of Rehabilitation Science and an Investigator with the CanChild

Centre for Childhood Disability Research, McMaster University, Hamilton, Ontario, Canada.

Daniela Rigoli, MA (PhD Candidate). Daniela is currently a Research Fellow in Psychology in the School of Psychology and Speech Pathology at Curtin University in Perth, Australia.

Marina M. Schoemaker, PhD. Marina is Associate Professor at the Centre of Human Movement Science, University Medical Centre Groningen, University of Groningen, Netherlands.

Scott Veldhuizen, MA (PhD Candidate). Scott is a research methodologist at the Centre for Addiction and Mental Health and a PhD student in the Department of Community Health Sciences at Brock University, St. Catharines, Ontario, Canada.

Brenda N. Wilson, MSc (PhD Candidate). Brenda is currently a Research Assistant Professor in the Department of Paediatrics at the University of Calgary and a Professional Practice Leader/Occupational Therapy with the Alberta Health Services in Calgary, Alberta, Canada.

Peter H. Wilson, PhD. Peter is Professor of Developmental Psychology in the School of Psychology at the Australian Catholic University in Melbourne, Australia.

Index

Lightning Source UK Ltd.
Milton Keynes UK
UKHW01f1317080618
323925UK00001B/57/P